THE RISE OF PSYCHO-PHARMACOLOGY

AND

THE STORY OF CINP

Edited by
Thomas A. Ban
David Healy
Edward Shorter

Animula
1998

Library of Congress Cataloging-in-Publication Data
    Ban T. A., Healy D., Shorter E. (eds):
    The Rise of Psychopharmacology. The Story of CINP
    Includes bibliographical references and indexes.
    ISBN 963 408 105 3

    1. Psychopharmacology. 2. History of 1950s and 1960s. 3. Collegium Inter-
    nationale Neuro-Psychopharmacologicum.

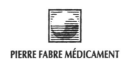

PIERRE FABRE MÉDICAMENT

Publisher: Animula Publishing House (Hungary) 1281 Budapest, POB 12
Printed in Hungary by Zrínyi Nyomda Co. Chief director George Vinkó. Budapest. 1156/11

TABLE OF CONTENTS

CINP STORY

MEMOIRS OF FELLOWS

THE COLLEGIUM

APPENDICES

EXTRACTS AND REVIEW

TABULAR PRESENTATIONS

INDEXES

PREFACE

Until the 1950s there was no such scientific discipline as psychopharmacology. Although the term "psychopharmacology" had been around since the 1920s, and physicians had prescribed psychoactive drugs for some time, nobody had any idea how the the drugs acted on the brain or how to design drugs that might actually help mental illness in a predictable way. Then in 1952 chlorpromazine entered the scene, and in 1958, the newly founded (in 1957) CINP held its first meeting in Rome. Forty years later, in 1998, the organization met for the 21st time in Glasgow.

In those forty years the foundation of psychopharmacology was laid. This volume is about the discipline's rise, to about 1970. Subsequent volumes will trace later events. Forty years after the founding of the organization with the clumsy latinate name of Collegium Internationale Neuro-Psychopharmacologicum (CINP), one sees what a tremendous difference in the treatment of mental illness the new science has made. Today drugs can keep in control some diseases which are based on pathological (mental) processing in the brain, just as digitalis keeps heart disease in control. And the story of these new drugs, as well as the underlying base of neuroscience on which the newer ones were developed, is virtually unknown.

Therefore there was a need for a book that would help to tell this epochal story. This is not a formal history of the founding of psychopharmacology, but a repertorium of the memoirs of those who were there. We have harvested anecdotal accounts from the pioneers of the field of the early days. Some of the authors are beautiful writers, others strain at their story. No matter. This is a sourcebook that others will want to use to find out how it once was, and through what difficulties the scientific field of psychopharmacology later came to blossom. Some readers will thrill to the story; others will want mainly to go back and see what actually happened. This book speaks to both.

Yet this is more than a source book. Many of these stories have relevance to current research, partly in keeping important scientific narratives from being forgotten, as for example the desipramine story, in the way that, for a century, digitalis was forgotten after William Withering discovered it late in the eighteenth century. But these stories illuminate current work also in showing how an organization matters: it can keep vested interests in check, or ensure that scientific standards are maintained in the quality and validity of the information communicated.

This book begins by letting the players of the day tell the main drug story: how the principal drug classes, such as the mood stabilizers, antipsychotics, anxiolytics and antidepressants were developed. Then the main builders of the underlying neuroscience frame come on stage and talk about their discoveries about the possible role of neurotransmitters in mental illness. At that point we hear from the national fields around the world. There are national idiosyncrases of multinational drug development: what happened in Czechoslovakia, in Britain, and elsewhere. Finally, we have at least presented the basic facts on the rise of the CINP itself, so that the readers interested in factors affecting – and controversies distracting – the organization can glimpse the point of departure. An appendix includes CINP-relevant extracts of material from the period which are not easily accessible for the English-speaking reader. It also lists the drugs involved and identifies the scientists and the clinicians participating in their development.

Several people aside from the editors helped put this book together. Elizabeth Hulse and Lynne Hussey served as subeditors. Sheryl Pearson gave support. Andrea Clark, the administrator of the History of Medicine Program at the University of Toronto, fielded faxes and phone calls from around the world.

Happily, the CINP has a History Committee, and the members of this committee eased the way for the appearance of the book. We especially acknowledge the past inspiration of Hanns Hippius and Oakley Ray. Claude de Montigny, President of CINP, was a bulwark of reliability.

But most of all , it is fair to say this book would never have seen the light of day were it not for the generous financial support of Pierre Fabre, Janssen Pharmaceutica and Research Foundation, Janssen Pharmaceutica Inc., and Janssen Pharmaceutica International in collaboration with Organon International. These firms, through their non-restricted publication grants, have been exemplary for their commitment to the dissemination of knowledge.

INTRODUCTION

This volume is based primarily on invited memoirs about the 1960s from CINP members who were part of those days. To characterize the decade by the term "rise" might not be as arbitrary as it seems, because it was during the 1960s that psychopharmacology developed a standard methodology, completed by 1970, for the preclinical and clinical evaluation of psychotropic drugs.

During the 1960s, research with the spectrophotofluorimetric method flourished, and by 1970 it had generated a wealth of information on neurochemical transmission relevant to psychotropic drugs. It was also during the 1960s that psychiatric rating scales were developed to detect the therapeutic activity and to demonstrate the efficacy of such drugs. By 1970 the first widely used assessment batteries for antipsychotics and antidepressants were in place.

During those years the membership of CINP grew steadily and reached by 1970 the critical mass needed to affect psychotropic drug development. During the 1960s psychiatrists also learned to accept the new drugs. By 1970 pharmacotherapy with neuroleptics and antidepressants had become the prevailing mode of treatment in schizophrenia and melancholia all around the globe. Psychopharmacology was indeed on the ascending side of its bell-shaped curve.

Since those exciting days thirty years have passed. Even the youngest of eyewitnesses is at least sixty years old. We have reached the limit in time for recapturing the mood, and not just the facts, of psychopharmacology in the 1960s by recording the accounts of those who lived it.

First-person memoirs of a period by the survivors have the charm of sometimes telling more about the people than the events. That is a bonus for biography. By ordering each topic chronologically, we make it easy for readers to reconstruct what happened. Each memoir is supplemented with the author's self-prepared biographic sketch and a brief "CINP biography" which includes his or her contributions to the proceedings of the first seven CINP congresses.

In the Appendix, some relevant information about drugs, CINP membership, and the like is given.

THE 1950s:
FROM PSYCHIATRY
TO
PSYCHO-
PHARMACOLOGY

On the eve of the introduction of effective psychotropic drugs, the psychiatric scene was characterized by widely divergent orientations in different parts of the world, e.g., Henry Ey's "organodynamic" approach in France, Wimmer's "psychogenetic" approach in Scandinavia. There was little common between the German "psychopathologists," the American "psychodynamicists," and the British "social psychiatrists." Accordingly, treatment kept by and large with the frame of reference of the psychiatry practiced in that country, thus being prevailingly "biological," "psychological," or "social."

Biological treatments in the 1950s consisted of psychosurgical (lobotomy), physical (electroshock, insulin coma), and pharmacological. Fever therapy was still conducted, as were pharmacologically-induced convulsions and toxic psychoses. Pharmacological treatments were restricted to the opiates for depression, and to the bromides, barbiturates, paraldehyde and chloral hydrate for day-time or night-time sedation. For the control of agitation, morphine with scopolamine, or hyoscine with apomorphine were available.

It was certainly not as a result of such medications, or of any of the other "psychological," or "social" treatments, that the census in psychiatric hospitals had already begun to decrease in the 1950s, prior to the introduction of the first neuroleptics.

Psychiatry was caught unprepared for the introduction of therapeutically effective psychotropic drugs. Because of suspicion and resistance in accepting the new drugs, it took a long time to demonstrate even the obvious effectiveness of chlorpromazine in the treatment of schizophrenia. Furthermore, some of the old pharmacological treatments based primarily on psychotherapeutic principles, such as chemically-induced abreactions with barbiturates or methamphetamine, as well as psycholytic and psychedelic therapies with lysergic acid diethylamide or psilocybin, lingered on for years after the introduction of the first set of new psychotropic drugs.

By contrast, basic scientists in neurophysiology and neurochemistry responded promptly and with open arms to the introduction of effective drugs in mental illness. They recognized without delay that psychotropics could provide the missing link for a neuroscience of which psychiatry is an integral part.

In the following, six memoirs will be presented which deal primarily with the 1950s. Four of the memoirs were written by psychiatrists, each characteristically working in a different frame of reference within his discipline; of the remaining two, one was a basic scientist, the other an internist.

TOWARDS FOOTINGS OF A SCIENCE: PERSONAL BEGINNINGS IN PSYCHOPHARMACOLOGY IN THE FORTIES AND FIFTIES

Joel Elkes

A PROGRAM ON "DRUGS AND THE MIND" - EXPERIMENTAL PSYCHIATRY IN BIRMINGHAM, ENGLAND

The inverted telescope of recollection is apt to diminish and obscure persons and events. However, in this instance, they remain clear, distinct, and warming to recall. I have referred to them more extensively in a recent invited address (1). It also carries a fuller bibliography.

The dialectic between Psychiatry and Molecules began quite early in my life. As a medical student at St. Mary's Hospital, London, in the thirties, I was deeply attracted to psychiatry. However, the excellent lectures and demonstrations in the local mental hospital left me bewildered, curious and hungry, and groping for a physiology and chemistry which at the time did not exist. Immunology was very strong at St. Mary's (where, some ten years later, Fleming discovered penicillin). So, one read wildly in immunology, particularly on Paul Ehrlich's ideas about cell surfaces, receptor configuration, specificity, side-chains ("Seitenketten") and the like. Soon, the lipoprotein structure of cell membranes became a consuming interest. I spent two gorgeous summers in the Department of Colloid Science at Cambridge under Sir Eric Rideal, spreading monomolecular films and reading on crystallography. Getting into micro-structures (membranes, organelles) became a persistent visual game. I did not know it then, but I was heading into pharmacology.

The opportunity came in 1941, when I accompanied my erstwhile chief and friend Alastair Frazer to Birmingham to help him found what, in retrospect, was to become a major department of pharmacology. Psychiatry was always beckoning in the background; but in those days, there were few bridges leading from cell biology to psychiatry, and it was not easy to convince university authorities that "Mental Disease Research" (as it was called) was a worthwhile enterprise. The leading laboratories were small, not very well equipped, and usually functioned

Joel Elkes is Distinguished Service Professor Emeritus at Johns Hopkins University, Baltimore, and Distinguished University Professor Emeritus in the University of Louisville. At present, he is Senior Scholar in Residence at the Fetzer Institute, Kalamazoo, Michigan. He founded the Department of Experimental Psychiatry in the University of Birmingham, England, in 1951, and subsequently (1957-63) served as Director of the Clinical Neuropharmacology Research Center, NIMH, Washington, D.C. He served as Psychiatrist-in-Chief and Director of the Department at Johns Hopkins between 1963 and 1975. After his retirement from Hopkins, he helped to create a program in Behavioural Medicine at McMaster University, Hamilton, Ontario, Canada, (1976-1981) and continued in cognate programs in the Department of Psychiatry, University of Louisville (1981-1994). In 1961, he was elected the first President of the American College of Neuropsychopharmacology.

Elkes was elected a fellow of the CINP in 1960. He presented a paper entitled "On the relation of drug-induced mental changes to the schizophrenias" at the 1st Congress.

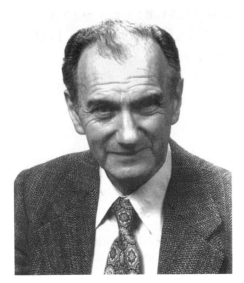

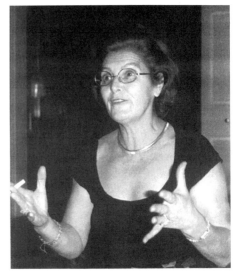

Joel Elkes   **Charmian Elkes**

outside universities, being mostly supported by local hospital boards. Yet, in retrospect, I was most fortunate. In Birmingham, I found acceptance of my interest in the chemistry of the brain, and, more importantly, while teaching conventional pharmacology I was allowed to stray. My colleagues and I strayed into the study of the cholinesterases, and the very powerful and specific anticholinesterases. We began mapping the distribution of these enzymes in the brain, noting their unevenness in the hope of finding a clue to the action of hypnotics. I was also fortunate in another respect. Tracking back to my days in physical chemistry, Bryan Finean (as my first PhD student) engaged in X-ray diffraction studies of living myelin, demonstrating clearly its ordered lamellar, paracrystalline structure (2). After two years of work in this field I found myself anchored. Neurochemistry extended its powerful pull, with psychiatry moving ever closer. At about this time (1945), another pivotal event took place. A small unit of "Mental Disease Research," loosely administered from the Dean's Office, became available. It fell under the aegis of the Department of Pharmacology, through the retirement of its director, Dr. A. Pickworth. I was put in charge of two rooms in the medical school. There was also some seed money. An enormous step in my life had been taken; I knew I was in biological psychiatry for good.

I began to read avidly, to train myself by seeing patients in the local mental hospital (the Winson Green Mental Hospital), and to familiarize myself with the drug treatments then available. The old reliable triad – bromine, chloral hydrate, and the barbiturates – was ever present, and the anti-epileptic drugs were coming into their own at the periphery. There was, of course, also insulin coma and ECT. Vast questions beckoned everywhere: I felt like a naturalist advancing into a strange continent. Deeply moved by what I saw and heard in the ward, I found myself discussing my bewilderment with Charmian, my late first wife, who was in general practice at the time. We talked into the night, pulled by the same curiosity. One day, after a meeting in London, we came upon reports on the effects of drugs on catatonic schizophrenic stupor. The syndrome was not uncommon in our mental hospital, and we were struck by the combination of mask-like rigidity, withdrawal, and cyanosis of the limbs. Quietly, Charmian suggested that we plan a study.

When we proposed this to Dr. J.J. O'Reilly, superintendent at Winson Green Mental Hospital (The Birmingham City Mental Hospital – now All Saints Hospital), he readily agreed and remained our supporter and friend in years to come.

Dr. O'Reilly put a small research room at our disposal and allowed us to choose patients, using our criteria; he also gave us nursing help. We used homemade gadgetry to measure "muscle tone" (i.e., rigidity) and foot temperature by thermocouple, and we also developed our own rating scales to measure change. The study taught us the enormous value of working in a realistic mental hospital setting. Sodium amytal, administered in full hypnotic doses intravenously, led to a paradoxical awakening of patients from catatonic stupor, a relaxation of muscle tone, and a rise in foot temperature. The effect of amphetamine was equally paradoxical. It led to the deepening of the stupor, an increase in muscle rigidity, and a deepening cyanosis. We also tried mephenesin, which had been shown by Frank Berger to be a powerful spinal internuncial neuron blocking agent and, through his prescient insights, later led to meprobamate and the whole family of anxiolytics. When tested in catatonic schizophrenic stupor, mephenesin produced marked muscle relaxation. There was, however, little effect on psychomotor response or peripheral temperature. The ability of patients to draw – for ten minutes, without prompting – while under the influence of drugs proved particularly interesting. Amytal markedly increased this ability, and amphetamine inhibited it. The experiments which we reported later (3) thus suggested *selectivity* in the action of drugs on catatonic stupor and raised the question of the relation of hyperarousal to catatonic withdrawal and, possibly, schizophrenia. Most important, however, these experiments established – at a tangible and a conceptual level – the need of working in parallel. The laboratory and the ward became ends of a continuum of related activities. I began to think of this continuum as *experimental psychiatry*.

At that time, then, there were two anchoring points for our work: neurochemistry, at the bench level, and human behaviour, as influenced by drugs. There was nothing in between, no indicator that could relate the effects of drugs on the brain to behaviour. I began to hunt again. The EEG was at that time coming into its own. Hill and Pond were publishing on the dysrhythmias, and Grey Walter and Gastaut were, in their own idiom, trying to relate functional states in man to EEG activity. And across the water there beckoned the great papers of Herbert Jasper and Wilder Penfield. I plumbed for the effect of drugs on the electrical activity of the brain in the conscious animal. There were very few data available in those days – except, a little later, those of Abraham Wikler and of James Toman's review (4). I obviously could not do it alone, and again, I was in the market for an associate.

I cannot recall now who told Philip Bradley about me or me about Philip Bradley, but I remember clearly his coming to my office and

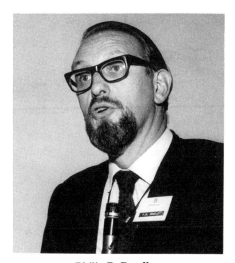

Philip B. Bradley

telling me of his experience and his interests. He had been trained in zoology and had carried out microelectrode studies in insects. He seemed interested in the problem, and a salary was available. So, after some consultation with Dr. Grey Walter, arrangements were made for him to spend some time with Walter to learn EEG techniques and then set up his own laboratory in the second of the two rooms of "Mental Diseases Research." This was duly done, and in 1948, Philip was working alongside us, developing his pioneering technique for recording electrical activity in conscious cats, a procedure that in those days (the days of sulfonamides – *not* penicillin) was quite a trick. The work proceeded well, and quickly established reference points for a pharmacology of the brain, inasmuch as it relates to behaviour. I still treasure a copy of Philip's thesis completed in October 1952 (5). It was a joy to see the clear and unambiguous effects of physostigmine, atropine, hyoscyamine, and amphetamine (and later, LSD-25) on the electrical activity of the brain in relation to behaviour. It was also particularly satisfying to find how these drugs grouped themselves in terms of their dependence on midbrain structures, and how information arriving at that time from Morruzzi and Magoun's (6) studies could be related to our own findings. There gradually emerged (and this was my own view) a concept of the presence of *families* of compounds that had arisen in the brain, in the course of chemical evolution. These compounds seemed chemically related to powerful neurohumoral transmitters familiar to us at the periphery. Three types of receptors, centering around members of the cholinester, the catecholamine, and later the indole family, were proposed (7, 8). Implicit in this concept of families of compounds was the notion of small regional *chemical fields* and of the interaction between molecules governing the gating, storage, and flow in self-exciting neural loops.

As we wrote at the time (9):

> It is likely that neurons possessing slight but definite difference in enzyme constitution may be unevenly distributed in topographically close, or widely separated areas in the central nervous system; these differences probably extend to the finest level of histological organization.... It would perhaps be permissible to speak of the operation of chemical fields in these regions. The agents in question may be either identical with or, more likely, derived from neuro-effector substances familiar to us at the periphery. Their number is probably small, but their influence upon integrative action of higher nervous activity may be profound. The basic states of consciousness may well be determined by variations in the local concentration of these agents.

It gives me special satisfaction to reflect on Philip Bradley's subsequent illustrious career and the influence he has exerted on the course of Neuropsychopharmacology in Europe and the world.

The third area to occupy us in those years concerned hallucinogenic drugs, which, from time to time, had been noted in literature. We began to read about them and formed a small discussion group to explore the possible relation of endogenously-produced hallucinogenic metabolites to schizophrenia. Hofmann's historic report to Stoll was written on April 22, 1943, and Stoll's paper on LSD-25 appeared in 1947 (10). We were immediately struck by the very low dose level, suggesting a specificity of very high order. Our own work in cats and a small number of human volunteers (of whom I was the first), using a single small dose (half a microgram per kilo) led us to conclude, later, that LSD-25 was acting on a serotonin-mediated receptor, peculiarly related to the afferent system (possibly the medial collaterals) (8) and exerting a selective inhibitory role on the organization of sensory information and the serial organization of information in time.

Thus, by about 1949-1950, three elements were in place in our small unit in Birmingham. There was a representation of neurochemistry; a laboratory for the study of electrical activity of the brain in the conscious animal, and there was Charmian's clinical investigation in the mental hospital. A *continuum* was in place. In our presentations and applications for funding, we referred to our program as a program of "Drugs and the Mind."

It is only fair to say that not everybody was friendly to our approach. The pharmacologists (with a few distinguished exceptions) regarded us as "odd men out" and we were strangers to the psychiatrists. But there was also solid support at the core. My chief, Alastair Frazer, was a staunch friend and supported us through thick and thin. I suspect, too, that he was a little proud to have our unit emerge in a large department preoccupied with lipid transport and fat absorption. And our Dean, Professor Leonard (later Sir Leonard) Parsons, gave us, at all times, the feeling that he truly understood what we were about. Sir Leonard was succeeded as Dean by Professor Arthur (later Sir Arthur) Thomson. When, on one particular occasion, I mentioned to him the need for more clinical facilities, he readily agreed. The Queen Elizabeth Hospital built us a small research wing adjoining the Medical School. But, more significantly, the Superintendent of the Mental Hospital, J.J. O'Reilly, put at our disposal an entire clinic, which had been used to house cases of chronic schizophrenia and organic psychoses. The house had at one time been the magnificent mansion of the Cadbury chocolate family. Over a period of nine months, it was steadily emptied (a result of deliberate policy of Dr. O'Reilly's), and sometime in 1952, we moved into a beautiful, well-equipped facility – standing among old trees with a rose garden at the back – and comprising forty-four beds, a day hospital, an out-patient clinic, and even an ethology laboratory, in which Michael Chance could carry out his pioneer studies on the effect of social setting on drug activity! When we were visited by the Rockefeller Foundation and the Medical Research Council (who supported us munificently), we could present a continuum extending from laboratories to clinic, and from the Medical School to the purview of the Regional Hospital Board.

In 1951, while in the United States on a Fulbright Fellowship to study psychiatry, I received a telegram informing me that I had been appointed the Head of a newly created Department of Experimental Psychiatry in the University of Birmingham. I returned humbled, thrilled, and bewildered by this extraordinary opportunity. A dream had come true.

We did not have to wait long for another major event. Sometime in late 1952, or early 1953, there walked into my office Dr. W.R. Thrower, Medical Director of Messrs. May and Baker. Dr. Thrower told me that May and Baker had acquired the British rights for chlorpromazine and presented me with Delay and Deniker's reports (11). They had a supply and could make up the necessary tablets. Would we care to perform a blind-controlled trial? Being very impressed by Delay and Deniker's pathbreaking studies, I said we certainly would and suggested that we would do so at the Winson Green Mental Hospital. Again, I asked Charmian whether she would be interested. She was, and it was she who assumed full responsibility for the management of what was to prove, I think, a rather important step in clinical psychopharmacology. For, as I think back on it, all the difficulties, all the opportunities, all the unpredictable aspects of conducting a trial in a mental hospital were to show up clearly in that early trial: the preparation of the ward, the training of the personnel, the gullibility of us all (the so-called "halo" effect), the importance of nursing attendants, relatives, and patients themselves as informants; the use of rating scales and the calibration of such scales – all these elements came into their own, once Charmian (and to a lesser extent I) were faced with the realities of working in a "chronic" mental hospital ward. I still remember the morning when we all trooped into the boardroom of the hospital, spread the data on the large oak table, and broke the code after the ratings and side effects had been tabulated. The trial involved 27 patients chosen for gross agitation, overactivity, and psychotic behaviour: 11 were affective, 13 schizophrenic, and 3 senile. The design was blind and self-controlled, the drug and placebo being alternated three times at six-week intervals. The dose was relatively low (250 to 300 mg per day). We kept the criterion of improvement conservative, which was reflected in our discussion. Yet there was no doubt of the results: 7 patients showed marked improvement; 11 slight improvement; there was no effect in 9 patients. Side effects were observed in 10 patients. Our short paper (12), which conclusively proved the value of chlorpromazine and was the subject of an editorial in *The British Medical Journal,* was a blind self-controlled trial. But it was more, for it was a statement of the opportunities offered by a mental hospital for work of this kind, the difficulties one was likely to encounter, and the rules that one had to observe to obtain results. As we wrote (12):

> The research instrument in a trial of this sort being a group of people, and its conduct being inseparable from the individual use of words, we were impressed by the necessity for a 'blind' and self-controlled design and independent multiple documentation. For that reason the day and night nursing staff became indispensable and valued members of the observer team. We were warmed and encouraged by the energy and care with which they did what was requested of them, provided this was clearly and simply set out at the beginning. A chronic 'back' ward thus became a rather interesting place to work in. There may well be a case for training senior nursing staff in elementary research method and in medical documentation. This would make for increased interest, increased attention to, and respect for detail, and the availability of a fund of information, all too often lost because it has not been asked for.

GROPING TOWARDS FOOTINGS OF A SCIENCE

By the mid-fifties, the good boot of empiricism had propelled our field mightily forward. New drugs were beckoning on the horizon and facts were hunting for an explanation. Yet the *science* of it all was sparse, a mere silhouette. New methods, new facts, new connections were needed to generate new hypotheses, to fill in details, and to give the field coherence and structure.

As we were working away in Birmingham, it became apparent to me that we were dealing with a science of a very peculiar kind. It was not a discipline in a traditional sense, but an *inter*science par excellence. It depended on the free flow of information between disparate fields; transdisciplinary communications were situated at the heart of progress. To be sure, the component fields were developing at different rates: but they induced questions between domains which proved provocative and catalytic.

The five areas which seemed important to us at the time were *functional neuroanatomy* (as exemplified by the work of Magoun, McLean, Nauta, Jung, and Olds); *neurochemistry,* particularly *regional neurochemistry* of the brain; *electrophysiology* of the brain, particularly in the conscious animal; *animal behaviour* studies; *human subject studies* and the refinement of the *clinical trial.* These seemed to be footings on which the new science could stand and grow. I have expanded on these concepts in an older review (13). Nowadays, of course, we could add molecular biology and genetics.

Equally important, as one thought of it, seemed the creation of environments which would facilitate such interdisciplinary conversation. This was not always easy, but possible, as I found out in later ventures at the NIMH and at Johns Hopkins.

INTO A WILDER FIELD: CONTACTS, MEETINGS, AND SYMPOSIA

It is hard to recapture the sheer elan and energy which developed in us all in those early fifties and the contacts which generated spontaneously as we went on in our work. The little handwritten blue airletters carried prepublication news, and were eagerly awaited. I vividly remember Hy Denber's first visit to us, soon after the publication of our chlorpromazine paper, and our discussion on dosage levels. There was an exciting correspondence with Nate Kline, whom I had first met in 1950, concerning reserpine. Later the Killams came, and a lifelong friendship ensued, and Jim Hance, who had worked for Phil Bradley and subsequently went to work with the Killams. Warren McCullough and Pitts visited us and fascinated our group with their mathematical models of self-regulation. Tinbergen (since a Nobel laureate) spoke on ethology at the Uffculme Clinic soon after it opened, and Leonard Cook, a most welcome visitor from Smith, Kline and French (SKF), shared with us some of the new and exciting techniques in the emerging field of behavioural pharmacology that he was developing. There were contacts with Ed Fellows, of SKF, who had introduced "Dexamyl," and David Rioch and Joseph Brady of the Walter Reed; later we contacted Jim Olds. Most importantly, the Macy Foundation began to organize its excellent Macy conferences on neuropharmacology, which brought us all together regularly. Also, in 1953, Hudson Hoagland organized an important interdisciplinary symposium at the Batelle Institute, at which we began, for the first time, to talk about the importance of social setting in relation to drug effects. This was called "sociopharmacology," a strange new concept to the orthodox pharmacologist. I had started to commute to the States regularly, visiting colleagues and comparing notes as the field was shaping. One such visit was of particular consequence: I believe it took place in 1952 or early 1953. A number of us met to discuss the need for an international symposium in neuro-chemistry, the first of its kind. Included were Seymour Kety, by that time Director of the Intramural Program for the NIMH; Heinrich Waelsch, Professor of Neurochemistry at Columbia; Jordi Folch-Pi, Director of the McLean Hospital Laboratories at Harvard; and Lou Flexner, Chairman of Anatomy at Pennsylvania . Also, I got in touch with Derek Richter and with Geoffrey Harris, who later was to emerge as a father of modern neuroendocrinology. As the theme of this symposium, we chose the "Biochemistry of the Developing Nervous System." As a place to hold it, we chose Magdalen College, Oxford. I was charged with being the Organizing Secretary, and I could not have done so without the devoted help of my British colleagues. The Symposium took place in the summer of 1954; sixty-nine colleagues from nine countries participated. It may very well be that at this Symposium the term "Neuro-chemistry" was used officially for the first time. As Heinrich Waelsch and I put it in our introduction to the Proceedings (14):

> ... We agreed, also, that from the start it would be well to consider the brain as a biological entity in all its complexity of morphology and function, rather than as a homogenate, or an engineering problem.

Three subsequent symposia reflected the momentum that was developing at this historic first meeting. The second on "The Metabolism of the Nervous System" was held in Aarhus, Denmark in 1956. The *Proceedings* were edited by D. Richter. The third on "The Chemical Pathology of the Nervous System" followed in Strasbourg, France, in 1958. The *Proceedings* were edited by Jordi Folch-Pi. The Fourth International Symposium centered on "Regional Neurochemistry." It was held in Varenna, Italy, in 1960. Seymour Kety and I edited the *Proceedings.*

Again, it is hard to convey the productivity that attended these meetings, as they steadily shaped some basic concepts in our field. Bit by bit, the footings of our new science were being put into place. Neurochemistry, and particularly the regional neurochemistry of the brain, was being related to electrophysiology; electrophysiology was being related to the emerging reward systems of Jim Olds, Joe Brady and Peter Dews. Behaviour analysis techniques were applied to the study of the effects of drugs on behaviour, and there was steady refinement of the clinical trial. In a word, things began to connect. In 1956, under the joint chairmanship of Jonathan Cole and Ralph Gerard, a milestone conference in psychopharmacology was held under the aegis of the National Research Council, the National Academy of Science, and the American Psychiatric Association (15), during which year also, Cole's Psychopharmacology Service Center was created – a step of enormous consequence for the future development of the field all over the world.

In 1957, the World Health Organization invited me to convene a small study group on the subject of "Ataractic and Hallucinogenic Drugs in Psychiatry." The following participated:

Ludwig von Bertalanffy, USA (Systems Theory)
U. S. von Euler, Sweden (Pharmacology)
E. Jacobsen, Denmark (Pharmacology)
Morton Kramer, USA (Epidemiology)
T. A. Lambo, Nigeria (Transcultural Psychiatry)
E. Lindemann, USA (Psychiatry)
P. Pichot, France (Psychiatry)
D. McK. Rioch, USA (Neurosciences)
R. A. Sandison, England (Psychiatry)
P. B. Schneider, Switzerland (Clinical Pharmacology)
J. Elkes, England (Rapporteur)

I wrote the report (16), which, incidentally, carried Eric Jacobsen's pioneer classification of the main drugs according to their pharmacological properties. In the meantime, the scientific command of the U. S. Air Force, through its principal representative in Europe, Colonel James Henry, had catalyzed meetings, at which the international implications of brain research became steadily more apparent. After preliminary meetings in 1958 and 1959, a number of us met at UNESCO House in 1960 to draft the Statutes and Bylaws of IBRO – the International Brain Research Organization. The disciplines of neuroanatomy, neurochemistry, neuroendocrinology, neuropharmacology, neurophysiology, behavioural sciences, neurocommunication, and biophysics were represented. Dr. Daniel Bovet and I represented Neuropharmacology in the first Central Council of IBRO. Our emerging field had now a major international presence.

TOWARDS THE CINP, THE ROME CONGRESS, THE NIMH, AND HOPKINS

In the Spring of 1955 or 1956 – I cannot remember which – Professor Ernst Rothlin and Mrs. Rothlin paid us a leisurely three-day visit in Birmingham. During our conversations, in which Charmian, Philip Bradley, William Mayer-Gross, and I participated, two broad ideas kept surfacing. One was the need for an international forum to discuss and serve the advances in our field. The other, the need for an international journal. I do not rightly recall whether the Latin name of *Collegium* was used in our discussion, but the need for an organization certainly kept recurring.

As for the journal, preliminary work had already been done. Willie Mayer-Gross had been in touch with R. Jung of Munich. Springer, the publishers had been approached and appeared interested. Further discussions involved Jean Delay, P. Deniker, P. Pichot of Paris, and most importantly, Abe Wikler of Lexington. It took quite a number of telephone calls and letters to persuade Abe to assume the co-editorship of this new journal. I served on the editorial board and still recall the excitement when the first slim yellow issue of *Psychopharmacologia* landed on my desk.

Perhaps this is also the place to emphasize the prescient vision of psychopharmacology that Abe Wikler had developed at the time. He saw, long before most of us, the true dimensions of the field, defining it beautifully in his book on the *Relation of Psychiatry to Pharmacology,* (17) now out of print. It set a standard of rigour and excellence – a standard he set for *Psychopharmacologia,* which continued as a model for years to come. Our contacts with the Rothlins and the Sandoz Group remained very much alive.

In 1957, at the invitation of Seymour Kety and Robert Cohen, I moved to the United States to establish the Clinical Neuropharmacology Research Center at St. Elizabeth Hospital, where Nino Salmoiraghi, Steve Szara, Hans Weil-Malherbe, Fritz Freyhan, and Floyd Bloom, joined us in rapid succession. Max Hamilton was our first visiting scholar. After I left (in 1963), Nino Salmoiraghi assumed the directorship. He was followed by Floyd Bloom and later by Richard Wyatt, the present incumbent.

Philip Bradley remained in contact with European colleagues. As he, Deniker, and Radouco-Thomas reported (17): At a meeting on psychotropic drugs in 1957 in Milan, "a small group of interested people representing pharmacology, psychiatry, psychology, and so on, held informal discussions and decided that regular opportunities should be provided for workers in the various fields of research and clinical investigation, to meet and discuss their common problems." The idea was taken further at the Second International Psychiatric Congress in Zurich in September of the same year (I could not attend, having just moved to Washington). It was at this Congress that our new *Collegium* was formally inaugurated, and it was Professor Trabucchi's invitation which led to our first Congress in Rome in 1958.

I attended the Congress, co-chairing the third Symposium and reading a paper on the "Relation of Drug Induced Mental Changes to Schizophrenia" (18) at the fourth. Across a span of nearly fifty years, one cannot help but be encouraged and thrilled by the vision of the organizers and the sheer span, grasp and inclusiveness of the program. For at what earlier international forum had the four footings of our science – neurochemistry, electrophysiology, animal behaviour, and the refinement of the clinical trial – been so skillfully juxtaposed? Where had one encountered papers on the measurement of subtleties of subjective experience in drug-induced states and discussed rating scales for subjective experience and objective behaviour? Or had been considered, in context, the huge policy implications of the psychoactive drugs for the mentally ill? I feel that by the end of the Congress, the silhouette had filled out and sharpened, presenting a new landscape in clear light. Biochemistry, physiology, psychology, and behaviour were looking each other in the face in a new kind of recognition. We had a map. It is exciting to recall this historic encounter.

As for my own paper (19), I could only submit an abstract – having been preoccupied with our newly-formed group in Washington. I presented an expanded version of the same ideas at the Third International Neurochemical Symposium in Strasbourg during the same year. In this paper (20), I examined schizophrenia as a possible disorder of information processing by the brain, drew attention to the possible place of subcortical structures (putamen, caudate, globus pallidus, and hippocampus) in the processing and misprocessing of such information, and considered the role of amines, particularly serotonin, norepinephrine, and dopamine in such misprocessing.

In 1963, I was invited to assume the chair at Johns Hopkins and the directorship of the Henry Phipps Psychiatric Clinic. But this "epistle" is already far too long, and I must defer details of this most fruitful and meaningful period to another occasion. Let me simply say that, at Hopkins we went on doing "more of the same." Sol Snyder began his pathbreaking neurochemical studies while still a resident, and now heads up the superb Department of Neuroscience at Hopkins. Joe Brady built primate laboratories for his far-reaching program in behavioural biology. Joe Coyle advanced developmental neurobiology in a way which inspired many residents to follow in his footsteps; he is now chief of Psychiatry at Harvard. Ross Baldessarini is director of the Mailman Laboratories at Harvard. "Uhli" Uhlenhuth, Lino Covi and Len Derogatis developed their rating scales and engaged in important outpatient studies. Uhli was also president of the ACNP at its twenty-fifth anniversary. Last but not least, reaching back to joint times at the NIMH, Floyd Bloom is now editor-in-chief of *Science.* There are many, many others one wishes to mention, but 'tis time to stop.

CLOSING

In 1961 the newly constituted American College of Neuropsychopharmacology did me the immense honour of electing me as their first president. Looking back on my year of service, I said (21):

> It is not uncommon for any one of us to be told that Psychopharmacology is not a science, and that it would do well to emulate the precision of older and more established disciplines. Such statements betray a lack of understanding for the special demands made by Psychopharmacology upon the fields which compound it. For my own part, I draw comfort and firm conviction from the history of our subject and the history of our group. For I know of no other branch of science which, like a good plough on a spring day, has tilled as many areas in Neurobiology. To have, in a mere decade, questioned the concepts of synaptic transmission in the central nervous system; to have emphasized compartmentalization and regionalization of chemical process in the unit cell and in the brain; to have given us tools for the study of chemical basis of learning and temporary connection formation; to have resuscitated that oldest of old remedies, the placebo response, for careful scrutiny; to have provided potential methods for the study of language in relation to the functional state of the brain; and to have encouraged the Biochemist, Physiologist, Psychologist, Clinician, Mathematician, and Communication Engineer to join forces at bench level, is no mean achievement for a young science. That a chemical text should carry the imprint of

experience, and partake in its growth, in no way invalidates the study of symbols, and the rules among symbols, which keep us going, changing, evolving, and human. Thus, though moving cautiously, Psychopharmacology is still protesting; yet, in so doing, it is, for the first time, compelling the physical and chemical sciences to look behaviour in the face, and thus enriching both these sciences and behaviour. If there be discomfiture in this encounter, it is hardly surprising; for it is in this discomfiture that there may well lie the germ of a new science.

In our branch of science, it would seem we are as attracted to soma as to symbol; we are as interested in overt behaviour as we are aware of the subtleties of subjective experience. There is no conflict here between understanding the way things are and the way people are, between the pursuit of science and the giving of service. So we must go on along lines we began: talk to each other, and keep talking. Psychopharmacology could prove a template for a truly comprehensive psychiatry of the future. We must train colleagues who do good science and, above all, who also *listen:* For, like it or not, our humanity will never leave us in our molecular search.

REFERENCES

1. Elkes, J. (1995). Psychopharmacology: Finding one's way *Neuropsychopharmacology* 12: 93-111.
2. Elkes, J. and Finean, J. . (1953). X-ray diffraction studies on the effects of temperature in the structure of myelin in the sciatic nerve of the frog. *Exp. Cell Res* 4: 69.
3. Elkes, J. (1957). Some effects of psychotomimetic drugs in animals and man. In *Neuropharmacology:Transactions of the Third Conference, New York. Josiah Macy, Jr. Foundation* 11: 205-294.
4. Toman, J., and Davis, J. P. (1949). The effects of drugs upon the electrical activity of the brain. *Pharmacological Reviews* 1: 425.
5. Bradley, P. B. (1952). Observations of the Effects of Drugs in the Electrical Activity of the Brain, Doctoral thesis, University of Birmingham, England.
6. Morruzi, G., and Magoun, H. W. (1949). Brainstem reticular formation and activation of the E.E.G. *Electroencephalography Clinical Neurophysiology* 1: 455.
7. Bradley, P.B., and Elkes, J. (1953). The effects of atropine, hyoscyamine, physostigmine and neostigmine on the electrical activity of the brain of the conscious cat. *J. Physiol.* (London) 120: 14.
8. Elkes, J. (1958). Drug effects in relation to receptor specificity within the brain: some evidence and provisional formulation. In G.Wostenholme, (ed.), *CIBA Foundation Symposium in Neurological Basis of Behaviour* (pp. 303-332). London: Churchill.
9. Bradley, P.B., and Elkes, J. (1957). The effects of some drugs in the electrical activity of the brain. *Brain* 80: 113-114.
10. Stoll, A. (1947). Lysergsäure-Diaethylamid - ein Phantasicum aus der Mutterkorngruppe. *Schweiz Arch. Neurol. Neurochirurg. Psychiat* 60: 279-323
11. Delay, J., and Deniker, P. (1953). Les neuroplegiques en therapie psychiatrique. *Therapie* 8: 347-364
12. Elkes, J., and Elkes, C. (1954). Effects of chlorpromazine on the behaviour of chronically overactive psychotic patients. *British Medical Journal,* 2: 560.
13. Elkes, J. (1955). The Department of Experimental Psychiatry, *University of Birmingham Gazette,* March 11.
14. Waelsch, H. (ed.). (1955). Biochemistry of the developing nervous system: *Proceedings of the First International Symposium in Neurochemistry* (p. 5). New York: Academic Press.
15. Cole, J., and Gerard, R. W. (eds.). (1957). *Psychopharmacology: Problems in Evaluation.* Washington, D.C.: National Academy of Science and National Research Council.
16. Elkes, J. (Rapporteur). (1958). Ataractic and hallucinogenic drugs in psychiatry. *WHO Tech. Rep. Series,* 152. Geneva: World Health Organization.
17. Wikler, A. (1957). *The Relation of Psychiatry to Pharmacology.* Baltimore: Williams and Wilkins.
18. Bradley, P. B., Deniker, P., and Radouco-Thomas, C. (eds.) (1959). *Neuropsychopharmacology,* 1, Proceedings of the First Meeting of the Collegium Internationale Neuro-Psychopharmacologicum, Rome, September 1958 (pp. vii-viii). Amsterdam: Elsevier.
19. Elkes, J. (1959). On the relation of drug-induced mental changes to the schizophrenias. In P. B. Bradley, P. Deniker, and C. Radouco-Thomas (eds.). *Neuropsychopharmacology,* 1 Proceedings of the First Meeting of the Collegium Internationale Neuro-Psychopharmacologium, Rome, September 1958. (p. 166). Amsterdam : Elsevier.
20. Elkes, J. (1961). Schizophrenic disorder in relation to levels of neural organization: the need for some conceptual points of reference. In M. Folch-Pi (ed.), *The Chemical Pathology of the Nervous System* (pp. 648-645). London: Pergamon Press.
21. Elkes, J. (1963). The American College of Neuropsychopharmacology: A note in its history and hopes for the future. *American College of Neuropsychopharmacology Bulletin,* 1: 2-3.

REMINISCENCE, 1958

Romolo Rossi

In 1958, when I was a twenty-four-year-old medical student in my fifth year at the University of Genova, the psychiatric ward of the Department of Neurology was a strange place. (There was no Department of Psychiatry at the university in the 1950s). There were rows of beds and near them, immobile people, seemingly petrified, with gloomy, hostile faces. A few smiled falsely and were over-pleasing, whereas others were strange and incomprehensible. Silence and immobility dominated the ward. Where was the unrest, the excitement, the agitation, the chaos, the turbulence, the out-of-control actions, the characteristics of insanity anticipated in my student eyes and in the eyes of the average person? Was this madness I was seeing ? Where was the inner turmoil that was supposed to be a part of mental illness? Where was the "ship of fools" of Hieronymus Bosch? Where was the world of Peter Brueghel? Where

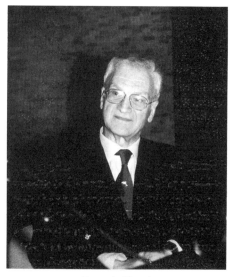

Romolo Rossi

was the bizarreness and irregularity? I failed to sense the immense suffering, the internal torment that this situation, frozen and still, kept hidden within itself. But the student that I then was, naive and inexperienced in medicine and life, came to understand Dante's intuition when he placed extreme suffering in the last circle of hell. That was where Lucifer endured his punishment in the midst of ice, immobility, and eternal cold. However, if the student quickly grasped that this frozen immobility was hell, he soon realized that there was also another madness, one of burning torment, shouting, and chaos. This madness however, was somewhere else. As soon as excitement appeared, as soon as the person became agitated, raised his or her voice, became aggressive, or sang loudly, he or she was transferred to another circle, the insane asylum, the Psychiatric Hospital, where the restless agitation of many similar persons created

Romolo Rossi is professor of psychiatry and director of the Department of Psychiatry at the University of Genova. He is a psychoanalyst and a past president of the Italian Society of Psychotherapy. In 1960 he studied the effect of imipramine and ECT in the treatment of depression.

Rossi was elected a fellow of the CINP in 1966. He coauthored papers on "Considerations on circulatory and psychopathological responses to stimulant drugs in psychiatric patients" (Fazio, Gilberti and Rossi) and on "Stimulation threshold in depression" (Gilberti and Rossi), at the 4th and 5th Congresses, repectively.

the exact counterpoint of the immobility seen at the psychiatric ward of the university clinic. Thus, the student saw that there were two types of madness: the frozen and the inflamed. They were handled in different ways and at different places. But overall there was the impotence, the helplessness of the doctor. Yet with the unconscious playing its tricks, the doctor, believed to be omnipotent, became presumptuous in a false attempt to interpret and explain what he could not treat. Sadness entered the heart of the student, who was not yet sophisticated enough to play such games.

All this discouraged the student. He was working hard to complete a thesis on the circadian variations of the symptomatology of episodic depression. He had little faith in "electroconvulsive therapy" (ECT), even if it were a matter of local pride in Genova, where Cerletti, who introduced this treatment, had once lived. Watching the administration of ECT was a disturbing and disquieting spectacle: patients lying in beds, one next to the other, comatose or in the grip of convulsions barely masked by muscle relaxants. ECT was given too widely in those years and without the clearly defined indications and procedures which characterize its use today.

Psychoanalysis of that period suffered from the vice of omnipotence. It could explain everything – the meaning of history, of art, of psychology, of sport. Since it was believed that it could cure every illness, the clinical indications for its use were almost without limit. It had magnificent theories and its techniques were employed as a magic key that could open all locks. As a result, its scientific credibility was lost.

What then was this small metal cylinder (I do not think that plastic was used in those days) filled with little red pills that had no name, only a particular code name, G22355, on the label? It was not that the student did not know the drugs that acted on the mind, or that he was unaware of the amphetamines and the barbiturates. It was not that he did not know about extraordinary substances that could induce convulsions and be used for shock therapy and substances which could induce catharsis and which could be used for diagnosing. It was the era of LSD, Ditran, JB329, narcoanalysis, and weckanalysis.

But this little bottle with its nameless pills was not taken very seriously. It was seen as just one more new treatment like the others in this stagnant pool of depression. It was perceived as a stone thrown into the water: it would produce concentric ripples that would then vanish, and all would be as before. How humble were our expectations! And how much greater was our excitement when, notwithstanding our prejudices and scepticism, it worked. The student, amazed, saw gloomy, rigid faces move and a smile appear. Slow, stiffened movements dissolved into emotional expressions and gesticulations. Halting and sparse language became fluent and lively, filled with colourful metaphors. Black, desperate feelings were transformed. Detachment from the world and a lack of interest changed into anticipation of the future.

All of this took place in a few days or weeks, and none of it by chance, as our statistics revealed. It was a return to life for which nothing could be substituted. One can understand the wave of emotion and the enthusiasm felt by the student of those days, who saw results never observed before, and which he had not even dared to hope for. He began to perceive gradually that things were about to change completely.

Psychiatry changed and became medicine; the student could walk into the psychiatric wards just as he walked into the ward of any other medical department. Having specialized and effective treatments, his discipline became a speciality and he no longer had to feel like an outsider. In all this he perceived, possibly a bit naively, that he was like the others, perhaps even better.

Psychiatry today, with its many different modes of effective treatments, is one of medicine's richest disciplines. Perhaps we do not understand the sense of pride that was felt at that time. As time passed, ECT was restored to limited use with well-defined indications; and psychoanalysis once again found its boundaries and regained its own large and specific area in understanding emotional disturbances.

As a student then, I barely believed what I saw, and it was only later that I would ponder my experience and put it in perspective. After that I would see, always with amazement, that crises of anxiety, phobias, and other symptoms which I had never expected to improve got better with the aid of these strange red pills. But what struck me the most was the change in expressiveness, in movement, and in interest in the future in melancholics.

All of this occurred before pharmacotherapy became institutionalized by controlled clinical trials, double-blind studies with crossover designs, which would seem grey, ordinary, and monotonous. What still stands out vividly in my memories is the changing face of depression, the smile that reappeared, the hint or sign of understanding that said, "I am no longer desperate." A philologist might have cited Greek mythology in reference to Tophronios and his healing den. For me, the student of those days, the nameless pill which brought about the change has remained very much alive. I will always remember it as G22355.

(Translated by Prof. C. P. Rosenbaum).

DELIRIUM TREMENS: THERAPY WITH LIVER EXTRACTS AND ITS CONSEQUENCES

Cornelis H. van Rhyn, Sr

After I qualified as a *zenuwarts* (neuropsychiatrist) in October 1949, I accepted a position at Brinkgreven psychiatric hospital as head of the male service. It was my predecessor, Nico Speyer, who introduced disulfiram for chronic alcoholics at Brinkgreven. As a result, by the time of my arrival the hospital had become a centre for alcohol-related diseases, such as Korsakoff syndrome and delirium tremens (DT). In the Netherlands, DT is not seen frequently; at Brinkgreven, we had only three to five cases of DT a year. Compared with other European countries, for example, France, Switzerland, Germany, Austria, that number was very low.

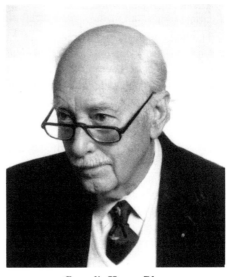

Cornelis H. van Rhyn

By searching for a possible biochemical explanation for DT, we found an abundance of information. Nevertheless, the treatment of DT remained difficult in the 1950s. There were several treatments, but each of them was merely symptomatic, directed at controlling one or another manifestation of the "psychosis." We used scopolamine, paraldehyde, and chloral hydrate for sedation, vitamin B complex for the prevention of the amnestic syndrome, and various other remedies including vitamin C, calcium, cortisone, intravenous saline, and so on. The psychosis (delirium) in most cases lasted seven to ten days, but sometimes much longer and in some cases it was followed by the development of Korsakoff syndrome. Prognosis was poor, fatal in five to twenty percent of the cases.

In 1952 Van der Scheer, a professor of psychiatry, visited us at Brinkgreven to discuss the need to treat the causes rather than the symptoms of psychoses. He reminded me of his article on the pathogenesis of DT, in which he postulated that DT is a disorder of the brainstem, probably induced by a liver disturbance. With his theory in mind, Van der Scheer encouraged me to try crude liver extract in therapy.

Cornelis H. van Rhyn was born in 1918. After studying medicine at Utrecht, he spent ten years as a clinical neuropsychiatrist. Between 1961 and 1988 he was in private practice as a psychotherapist in Enschede. He now lives in an old farmhouse in the Ardèche department, France.

Van Rhyn was a founding member of the CINP. He presented a paper on "Experiments in Parkinsonism" at the 1st Congress.

Three kinds of liver extracts were available at the time in the Netherlands: Pernaemon Crudum (Organon), HeparRaForte (Philips-Roxane), and a German preparation. After being assured that none of these extracts contained "particles" which would preclude their intravenous use, we decided to administer 1 ml of HeparRaForte, the preparation we had on stock at the hospital, to the first DT patient admitted to my service. Five minutes after the first, we gave the patient a second (2 ml) injection, and after another five minutes, a third (3 ml). The results were dramatic: within half an hour hallucinations were removed, tremor was reduced and consciousness was restored!

The next patient admitted to my service with DT died of acute cardiac insufficiency before we could treat him. An autopsy showed hypertrophic liver cirrhosis (with icterus), splenitis, and pleural and peritoneal hemorrhages. Subsequently, however, we had no case of death in a series of 20 patients treated with HeparRaForte. In fact, most of the patients responded within hours. Recovery was complete ("full"); none of the patients developed Korsakoff syndrome.

My findings with liver extract were verified by Idema and Beck, working in Enschede, at a hospital similar to ours. Instead of HeparRaForte, however, Pernaemon Crudum was used, one of the other liver extracts available in the Netherlands. Idema and Beck treated six patients with dramatic results. Their success in treating DT with Pernaemon Crudum was so great that in the years which followed we did not have any patients with DT from the region served by the Enschede hospital.

Then suddenly, HeparRaForte lost its therapeutic effects. We also noted that its colour was lighter than before. It appeared that HeparRaForte was altered without any notice given by Philips-Roxane. Even our repeated requests for information remained unanswered until in response to Professor Sorgdrager's threatening letter, the company admitted that HeparRa-Forte was diluted with folic acid to reduce the pain of parenteral injections. By that time we knew something like that had happened from the "gold chlorid chromatogram" of the substance (done by my friend Piet Sorgdrager), but it did not matter any longer. We had already shifted from HeparRaForte to Permeanon Forte (which had to be given in "double doses" to attain similar therapeutic effects) with the assurance from Organon, the manufacturer of the substance, that no folic acid would be added to it.

I summarized my observations about the use of crude liver extracts as follows:

(a) crude liver extract is therapeutically effective in DT;
(b) the specific qualities of crude liver oil are blocked by folic acid; and
(c) the liver enzyme, xanthine oxidase and folic acid are antagonists.

In the 1950s there was little information about xanthine oxidase, presumably responsible for the therapeutic effects of crude liver extract in DT. More recently, via the Internet I have found more than sixty publications on it, but none of them provided a direct answer to the question, "Why does xanthine oxidase have a therapeutic effect in delirium tremens?" On the other hand I did find out that xanthine oxidase is highly active in the liver of the fetus and that its activity diminishes gradually after birth. While this would explain why twice the dose was needed from Pernaemon Crudum (whose preparation was extracted from the liver of adult cows), than from HeparRaForte, (extracted from new born calves), it did not give any clues as to why xanthine oxidase would have a therapeutic effect in DT.

One possible explanation for the therapeutic effect of crude liver extracts in DT is that xanthine oxidase decreases (by oxidizing) acetoin – a condensation product of two toxic acetaldehyde molecules – and thereby reduces its toxic effects on the brain stem, responsible for delirium. This theory is based on findings that in chronic alcoholism there is an equilibrium between acetoin and alcohol and acetaldehyde, which is offset by the sudden withdrawal of alcohol. This explains why the dilution with folic acid, an antagonist of xanthine oxidase, interferes with the therapeutic effect of crude liver extracts in DT. It is also in line with Professor Van der Scheer's contention that all mental and somatic symptoms of delirium can be explained by the "chronic toxicity" of the brain stem.

This paper was written in honour of the late Professor Van der Scheer by a grateful Cornelis van Rhyn.

PERSONAL REMINISCENCES OF THE EARLY DAYS OF PSYCHOPHARMACOLOGY

Gerald J. Sarwer-Foner

As founder and editor-in-chief of the undergraduate medical journal of the University of Montreal, *La Revue Médicale de l'Université de Montréal,* I assigned various collaborators to review journal articles, allotting some to myself. Thus, in the 1947 and 1948 issues of *La Semaine des Hôpitaux de Paris,* the medical journal of the University of Paris Hospitals, I read Henri-Marie Laborit's early work on his "lytic cocktail," for use in the neurosurgery of highly vascular gliomas. This, of course, unbeknown to me at the time, was also the first reported use of an aliphatic phenothiazine, promethazine, to tone down the cortical activity of patients to whom it had been given in combination with other medicines. Years later when I met Henri-Marie Laborit at a Paris CINP meeting, he was astounded that I knew these early papers, exclaiming, "My God, I am so happy that somebody read them then."

I had trained in psychiatry after completing my internship, as a Senator Fulbright Fellow in 1951 to 53 at Butler Hospital, Providence, Rhode Island, with David Graham Wright and his team of excellent practitioners in the humane treatment of psychosis (to which were added the wisdom of such psychoanalytic greats as Gregory Zilboorg); and at the Department of Psychiatry, Western Reserve University Medical School, Cleveland, Ohio, under Professor Douglas Bond. I was absorbing much of psychodynamics, the continuation of "moral therapy" in addition to the existing biological therapy of the time.

I returned to Montreal in 1953 to complete my psychiatric training with Dr. Travis Dancey and his team at Queen Mary Veterans Military Hospital, and in Professor D. Ewen Cameron's Department of Psychiatry at McGill. Here, I experienced what a well-staffed and -equipped, university general hospital psychiatric unit could offer its patients, both for treatment and research. We had one physician per five patients, and one nurse, occupational therapist, physical-training instructor per two or three patients (though they weren't assigned on that basis). We also had excellent clinical psychologists for psychological testing and research studies. I started my clinical research in this setting with an understanding director of the department who was sympathetic to the inclusion of multiple observers of the patients' progress as well as to patient responses to "organic" and psychotherapeutic treatment.

Gerald J. Sarwer-Foner is Professor of Psychiatry and Behavioral Neurosciences at Wayne State University Medical School in Detroit, Michigan, and Professor and past Chair of Psychiatry at the University of Ottawa Medical School. He is a psychopharmacologist as well as a psychiatrist, training psychoanalyst, and forensic psychiatrist. Sarwer-Foner established the psychodynamic action of psychotropic medication, and was a pioneer in the combined use of psychotherapy and pharmacotherapy.

Sarwer-Foner was elected a fellow of the CINP in 1962. He presented papers on "Some psychodynamic and neurological aspects of paradoxical behavioural reactions" and on "Accumulated experience with transference and countertransference aspects of psychotropic drugs" (Sarwer-Foner and Kerenyi) at the 1st and 2nd Congresses.

I received my McGill diploma in psychiatry in 1955. In the same year I also qualified as a psychiatric specialist of the Royal College of Physicians and Surgeons of Canada. Subsequently, I became consultant in psychiatry to Queen Mary Veterans, to be appointed as director of psychiatric research, as the research at the service developed in amplitude.

The Department of Psychiatry at McGill was becoming one of the world's largest training centres and was thick with talent. Heinz E. Lehmann was, in the mid-1950s, clinical director of the University Mental Hospital, the Verdun Protestant Hospital (today the Douglas Hospital). He was always interested in research as he treated the mental hospital patients. He and a psychiatric resident of the time, Gordon E. Hanrahan, published the first North American paper on the use of chlorpromazine in 1954, which is deservedly remembered and cited. Because of this, another McGill paper of the time, from the Allan Memorial Institute, is poorly remembered; but had Professor Lehmann's paper not appeared when it did, Hassan Azima and William Ogle's paper published four months later might have been the first North American publication on chlorpromazine in psychiatric patients. N. William Winkelman, Jr., of Philadelphia, was actually the first in North America to obtain chlorpromazine from the pharmaceutical company, but was slow completing his studies, publishing considerably later.

Bill Ogle joined me as our first research fellow in studying reserpine, the second neuroleptic drug to appear. It was just about the time that we prepared a paper for presentation at the Allan Memorial Institute of the Royal Victoria Hospital that Nathan Kline of New York published his first paper on reserpine. Kline, a psychiatrist with research experience in psychology and neuroendocrinology, Hassan Azima, a psychiatrist at the Allan Memorial Institute, and I were invited in 1954 to present our findings on reserpine at the New York Academy of Sciences. The presentations were interesting in that they not only compared the results of reserpine with chlorpromazine, but also the results of reserpine in different settings, i.e., at state mental hospitals (Lehmann; Kline), at a psychiatric unit in a general hospital (Sarwer-Foner), and at a psychiatric institute section of a general hospital (Azima). Kline was pleased with my work and interested in our approach. Our meeting at the New York Academy led to a lifelong friendship.

Much research in the new discipline of biological psychiatry covering EEG (Charles Shagass), psychophysiology (Bob Malmo), neurochemistry (Theodore Sourkes), and neuroendocrinology (Robert Cleghorn) to mention just some, was already well established and growing at McGill in the mid-1950s. These existed side by side with stimulation from other departments of McGill, for example, Herbert Jasper's Electrophysiology Deparment in Wilder Penfield's Montreal Neurological Institute, and Donald Hebb's Department of Psychology.

My own work led very rapidly to the publication of a series of papers between 1954 and 1961 (1, 2) that created the first studies of the "target-symptom approach" to psychopharmacology, of the combined use of psychotherapy and psychotropic medication, and of the psychodynamic action of drugs. To the latter, Azima (3) and Winkelman, and later Mortimer Ostow of New York, each contributed his own views. Fritz Freyhan originally coined the name "target symptom approach" for our work, as compared to the "antipsychotic approach (3)."

As my papers appeared during the mid-1950s, the New York State Hospital System of some 200,000 patients, then the largest in the world, had become fascinated by the early results of chlorpromazine and reserpine. They appointed Dr. Henry Brill, an experienced hospital superintendent and assistant commissioner for mental health, to supervise the coordination and establishment of neuroleptic treatment in that system. He fostered the organization of state

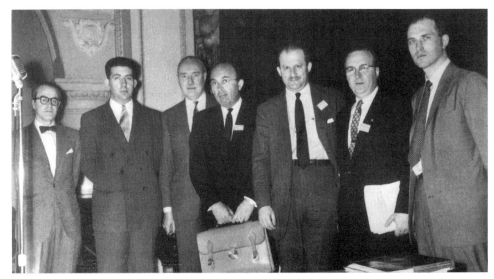

From left: Fritz Freyhan, Gerald J. Sarwer-Foner, W. Clifford M. Scott, Herman C. Denber, William Winkelman Jr., Alexander Gralnick and Bruce Sloan

hospital research units, as for example the ones directed by Nathan Kline, Herman C. B. Denber, Sydney Merlis, Anthony Sainz, to mention only a few.

I asked Professor Ewen Cameron, at the time the chairman of the Department of Psychiatry at McGill, to invite Pierre Deniker to lecture at McGill when he was in New York in 1955, and again when he was there to receive the Lasker Award. Deniker did so with great success, employing his usual charm and humour. In my home (where he showed my young son his Lasker Award statue) and at a dinner I gave in his honour attended by many of our McGill researchers, he regaled us with stories of fascinating experiences replete with Gallic quips. Deniker and I had corresponded and met in person on several occasions and had become good friends.

Because I spoke English and French, Jean Delay asked me whether I would interpret for him when he met with Nathan Kline at the Second World Congress of Psychiatry in Zurich in 1957. I agreed and stood by, with silent amusement, as Delay demonstrated that he did not need an interpreter, expressing himself vigorously and cogently without my intervention. Kline, with the collaboration of Delay and Heinz Lehmann, had organized a large Psychopharmacology Symposium for this meeting and had all the active researchers there, including myself, Azima and Cleghorn from McGill, as well as a full roster of basic science researchers and distinguished European and British professors.

Subsequent to the 1957 World Congress, Hy Denber urged me to hold a meeting in which all aspects of the use of neuroleptic medication could be explored. I organized this at Queen Mary Veterans Hospital (Montreal) in 1958 along the lines of the British learned societies of old. Here small groups of eminent colleagues met to hear stimulating presentations, to which they responded in lengthy discussion periods. This was a huge success, and the discussions, having been tape-recorded, were published in the book, *The Dynamics of Psychiatric Drug Therapy*, in 1960 (5). Gerald Klerman presented his first psychiatric paper here and Al DiMascio was an early participant.

The 1958 Montreal meeting had an unintentional effect: the participants loved the format and the exchanges and voted to hold a second meeting at Harvard to be chaired by Milton Greenblatt; this was also very successful and led to a third, chaired by H.C.B. Denber, and to many others in subsequent years. Because it was a nameless group with no structure other than the desires of the members who participated, a wit called it, "The Group Without a Name Research Society." Later, for reasons of ease in obtaining hotel accommodations for an organized body, it became known as the "Group-Without-A-Name International Psychiatric Research Society." The group met annually for many years and contributed notably to the literature. Most of the people who took part in this research became well-known. Initially we were a small enough group to be easily accommodated at small meetings.

I was thirty years old in 1955 when my first published papers appeared. Roy Grinker, then editor of the prestigious *AMA Archives of Neurology and Psychiatry,* grabbed me after one of my presentations at the American Psychiatric Association and, in his kindly but imperious way, informed me that he was publishing my paper in the *Archives.*

Our work was widely recognized – initially perhaps more in the United States, Great Britain, France, and Europe than in Canada, where the young Canadian Psychiatric Association was meeting its first challenges. In France, Professors P. Lambert and J. Guyotat in Lyons and Chambéry confirmed our work. Professor P. Pichot, a former teacher of Azima, knew his work better than he knew mine. Other European academics followed our work as well, and as a very young and academically junior man, I got to know many of the senior people in psychiatry.

Along with Brian Hunt and Hassan Azima, I was a student of the first class of the new Canadian Institute of Psychoanalysis in Montreal from 1958 to 1962. I was asked to lecture on my work to Martin Wangh's Committee on Psychotic Emergencies of the New York Psychoanalytic Institute, despite being still a student.

In the space allotted I have tried to reminisce about my contacts with the very early contributors to neuropsychopharmacology. Much could be said about the larger second wave of clinicians and researchers which appeared as this field developed.

REFERENCES

1. Azima, H., Sarwer-Foner, G.J., (1961) Psychoanalytic formulations on the effects of drugs in pharmacotherapy, *Rev. Canad. Biol.,* 2:603-614.
2. Sarwer-Foner, G.J. (1957) Psychoanalytic theories of activity-passivity conflicts and the continuum of ego defenses:experimental verification using reserpine and chlorpromazine, *A.M.A Arch.Neurol.Psychiat,* 78:413.
3. Sarwer-Foner, G.J. (1964), On the mechanisms of action of neuroleptic drugs: a theoretical psychodynamic explanation, The Hassan Azima Memorial Lecture. 18th Ann Meeting, Soc. of Biological Psychiatry, Atlantic City, N.J., June 7-9, 1963, In J. Wortis (ed), *Recent Advances in Biological Psychiatry,* Vol. 6, (pp. 217-233) New York: Plenum Press.
4. Sarwer-Foner, G.J. (1989) The psychodynamic action of psychopharmacologic drugs and the target symptom vs. the antipsychotic approach to psychopharmacologic therapy: thirty years later, Read at History of Psychiatry Section, World Psychiatric Association Annual Meeting, Quebec City, Oct. 2-4, 1985. *Psychiatr. J. Univ. Ottawa.* 14 : 268-278
5. Sarwer-Foner, G.J., (ed.) 1960. *The Dynamics of Psychiatric Drug Therapy.* Springfield, Charles C. Thomas, (642 pages).

THE INTRODUCTION OF MEGAVITAMIN THERAPY FOR TREATING SCHIZOPHRENIA

Abram Hoffer

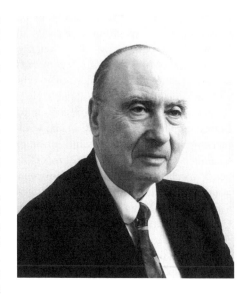

Abram Hoffer

In 1950 I joined the Psychiatric Services Branch of the Saskatchewan Department of Public Health, located in Regina (Saskatchewan, Canada). I had received my PhD from the University of Minnesota (USA) in 1944 and my MD from the University of Toronto (Ontario, Canada) five years later. My job at the Department of Public Health was to create a psychiatric research unit. In order to learn psychiatry I became a resident and four years later received my specialist certificate (to become a fellow in the Royal College of Physicians and Surgeons, Canada) in psychiatry. In 1951 I visited almost all of the research centres operating at that time in Canada and the United States in order to find out what was being done in psychiatric research. During my visit to one of the centres I was shown the site, with a builder's shack on it, that was later to become the National Institutes of Health in Bethesda, Maryland.

Because of my training in biochemistry, I was oriented towards the biological sciences. After I began working with schizophrenic patients, it became clear to me that this was essentially a biochemical disorder that induced major psychological symptoms in its victims. These patients occupied half of all the psychiatric beds in our province, and there was no effective treatment.

Fortunately, Humphrey Osmond joined us to become superintendent of one of our two mental hospitals in Saskatchewan. He brought with him the idea that in the body of a schizophrenic patient there might be a substance related to adrenaline with the psychological properties of the hallucinogen mescaline. He and John Smythies had studied mescaline psychosis and had concluded that there were many similarities. This idea appealed to me, and the three of us soon formulated the adrenochrome hypothesis of schizophrenia. This hypothe-

Abram Hoffer was born in rural Saskatchewan in 1917, the son of pioneer farmers. After receiving his PhD in agricultural biochemistry and his MD, he directed psychiatric research in the province of Saskatchewan. He is the author of sixteen books and more than five hundred research papers.

Hoffer was one of the founders of the CINP.

sis, although ignored for a long time by psychiatry, proved prescient and determined the path of our research for the next thirty years. It is now coming back into orthodox psychiatry since adrenochrome has been shown to be present in the body, and its first reduction product, adrenolutin, is relatively easily measured in the blood.

The adrenochrome hypothesis directed our attention to the use of megavitamin therapy. We reasoned that nicotinic acid or nicotinamide might decrease or inhibit the formation of adrenochrome by decreasing the formation of adrenaline from noradrenaline, and that ascorbic acid, a water-soluble antioxidant, would decrease the oxidation of adrenaline. Vitamin C was then known to be a powerful antioxidant and had been used to stabilize adrenaline solutions.

Our first pilot trials with megavitamin therapy were positive, and we followed up these trials with the first series of double-blind, placebo-controlled prospective studies in psychiatry, completing six double-blind clinical trials by 1960. Vitamin B-3 (nicotinic acid and nicotin-amide) was the first chemical to be tested in double-blind studies in psychiatry. We doubled with Vitamin B-3 treatment the two-year recovery rate of acute schizophrenic patients, from 35 to 75 percent. The double-blind approach is not very elastic, and as we had designed our first series of studies before the tranquilizers became available, we ran the clinical trials without these drugs.

My adoption of the double-blind methodology was forced. We had applied for a research grant from the federal government in 1952 in order to test yeast nucleotides for treating schizophrenia (a treatment that was not found to be therapeutically effective) and Bud Fisher, who was statistical adviser to the government of Canada in Ottawa at the time, recommended that we use the double-dummy design, which had been developed in England a few years earlier. I was familiar with the design from my studies in agricultural biochemistry while I was working for my PhD. We agreed to use the method because it was clear that if we did not, we would not receive the grant. On Fisher's advice we randomized our patients and treated them with either the active substance or a placebo, following the procedure now hallowed by long usage. Since we published an account of our work in the *Menninger Bulletin* in 1954, it is possible that the double-blind method would have reached psychiatry somewhat later if we had not used it when we did.

Today I am convinced that the double-blind is a "dud" method, used only by clinicians and administrators who have a lot of money and little imagination. It is a method which has never been validated, an emperor without clothes. I have been pointing this out for many years, but few see the naked emperor – the retrospective, double-blind, placebo-controlled experiment. I suspect that it is useful only after one already knows that a compound works, and that it is employed today mainly in order to get published and to satisfy funding agencies when one applies for grants.

I was aware of the important role played by drugs, especially the antidepressants, and had begun to use them as soon as they became available. I was using lithium long before it came on the market, by making capsules from pure lithium salts. But my role in the development of tranquilizer treatment was very minor. I was too preoccupied with nutrition and megavitamin therapy.

By 1955, information about the efficacy of chlorpromazine had filtered into Saskatchewan. In our research we were interested in any therapy that might help our patients, but we had not made any provision for using the new drugs in our controlled studies. It soon became apparent that chlorpromazine was a powerful tranquilizer which rapidly controlled agitated and psycho-tic behaviour. In sharp contrast, vitamin therapy was slow and required a good deal of patience on the part of the therapists. When no drugs were available, there was no alternative to patience, but when chlorpromazine and other tranquilizers appeared, psychiatrists preferred to use them rather than to wait. I soon found that a combination of tranquilizers and megavitamins worked quickly. I was able to see the rapid effect of the drugs, together with the slow but sure therapeutic effect of the vitamins. Eventually, in most patients it was possible to discontinue the drug and to keep patients well on the megavitamins alone.

My early work with Osmond was very exciting and, in my opinion, productive. We travelled many miles together, attending meetings and seeking research grants. But we also received much unwelcome attention simply because we were doing something different. No matter how well we presented our material or emphasized its scientific aspects, it was rejected out of hand. On one occasion, a psychologist from Los Angeles came to one

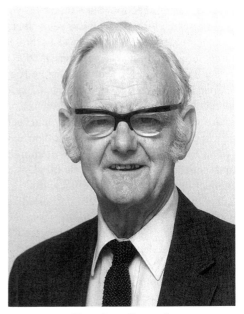

Humphrey Osmond

of our meetings in Saskatchewan. While he was drunk and belligerent, he asked me to explain the adrenochrome hypothesis. I tried to do so, but he would not listen and kept breaking in. After a few minutes I asked him what kind of evidence I would have to present to convince him. He replied that no amount of evidence would ever do so – *in vino veritas.* He, in fact, represented the common psychiatric opinion of megavitamin therapy at that time and even today.

But we were consoled by the most important fact of all: our patients responded well, became normal and were able to resume their practice, regardless of whether their profession was law, medicine, or even psychiatry. One of my patients who recovered on megavitamin therapy became a psychiatrist and later president of a large psychiatric association. (Coincidentally, the association was busy for some time attacking us for our work on megavitamin therapy.) I have seen few similar recoveries when such patients were treated with drugs only. We were also given strong support by a few famous physicians and scientists, such as Nolan D.C. Lewis, Heinrich Klüver, Linus Pauling, Sir Julian Huxley, and Walter Alvarez.

Our work contributed indirectly to the development of psychopharmacology. During the Second World War, biological psychiatry had almost vanished because of the rising influence of psychoanalysis (which swept the field by 1960), a shortage of research funds, and preoccupation with the war effort. In the United States, biological psychiatry was kept alive by Nolan Lewis, chair of the dementia praecox committee of the Scottish Masons Rites. Their committee met once a year in New York and distributed small grants to various groups doing biochemical research in the field. In 1952 Osmond and I appeared before the committee, and for the first time, in the Canada Room of the Waldorf Astoria, we outlined our adrenochrome hypothesis. (In October 1997, I addressed a large group of physicians, nutritionists, and others

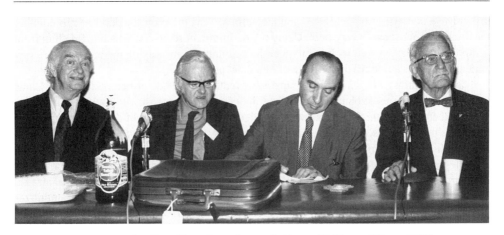

From left: Linus Pauling, Humphrey Osmond, Abram Hoffer and Roger Williams

from Japan, who had flown to New York to hold a two-day symposium. That occasion reminded me of my experience in the hotel so many years earlier.)

We did not receive a grant, but we were encouraged to continue our investigations, which later, in 1954, led to a large grant from the Rockefeller Foundation over a six-year period. J. Weir, medical director of the foundation, told me that ours would be the last grant the foundation would give to psychiatry. He added that the foundation had provided large grants to the Ivy League universities to establish chairs in psychoanalysis, but on reviewing the outcome of these grants, it had concluded that the money had been wasted. Weir also told me that if the results of our research were positive, the foundation might come back into the field again. One condition was attached to the grant we received: I had to become a Rockefeller Travel Fellow and spend three months visiting psychiatric centres in Europe.

The development of the idea of "model psychosis" – the idea that hallucinogens such as mescaline and LSD could produce in normal people a condition similar to that induced by the schizophrenic process – was the second major change that paved the way for the eventual resurgence of biochemical psychiatry. Arising from this work was the concept of "psychedelic therapy," a term coined by Humphrey Osmond and announced at a meeting of the New York Academy of Sciences in 1957. Psychedelic therapy was banished to the streets after 1960, but it is slowly finding its way back into scientific psychiatry.

Thus, there have been two parallel pathways in modern pharmacotherapy in psychiatry. There was the tranquilizer pathway, fuelled by massive advertising on the part of the drug companies to promote a patented compound that was a good sedative, but did not have the disadvantages of the barbiturates. This has become the dominant movement in modern psychiatry. The main effort of the drug companies today is to find a better drug, one that is more effective and less toxic. Unfortunately in schizophrenic patients, tranquilizers, although helpful, do not in most cases lead to complete recovery. They reduce the frequency and intensity of the symptoms, but at the price of side effects, including tardive dyskinesia and the, to my mind even more pernicious, "tranquilizer psychosis." I believe that it was Mayer-Gross who once remarked that tranquilizers replaced one psychosis with another; he was quite right. The "tranquilizer psychosis" is characterized by the same symptoms present in the original psychosis, but attenuated by the drug, together with the superimposed symptoms of apathy, difficulty in concentration, and muscular side effects. The price for the comfort provided by the drugs is in most cases very high. Using my definition of recovery, which is freedom from symptoms, getting on well with family and the community, and paying income tax, very few patients on drugs alone reach this state of health, even today.

The other pathway in pharmacotherapy was eventually named "orthomolecular" by Linus Pauling in his famous 1968 paper published in *Science*. Pauling became interested in mega-vitamin therapy, and this other pathway was developed by a couple of dozen American and Canadian psychiatrists, some familiar with our book *How to Live with Schizophrenia*. He reversed his earlier decision to retire and accepted a position at the University of California, San Diego, as a Distinguished Professor of Chemistry. But he was attacked with great vigour and enthusiasm by the psychiatric establishment, led by the National Institute of Mental Health.

Unfortunately, the orthomolecular pathway has been overshadowed by the tranquilizer pathway in spite of the fact that by 1985 about 100,000 schizophrenic patients were treated with the orthomolecular approach without a single patient developing tardive dyskinesia. Vitamins can't be patented and have no vigorous and wealthy parents to promote their use. They do work well together, but only recently is there a universal recognition of this. Today the International Society of Orthomolecular Medicine has seventeen affiliated member countries. In Brazil alone there are between five and six thousand orthomolecular physicians.

The major contributions that I and my colleagues made were, I think, the following: the introduction of megavitamin therapy, now considered the beginning of the new paradigm in medicine – that is, the use of vitamins as therapy and not just for the prevention of illnesses; the generation of biochemical hypotheses about the cause of schizophrenia; the provision of evidence for the important role that biochemical abnormalities play in creating schizophrenia, which over the past ten years has become much more acceptable; and lastly, psychedelic therapy.

THE BEGINNING OF PSYCHOPHARMACOLOGY
A Personal Account

Leo E. Hollister

In 1952 I had no idea of becoming a psychopharmacologist. That was the year I joined the staff of a psychiatric hospital as an internist with responsibility for the medical needs of psychiatric patients. It soon became apparent that mental illnesses, especially schizophrenia, were among the most disabling afflictions known. Nonetheless, my primary therapeutic interest remained hypertension. From the time of my internship until then, I had tried many proposed treatments for this disorder, none with much success. Thus when, in 1953, a representative from CIBA Pharmaceuticals told me about a new drug, reserpine, which had been reported to be effective, I grabbed at the chance. Sure enough, after treating twenty or so patients, I became convinced of its efficacy.

When the CIBA representative returned to see me later the same year, he told me that the drug had also shown some efficacy in treating schizophrenia. I knew little about that disorder, but thought that our staff psychiatrists should take a look at this new treatment. I approached the chief of psychiatry with

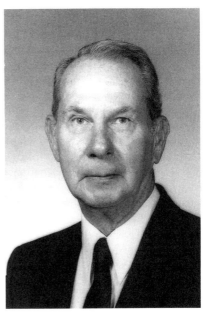

Leo E. Hollister

the notion, but he gently pooh-poohed the idea of any drug being useful, since so many previous ones had failed. With his assent, I decided to look into the question myself. Since many of the staff were now personal friends, as well as golfing buddies, there was no problem getting their cooperation. Studies began on my medical ward with either the drug or a placebo, and patients were then returned to their psychiatric wards for evaluations.

Leo E. Hollister, one of the pioneers in the use of psychotropic drugs, has been a psychopharmacologist for forty-five years. He is the author of over four hundred original contributions, as well as numerous book reviews, chapters in books, and other publications.

Hollister was elected a fellow of the CINP in 1958 and served as president on the 11th executive. He presented papers on "General review of complications of psychotherapeutic drugs," on "Relationship between blood levels of centrally-acting drugs and clinical effects," and on "Combinations of psychotherapeutic drugs" at the 5th, 6th, and 7th Congresses, respectively.

Initially, we did not see much in the way of improvement. However, CIBA had sent a research physician, Dick Roberts, to the west coast to oversee studies with the drug. He indicated that the doses for hypertension we were using were too low. When we switched to larger doses, in the order of 3-5 mg/day, we saw definite improvement among those treated with the active drug as compared with patients who received the placebo.

In June of that year, the American Medical Association had its annual meeting, which in those days was a big affair. I found an exhibit on the use of chlorpromazine in schizophrenia, presented by Mark Altschule, a Harvard professor of medicine, and Willis Bower, a psychiatric resident. I was familiar with Altschule's work in internal medicine and was therefore somewhat surprised at this exhibit. However, his wife suffered from the disorder, which accounted for his interest in the new drug.

Encouraged by the results they reported, I soon started trials of chlorpromazine in the same fashion as I had with reserpine. Patients were randomly assigned to the active drug or placebo, started on treatment with intramuscular doses followed by oral doses, and then returned to their psychiatric wards for blind evaluation (the physicians on these wards had no knowledge of whether their patients had received the active drug or the placebo). These were, I believe, the first studies of the now-standard parallel-group, double-blind controlled design with random assignment of patients. Meanwhile, to investigate the depression-eliciting properties of reserpine, I treated nineteen normal subjects with the drug in doses no higher than 1 mg/day and proved that, in contrast to those who had received the placebo, a sizable number developed symptoms of mental depression.

At the end of 1954 the American Association for the Advancement of Science (AAAS) held its annual meeting in Berkeley, California. I was invited to be part of a group that presented findings on the new psychotherapeutic drugs. Among the others were Nathan Kline, reporting on studies with reserpine, John Kinross-Wright, describing his work with chlorpromazine, and Murray Jarvik, reporting on LSD. In a single paper, I presented all three controlled studies that we had completed to that point. In those days I was quite naive. I thought that once something had appeared in print, regardless of the vehicle, it became part of general knowledge. As it turned out, I never published any of these studies elsewhere. The AAAS book was finally issued in 1957, and the total number of copies in circulation was probably less than two hundred. So my naivety managed to hide my light under a bushel.

One of the patients we treated in the early studies was a young Armenian man who had been severely schizophrenic for some years. He typically assumed a fetal position. I had tried everything possible with him, but nothing made him move until he received reserpine. He finally improved enough to be discharged from the hospital and to resume his former hobby of photography. When the Russian Sputnik flew in 1959, he took the best photograph of it, which was published with his credit line in *The Encyclopedia Britannica*. About twenty-five years later, while I was making medical rounds in the coronary care unit, I heard my name called out. Sure enough, it was the Armenian, who had suffered a myocardial infarct. We had a pleasant conversation during which it became apparent that he was still psychotic, though not badly so. This example shows both the hope that these drugs could inspire – patients saved from a potential lifetime of hospitalization – and the disappointment of no full recovery.

In mid-1955 I was invited to the second New York Academy of Sciences (NYAS) conference on reserpine, one devoted entirely to its psychiatric use. My paper, which reported our controlled studies, caught the fancy of the press and was given nationwide publicity over the wire services. Upon my return home, my office was inundated with mail from desperate people offering to bring me their afflicted loved ones. I answered each letter, telling them that there were no secrets in medicine and that this treatment should be available in their home territory. This was my first encounter with the enormous power of the press, which is often used so recklessly.

Thus within three years, from being someone who had no interest in psychopharmacology, I had become nationally known. As before, I published only in

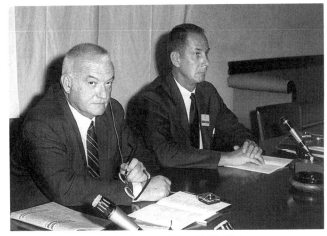

Pierre Deniker and Leo E. Hollister

the *Annals* of the NYAS, which appeared in 1959. Part of my anonymity was the result of some uncertainty in my own mind about my role in a field in which I had no formal training. Perhaps it was a touch of the "imposter syndrome." It was not until I became a member of the Veterans Administration Cooperative Studies and of Chemotherapy in Psychiatry in 1957 that I finally believed I had some role to play in the accurate clinical evaluation of these drugs. The VA studies pioneered the large-scale multiclinic research that was later emulated by the National Institute of Mental Health and a couple of state hospital systems.

Nonetheless, I remained pretty much on the sidelines for a few more years. I somewhat reluctantly joined the American College of Neuropsychopharmacology, waiting until the third annual meeting before I attended (I have not missed one since). Similarly, although I joined the original roster of the Collegium Internationale Neuro-Psychopharmacologicum (CINP), my first congress was the fourth, and I did not appear on the program until the fifth. I find it somewhat remarkable, in retrospect, that I eventually became president of both these fine organizations.

By the end of the 1950s I was completely hooked on clinical psychopharmacology. In collaboration with John Overall, a psychometrician and biostatistician, I embarked on a series of drug evaluations with special emphasis on discovering which types of patients (using factor analytic techniques) were most amenable to treatment with specific drugs. Although we found that the best results among depressives were obtained in those who most clearly showed endogenous depression, we were unsuccessful in delineating such groups of responders to antipsychotics.

Meanwhile, having been discouraged by the nature of studies done on LSD up until 1960, I started systematic evaluations of so-called psychotomimetic drugs, including their potential therapeutic uses. This research led to a series of studies on cannabis and its constituents, which continued until fairly recently. I was helped enormously by Hampton Gillespie in carrying out the marijuana studies and enjoyed the excellent collaboration of the Swedish group headed by Stig Agurell. My affiliation with the Committee (later College) on Problems of Drug Dependence began during this period, and I served as chairman of the group for several years. In the 1970s, with the able assistance of Kenneth Davis, we began studies on the cholinergic hypothesis of Alzheimer's disease, as well as on the potential role of acetylcholine in other disorders. With another able student, John Csernanasky, during the 1980s, studies were launched on some of the more basic aspects of schizophrenia. Many of us owe so much to our students and colleagues.

Since then, a new generation of investigators have appeared who are able to use the tools now available to explore the complexities of the mind and the drugs that affect it. I well remember watching Bill Oldendorf in 1960 demonstrate how, with an X-ray unit running on a circular model-train track, one could obtain X-ray photographs of the contents of a phantom head. Who could have guessed that the discovery of computerized tomography – and other forms of scanning – would advance our field so greatly? The techniques of molecular medicine, which began in 1949 with the demonstration by Itano and Pauling that sickle-cell anemia is due to aberrant amino acid substitutions on the hemoglobin molecule, has had a major influence on psychiatric investigations. Our older approaches now seem so primitive.

The luckiest people, in my opinion, are those who thoroughly enjoy their work and experience much intellectual stimulation from it. I count myself among them for having been privileged to work in the field that I accidentally entered. Although I have probably contributed some grains of sand and a few pebbles to the edifice of knowledge, my greatest regret is not having been able to provide some of the boulders, such as those added by other members of the CINP. Our field should become more exciting in the future, so that when the organization celebrates its centenary, rather than its fortieth birthday, most of our goals in alleviating mental illnesses will have been realized. But I would also have predicted that outcome forty years ago.

THE MAINSTREAM
OF
DRUG DEVELOPMENT

The 1960s started with a positive note. The therapeutic effectiveness of chlorpromazine and four other phenothiazine neuroleptics (mepazine, perphenazine, prochlorperazine, and trifluoperazine) was convincingly demonstrated in the treatment of schizophrenia by the United States Veterans Administration Collaborative Studies. Pharmacotherapy of schizophrenia was no longer just a matter of faith.

By the mid-1960s the effectivenesss of the neuroleptics in schizophrenia had been established, followed by the demonstration of the effectiveness of antidepressants in depression. By the end of the decade the proven therapeutic activity of lithium had been extended from the control of manic excitement – already established in the 1950s – to the maintenance and prophylactic treatment of bipolar manic-depressive disease.

The impact of psychopharmacology on psychiatry was soon visible. While the theoretical framework of psychiatry remained splintered among the various psychiatric schools, the essential features of psychiatric treatment were becoming increasingly similar all around the world.

A consequence of the rise of psychopharmacology was a rapid increase in the number of psychotropic drugs. By the end of the 1960s, well over eighty psychotropics had been studied clinically, and about fifty were available in one country or another for clinical use (Appendix 2.1). There were also well over sixty companies marketing more than one or two of these drugs in different variations (Appendix 2.2).

The steady flow of new drugs stimulated neuropharmacological research, leading by the mid-1960s to neurochemical theories about the mechanism of action of antidepressants and neuroleptics. The theories spilled over into speculations (often referred to as hypotheses) about the pathomechanism of mental illness, e.g., the ill-fated catecholamine hypothesis of depression or the durable dopamine hypothesis of schizophrenia. The need to decide promptly whether to proceed or stop at various stages in the development of a new molecule led to the development of new animal pharmacological tests and screening batteries, and to the furthering of clinical neurophysiological methods, e.g., the quantitative EEG. By 1970, to meet the needs for the rapid demonstration of the efficacy of a new psychotropic, two major sytems for the clinical evaluation of psychotropics were in place: the AMDP System, created by academics in the German-language area, and the ECDEU-BLIPS System, developed by the Public Health Service in the United States. AMDP stands for Association for the Development of a Methodology for Documentation and Assessment in Psychiatry; and the ECDEU-BLIPS, stands for Early Clinical Drug Evaluation Units-Biometric Laboratory Information Processing System.

In the following, a series of memoirs will be presented under the subheadings of Development of Drugs, Neurochemical Underpinnings, Pharmacological Profile, Neurophysiological Profile, and Clinical Profile. The contributions under the heading Development of Drugs include a paper on views of psychotropic drug development in the 1960s, and a paper on the regulatory framework of psychotropic drug development in the United States. The contributions under Neurochemical Underpinnings include a paper focused on the technological developments, e.g., spectrophotofluorimetry that opened the path to the mainstream of neurochemical developments relevant to the action of psychotropic drugs.

Development of Drugs

DRUGS AND INDUSTRY

David Healy

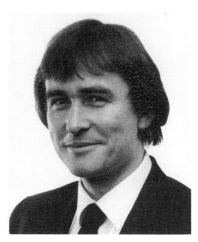

David Healy

The CINP was founded on the initiative of Ernst Rothlin from Sandoz, who was its first president. Early meetings were extensively supported by the pharmaceutical industry, especially the Swiss companies. Many of the clinicians and basic scientists who attended did so with industry support. Industry stood to gain by educating and influencing a cadre of clinical psychopharmacologists, who would in turn influence the prescribers in all countries worldwide. It also stood to gain in that the early discoveries of neuroleptics, minor tranquilizers, and antidepressants had all been serendipitous and there was an urgent requirement to establish the bases on which psychotropic agents worked, so that both therapeutics and drug development might become rational. The early days of the CINP, therefore, were inextricably bound up with the interests of the pharmaceutical industry, even if obviously industry-sponsored symposia were much less conspicuous during the 1960s than they have been in the 1990s. Attempting to recover the landscape of the 1960s is, however, difficult since so many fundamental assumptions have changed.

The 1960s were a decade in which the atmosphere in psychopharmacology mirrored the larger culture of the Western world. This was an era of hope and optimism, when presidential statements at CINP meetings could chart genuine progress made and anticipate the resolution of important issues, when no one was ashamed to speculate on what the effects of psychotropic drugs might reveal about the relationship of the mind to the body. The debates at the 1960, 1962, and 1964 meetings between Lewis, Shepherd, Freyhan, Brill, Kline, Roth, Lehmann, Delay, Deniker, the young Kielholz, Hippius, Angst, and others on issues to do with specific and non-specific factors in pharmacotherapy, as well as the target symptoms of psychotropic agents, had a brilliance and sophistication often absent from later debates. That brilliance did not come only from clinicians; in Birmingham in 1964, significant contributions were made at plenary and free-communication sessions by Pletscher of Roche, Janssen, Stille of Wander,

David Healy is currently director of the North Wales Department of Psychological Medicine, formerly secretary of the British Association for Psychopharmacology. His most recent book, *The Antidepressant Era,* (Harvard University Press, 1997) is a history of antidepressants. He has also contributed two books of interviews with major figures in the field of psychopharmacology (*The Psychopharmacologists*, Vols. 1 and 2), including a number who have contributed to this volume. His other research interests touch on cognitive neuropsychiatry and circadian rhythms.

Healy was elected a fellow of the CINP in 1994.

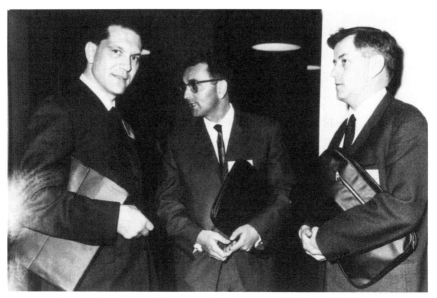

From left: Raymond Battegay, Jules Angst, and Walter Pöldinger

Theobald of Geigy, Cerletti and Taeschler of Sandoz, Petersen of Lundbeck, Hoffmeister and Kreiskott of Bayer, and Cook of Smith, Kline and French. (Significantly, perhaps, apart from SKF, the input from American companies was minimal. Efforts were being made to understand at a fundamental level what psychotropic agents were doing and what the implications of their therapeutic effectiveness were for our notions of mental illness and rational therapeutics. Yet, retrospectively, there was little progress; the issues remained unresolved and, perhaps more important, unaddressed today.

There were two engines of drug development in this period. One was simple animal models, such as the reserpine test for antidepressant activity introduced by Costa and Garattini in 1960, and the amphetamine-induced stereotypy model, which had been used by Janssen in the 1950s but became more widely employed during the 1960s under the influence of Randrup and Munkvad (1). While relatively simple procedures such as these were used for rapid screening purposes, a program of behavioural-biology research grew up within the laboratories of different pharmaceutical companies aimed at understanding in greater detail what the various agents did and what abnormalities of learning or neurobiology might underpin disease processes (2). Pharmaceutical companies had large numbers of compounds on their shelves, and the clear lesson from the development of chlorpromazine, which had generated $75 million for Smith Kline and French in 1955, was that there was a lot of money to be made by companies if they could detect therapeutic effects. The work of Leonard Cook at Smith, Kline and French and Alexandra Delini-Stula and others at Geigy Pharmaceuticals gives a good indication of the way developments were going (3, 4, 5).

The other engine of development came from clinical feedback. Investigators such as Guyotat and Lambert (6) in France in 1959 had suggested, for instance, that it might be worth constructing molecules with some of the properties of both the antidepressant imipramine and the neuroleptic levomepromazine. Suggestions such as these led to experiments with molecules and in this case to the production of an agent with the nucleus of an iminodibenzyl and the side chain of levomepromazine – trimipramine. As was hoped, this compound was distinctively different in its clinical actions from other antidepressants available at the time, but only in the 1990s has it become clear that it is far more distinctively different in the receptor profile of its activity than anyone at the time had any inkling.

The development of trimipramine was paradigmatic of much else. The use of clinical feedback methods such as this, and models such as the reserpine test, led to charges in the 1970s and 1980s that drug development had become a "me too" process. The charge was that pharmaceutical companies were making minor manipulations to existing molecules in order to get around the patent laws and that there was a lack of genuine innovation. For a long time, it was difficult to argue against this criticism, given that the structural formulae of the various tricyclic antidepressants indeed appeared to differ only in terms of minor chemical features. From the vantage point of the 1990s, however, it is now clear that desipramine (a noradrenaline reuptake inhibitor – NARI), imipramine (a serotonin and norepinephrine reuptake inhibitor – SNRI), clomipramine (which is close to being a selective serotonin reuptake inhibitor – SSRI), trimipramine (a noradrenergic and serotonin selective agent – NASSA), and opipramol (active on sigma receptors), for instance, all differ dramatically in the neurobiological effects that they exert, to the extent that all five agents, were they to be introduced now, would warrant different acronyms to reflect their differential effects on noradrenergic, serotonergic, or other systems. This astonishing diversity has taken three decades of "rational" development to reproduce, a fact that starkly raises the question of whether modern methods provide much of an advance over older ones.

The catecholamine hypothesis of affective disorders and the dopamine hypothesis of schizophrenia, introduced at the Washington CINP Congress in 1966, marked a turning point in two respects (8, 9). Following the emergence of these hypotheses, one sees a decrease in emphasis on the behavioural effects of both neuroleptics and antidepressants, and an increase in emphasis on the supposed cures that these agents will bring about. Before, psychotropic drugs had been seen as affecting target symptoms or syndromes. But now, debates vanish about what drugs should do in order to make patients well. The assumption appears to have become that the drugs cure diseases rather than bring about functional changes, and the goal of drug development is to pinpoint the common mechanism of different classes of neuroleptics or antidepressants, the belief being that this might in some way be linked to the lesions in these disorders (10). This change in assumptions was fuelled by the fact that, in terms of drug development, towards the end of the 1960s it became possible to screen for biochemical changes in the brain following psychotropic drug administration in animals. Tests on the effect of agents on reuptake systems began to be introduced as a means of screening for new agents. This development was to culminate in the mid-1970s with the beta receptor downregulation hypothesis of antidepressant action and the dopamine receptor hypothesis of schizophrenia.

In the early 1960s it was still possible for companies to take out process patents on agents rather than compounds or use patents. One sees, therefore, amitriptyline being developed by Merck, Roche, and Lundbeck concurrently. Take, for example, the demise of reserpine. It had been introduced in the 1950s. In the first CINP meeting, LSD, chlorpromazine, and reserpine, in that order, were the three most commonly cited entries in the index. In a prospective, randomized, placebo-controlled trial, reserpine had been shown to be useful for anxious depressions. Many clinicians commented that their patients did well indeed. Yet reserpine caused akathisia, which appears to have been associated with suicide attempts (11). These led to a concern about its use and to its effective demise. By the mid-1960s the number of references to reserpine in the index had shrunk to four or five.

To understand this demise, however, one must appreciate that in the early 1960s twenty-six different versions of reserpine were on the market. Accordingly, no one company had as great an interest in maintaining the compound's market share as, for instance, Eli Lilly has had in the 1990s in defending fluoxetine,which has also been associated with akathisia and the emergence of suicidal ideation. Fluoxetine notably "fails" the reserpine screening test, which suggests that this test, rather than testing for antidepressant activity, may have acted to ensure that the 1960s generation of antidepressants were less likely to cause akathisia than many subsequently developed compounds. But in addition, the fact that since the mid-sixties one company gets to own a drug exclusively means that drug development has depended to an ever greater extent on the market interests of that company and not on the interests of independent scientists, who can access the drug whether or not a company supports what they are doing.

In 1960-62 the thalidomide disaster struck, leading to the adoption of the 1962 amendments to the Food and Drug Act in the United States. These amendments maintained the prescription-only status of psychotropic agents in the face of considerable opposition (thalidomide had been available over the counter in parts of Europe). They put a premium on the use of placebo-controlled, randomized trials for testing clinical efficacy and also on developing agents for disease indications (12). The placebo-controlled clinical trial did not affect drug development until the 1970s. The clinical trial enters the index of CINP meetings only in 1970, although it enters as the most commonly cited entry at that meeting. Throughout the sixties, companies still depended on, and laid more weight on, the opinions of experienced investigators than they did on the results of controlled trials. It was only subsequently, in the 1970s, that the multicentred study began to come into its own. And it was not until the 1980s, as a result of the weak treatment effects of the antidepressants in particular, that the necessity for placebo controls was fully appreciated, which in turn meant the development of the multinational clinical trial. In the process, the independent clinical trialist had been eclipsed. The proceedings of CINP meetings in the 1960s still reveal trials done by independent or single investigators or small groups of investigators. Even in 1970 the majority of trials involved individual investigators testing drug combinations against their single components. There are few reports of double-blind, randomized, placebo-controlled trials of the kind we are familiar with today. The voices of experienced clinicians still carry weight, but the eclipse of these voices since 1970 has perhaps contributed in part to the atrophy of debate on the clinical significance of psychotropic compounds that begins to set in by that year.

In addition, retrospectively, it seems that after 1962 a mood developed which viewed with suspicion any use of psychotropic agents other than therapeutic. Given the thalidomide problems and the excesses of the psychedelic culture in the United States in the 1960s, this is perhaps understandable, but the changing state of affairs led Werner Janzarik in 1976 to bemoan the triumph of empiricism over theoretical development. Whereas the model psychoses and the implications of psychotropic drug effects for psychopathology were much discussed at early meetings, by the late meetings of the period, discussions in this area had all but ceased. By the time of the 1970 meeting in Prague, neurobiological investigations had begun to dominate. It requires only the addition of clinical trial results of the modern kind to produce the program for a 1990s-style CINP meeting, a meeting full of neurobiological and clinical data, but devoid of any effort to integrate these data sets into a coherent whole.

It would seem that there has been something of a fall from grace. Neither the clinicians' nor the drug developers' early hopes have been fulfilled. The group who have gained most significantly have been the molecular biologists. Where neurobiology is present in the early meetings, it is overwhelmingly in the molar vision of neurophysiology, rather than the molecular viewpoint of biochemical metabolite measurements or receptor binding or cloning. The term "receptor" is all but absent from the indices of CINP meetings through the 1960s. By 1970, however, the dominance of neurophysiology has begun to slip, and while studies on the molar effects of drugs on the behaviour of animals are still present, the molecular viewpoint is beginning its climb to ascendancy. No one in that year spoke out against the diversion that such developments were likely to entail.

But the extent to which we have been diverted becomes clear if one considers a beautiful quotation from Taeschler of Sandoz in 1964: "Finally let me extend my remarks on the pharmacology of the antidepressants to the larger field of psychopharmacology ... I have tried to put forward some evidence to the effect that observable drug-induced mood-lifting can best be explained in terms of a polyvalent action pattern rather than of a single pharmacological effect ... Such a concept is indeed valid for other drug-induced psychic changes. Closely related drugs may well prove to elicit qualitatively different effects depending on the quantitative distribution of their various pharmacological properties. This ... is a task that will require more of our attention in future" (13). If supplied with this quotation unreferenced and asked to make an attribution, most modern psychopharmacologists would be likely to opt for Carlsson circa 1990. Coming first in that year, such a comment would have been seen as prescient in the light of recent developments. Suitably adapted, it could provide the marketing copy for the generation of antidepressants and antipsychotics emerging in the latter half of the 1990s. Coming first in 1964, however, Taeschler's summing-up suggests that our primary achievement has been the reinvention of the wheel. One might even suggest that going "back to the future" to read the proceedings of CINP meetings in the 1960s would prove illuminating.

REFERENCES
1. Randrup, A., and Munkvad, I. (1965). Pharmacological and biochemical investigations of amphetamine-induced abnormal behaviour. In D. Bente and P. B. Bradley (eds.), *Neuropsychopharmacology* (vol. 4, pp. 301-303). Amsterdam: Elsevier
2. Brady, J.V. (1998). The origins of behavioural pharmacology. In D. Healy (ed.) *The Psychopharmacologists (Interviews)* (vol. 2). London: Chapman & Hall.
3. Cook, L. (1965). Behaviour changes with antipsychotic drugs in animals. In D. Bente and P.B. Bradley (eds.), *Neuropsychopharmacology* (vol. 4, pp. 91-99). Amsterdam: Elsevier.
4. Cook, L. (1998). Chlorpromazine and behavioural pharmacology. In D. Healy (ed.), *The Psychopharmacologists* (vol. 2). London: Chapman & Hall.
5. Delini-Stula, A. (1996). The changing face of psychotropic drug development from 1965-1995. In D. Healy (ed.), *The Psychopharmacologists (Interviews)* (pp. 425-440). London: Chapman & Hall.
6. Guyotat, J., and Lambert, P.-A. (1964). Un nouvel antidépressif dérivé de l'Iminodibenzyl: la Trimeprimine. In P.B. Bradley, F. Flügel, and P.H. Hoch (eds.), *Neuropsychopharmacology* (vol. 3, pp. 290-294). Amsterdam: Elsevier.
7. Van Rossum, I.M. (1967). The significance of dopamine receptor blockade for the action of neuroleptic drugs. In H. Brill, J.O. Cole, P. Deniker, H. Hippius, and P.B. Bradley (eds.). *Neuropsychopharmacology* (pp. 321-329). Amsterdam:Excerpta Medica.
8. Schildkraut, J. J., and Durrell, J. (1967). The effects of imipramine on the urinary excretion of catecholamine metabolism in depressed patients. In H. Brill, J.O. Cole, P. Deniker, H. Hippius, and P. B. Bradley (eds), *Neuropsychopharmacology* (pp. 352-359). Amsterdam: Excerpta Medica.
9. Eccleston, D. (1971). Biogenic amines and the affective disorders. In O. Vinar, Z. Otava, and P. B. Bradley (eds.), *Advances in Neuropsychopharmacology* (pp. 79-89). Amsterdam: North Holland Publishing Co.
10. Healy, D., and Savage, M. (subm.), Reserpine Exhumed.
11. Healy, D. (1997). *The Antidepressant Era*. Cambridge, Mass.: Harvard University Press.
12. Taeschler, M. (1965). Pharmacological aspects. In D. Bente and P.B. Bradley (eds.), *Neuropsychopharmacology* (vol. 4, pp. 197-202). Amsterdam: Elsevier.

DRUG DEVELOPMENT: REGULATIONS

Louis Lasagna

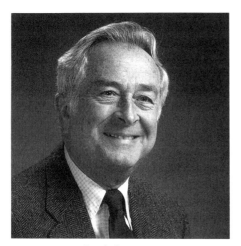

Louis Lasagna

The 1950s and 1960s were a remarkable time for the launching of new psychopharmaceuticals. Chlorpromazine (CPZ), for example, was synthesized in France in 1950, with the first clinical publications appearing in 1952. It not only controlled mania and psychotic agitation, but also decreased aggressiveness and delusions in schizophrenics, leading to the coining of the word "neuroleptic." The drug was introduced in Canada and the United States in the 1950s. The advent of haloperidol provided a successor to CPZ, and gradually took over the CPZ market during the period from 1959 to 1978.

New anxiolytics also were marketed during these decades, the first being meprobamate in 1955, its launch marked by the publication of articles describing research that could pejoratively be called anecdotal (or "naturalistic") today, but which were nonetheless extremely positive about the drug's benefits for anxious patients. Ultimately, meprobamate was replaced by the benzodiazepines, first chlordiazepoxide and then diazepam, both of which were enormously successful worldwide. The modern antidepressant story began in 1957 with imipramine, followed by the monoamine oxidase inhibitors (MAOIs). Lithium for the treatment of mania also surfaced in the 1950s.

What is striking about these additions to the pharmacotherapeutic armamentarium was the role played by old-fashioned clinical observation. The agents mentioned above were usually first identified by competent physicians who were alert enough to recognize therapeutic activity when they saw it. The era of randomized controlled trials had begun in the 1940s in the United Kingdom with streptomycin for tuberculosis, but general articles covering the philosophy and mechanics of such trials and recommending their use were still appearing in the 1950s (1); they urged a greater role for such evidence in drug development and regulation.

In the United States, it was not until 1962 that federal legislation was passed to empower the Food and Drug Administration (FDA) to require convincing evidence of efficacy as a

Louis Lasagna is a fellow and past president of the American College of Neuropsychopharmacology. He is Dean of the Sackler School of Graduate Biomedical Sciences and Academic Dean of the School of Medicine, Tufts University, in Boston, Massachusetts (USA).

prerequisite for marketing approval (2). Prior to that time the agency was legally limited to considering the evidence on safety, but the few doctors in the FDA (certainly less than a dozen – the exact number is debated), as far as one could tell, looked at the efficacy side only because allowable toxicity obviously could not be judged without an appreciation of what therapeutic benefits might ensue. The 1962 amendments (often referred to as the Kefauver-Harris Amendments) changed the regulatory demands for all time.

The interest of the U.S. Congress in pharmaceutical matters had begun in 1958 when a congressman named Blatnik held four days of hearings generally critical of the promotion of tranquilizers. But the attack was mounted in earnest on December 7, 1959, when Senator Kefauver began hearings that went on for twenty-six months, with testimony that filled 12,885 pages of government records. His concerns at first centred on possible collusion between drug companies with regard to the price of drugs, suboptimal industrial competition, excessive profits from the sale of medicines, and the failure of physicians to prescribe cheaper generic versions of drugs. With the passage of time, however, Kefauver's staff added new concerns to their agenda: patent-derived exclusivity, improper drug promotion, the lack of informed-consent procedures in the study of experimental drugs, and the need for convincing data on efficacy as well as safety.

In the course of the several drafts that the legislation ultimately went through, there was considerable discussion as to what constituted "substantial evidence" for supporting therapeutic claims. "Qualified experts" were clearly to be involved in the decisions, and Congress definitely had in mind non-governmental experts, not the opinions of FDA employees, as has become the rule. A distinction evolved between the terms "preponderant evidence" and "substantial evidence." Congress wisely realized that experts could differ, and it therefore recommended that if effectiveness was supported by "a responsible body of opinion," even if a minority point of view, a drug should be marketed. There was no congressional support for the view that a new drug had to have *greater* efficacy than already available drugs as a requirement for regulatory approval.

Despite the years of hearings and lengthy deliberation, the final bill seemed sure to die for lack of congressional support until the thalidomide tragedy surfaced, with testimony presented to Congress about the pathetically deformed phocomelic infants in Europe whose mothers had taken the drug early in pregnancy. The attendant publicity was abundant and dramatic, and S.1552 passed both houses of Congress unanimously, an exceedingly rare outcome for Washington legislation.

Despite the role of thalidomide in reviving the moribund Kefauver-Harris Amendments, the bill actually had nothing to do with teratogens per se. What *did* it put into law? The main points were

1. a tightening of federal control over the pharmaceutical industry's activities in interstate commerce;
2. the addition of a requirement for evidence of effectiveness for regulatory approval and marketing, in addition to the evidence of safety required by the 1938 statute;
3. the involvement of the FDA at the very start of clinical testing, to assess the adequacy of the preclinical safety studies, the investigators who would conduct the research, and the protocols proposed; in addition, informed consent was required for all clinical research, a change without precedent in U.S. law;

4. power for the secretary of Health, Education and Welfare (HEW; now Health and Human Services) to take a drug off the market without delay if it was judged to pose an "imminent hazard" to the public;

5. the secretary of HEW would henceforth play a role in the review and designation of generic drugs and was to ensure that drug labels carry such official names as well as the brand names;

6. drug advertising was to list all ingredients and a "brief summary" of safety data, as well as expected therapeutic benefits.

Since 1962 the drug development process has become more complicated, slower, riskier, and more expensive. It now takes ten to fifteen years from discovery to marketing, and only one in four or one in five drugs taken into humans ever achieves regulatory registration. Even with cautious, competent, and conservative regulatory agencies, drugs are occasionally withdrawn from the market, usually because of rare serious adverse events (4 percent of approved drugs in the United Kingdom, 3 percent in the United States) (3).

"Evidence-based medicine" has become synonymous with randomized, double-blind, placebo-controlled trials, even though such trials usually fail to tell the physician what he or she wants to know (4) – which drug is best for Mr Jones or Ms Smith, not what happens to a non-existent "average" patient. These developments (and such phenomena as "intent-to-treat analyses"), while reducing the likelihood of type I (false positive) errors, have probably increased the likelihood of type II (false negative) errors and have posed some ethical conflicts (5).

The decades since the 1950s and 1960s have thus seen a revolution in the regulation of pharmaceuticals. We will continue to get leads from unplanned "old-fashioned" clinical observation, but the days when a drug company would go to skilled and sophisticated psychiatrists, give them a supply of a new drug, and ask them to "try it on some different patients" seem gone forever. Is this a cause for celebration or depression, since preclinical data can rarely answer the question, what psychiatric illness will respond?

REFERENCES

1. Lasagna, L. (1955). The Controlled Clinical Trial. *Theory and Practice* 1: 353-367.

2. Lasagna, L. (1989). Congress, the FDA, and new drug development. *Persp. Biol. Med.*, 32: 322-343.

3. Bakke, O.M., et al. (1995). Drug safety discontinuations in the United Kingdom, the United States, and Spain from 1974 through 1993: a regulatory perspective. *Clin. Pharm. Therap.*, 58: 108-117.

4. Hill, A.B. (1966). Heberden Oration, 1965: Reflections on the controlled trial. *Ann. Rheum. Dis.*, 25: 107-113.

5. Lasagna, Louis. (1997). Scientific and economic threats to ethical drug development. *Reg. Affairs Focus*, 2: 9-10.

AS I REMEMBER

Frank M. Berger

I am honoured to have been asked to contribute to this volume, and I have much pleasure in recalling the excitement of events that commenced in England more than fifty years ago. I am a Czech by origin and a microbiologist by training. After obtaining my MD degree from the University of Prague in 1937, I worked as a bacteriologist at the Czechoslovak National Institute of Health in Prague. When my homeland was occupied in 1939, I moved to England, where I worked first as a physician in a refugee camp and later as a resident in a hospital for infectious diseases and as a bacteriologist in the West Riding of Yorkshire Laboratories in Wakefield. While there, I developed in 1944 a method for the purification of penicillin (1).

As a result of the attention that this work attracted, I was offered a position in the pharmaceutical industry. My task was to try to develop non-toxic antibacterial agents that would inhibit the growth of gram-negative microorganisms causing enzymatic destruction of penicillin. The only compound known at that time which had some marginal properties of this type was a substance called phenoxetol, the phenyl ether of phenol. Thus it seemed appropriate to examine the antibacterial and pharmacological properties of compounds structurally related to phenoxetol. The family of alpha-substituted ethers of glycerol was selected and synthesized by W. Bradley, the chief chemist, and evaluated by me. This is how I described the effect of these compounds in the first publication on this subject in 1946: "Administration of small quantities of these substances [the alpha-substituted glycerol ethers] to mice, rats or guinea pigs caused tranquilization, muscular relaxation, and a sleep-like condition from which the animals could be roused (2)."

I was deeply impressed with the tranquilization and muscle relaxation produced by these compounds and sensed that they might have important applications in clinical medicine. I selected for further study the 3-(2-methylphenoxy)-1,2-propanediol because it possessed the most intense muscle-relaxant action and had the widest margin between doses producing reversible muscular paralysis and death. This compound was named myanesin and subsequently assigned the generic name mephenesin. I set out the task to find its mode of action, and after much experimentation, I showed that it had a selectively depressant effect on the interneurons. This conclusion was made because mephenesin depressed the hyperexcitability of spinal reflexes without affecting normal reflex action. Symptoms of hyperactivity, such as reflex hyperexcitability, tremors or convulsions, whether produced by poisons such as strychnine or light anesthesia, could be inhibited with a small dose of mephenesin, which had

Frank M. Berger was born in the Czech Republic in 1913. He discovered mephenesin, the first skeletal muscle relaxant with tranquilizing properties, in 1945. After elucidating its mode of action and metabolism, he used this knowledge to develop meprobamate in 1952, the first anti-anxiety tranquilizer and the precursor of all drugs of this kind.

Berger was elected a fellow of the CINP in 1966. He presented a paper on "The antidepressant action of certain tranquilizers and its reinforcement by anticholinergic drugs" (Berger, Kletzkin and Margolin) at the 5th Congress.

no effect on normal reflexes and voluntary muscle power. These observations suggested that the drug might be useful in the treatment of spastic and hypertonic conditions (3). Mephenesin was soon (1948) shown to be clinically effective in these conditions by Schlesinger and colleagues (4) and others.

I arrived in the United States in October 1947, having accepted a position as assistant professor of pediatrics at the University of Rochester Medical School. I soon learned of Schlesinger's work and set out to investigate the oral effectiveness of mephenesin in spastic and hyperkinetic disorders (5). It proved quite effective in these conditions, but its duration of action was too short to be of practical value. Nevertheless, myanesin was put on the market in 1948 under the trade name Tolserol by E. R. Squibb. I was impressed with the state of well-being and mild euphoria produced by the drug for one to two hours following its administration. Perhaps this was the reason why mephenesin, in spite of its low activity and short duration of action, became one of the most frequently prescribed drugs in 1949.

However, it became clear to me that a product with this type of activity but possessing a longer duration of action was needed. To obtain such a compound, two different approaches were pursued. The first approach was based on the screening of compounds chemically related to mephenesin with the aim of finding a longer-acting congener. These efforts proved unsuccessful. The second approach consisted of attempts to slow down the metabolism of mephenesin. It was during this research that it became recognised that mephenesin was rapidly oxidized to its biologically inactive lactic acid homologue (6). As a result of this knowledge, it appeared of some promise to attempt to block the terminal hydroxyl group of mephenesin so that it would not be accessible to the action of oxidizing enzymes. Following this reasoning, the acid succinate of mephenesin was prepared (7). This compound produced effects qualitatively similar to, but less intense than, those produced by mephenesin. The pharmacological properties of carbamate esters of mephenesin and closely related compounds were also investigated and found to be of no practical interest.

At about this time I was approached by Carter Products, which also owned a small, financially unsuccessful subsidiary called Wallace Laboratories. Mr Hoyt, the owner of the firm, wondered whether I would be interested in trying to develop novel pharmaceutical products. I was, although accepting his offer involved leaving my dearly loved academic position at the University of Rochester Medical School. I joined Carter Products in June 1949 as Director of Research and was kept busy setting up an animal house and a pharmacological laboratory. I was soon able to continue my efforts directed at obtaining a longer-acting mephenesin, thanks to the assistance of B.J. Ludwig, the chief chemist at Carter Products. He synthesized many compounds of potential promise and first prepared meprobamate in May 1950 (8). The original patent application for the drug was filed on July 29, 1950, but later abandoned. A continuation-in-part patent application was filed on August 3, 1953 and issued on November 22, 1955. Meprobamate was first marketed in July that year by Wallace Laboratories as Miltown and by Wyeth Laboratories as Equanil.

The pharmacological properties of meprobamate were first mentioned in a paper entitled "The anticonvulsant activity of carbamate esters of certain 2,2-disubstituted-1,3-propanediols" (9). At that time it was assumed that all compounds of this type had a mephenesin-like type of activity. The evaluation of the anticonvulsant activity was considered to be the easiest way to assess their potency and duration of action. The paper shows that, of all of the propanediols that were investigated, meprobamate, the 2-methyl-2-n-propyl-1.3-propanediol dicarbamate, possessed the strongest and longest-lasting anticonvulsant action. The paper ends with the following prophetic statement: "A fuller pharmacological study of these or related compounds may uncover compounds with interesting central depressant properties."

I had been wondering, of course, whether the tranquilizing properties that made mephenesin so interesting would also be present in meprobamate. As I did not know of a reliable way to investigate this in animals, I approached Dr. Lowell Selling of Orlando (Florida) to study the action of meprobamate in humans. Before a clinical evaluation could start, it was necessary to obtain the compound in larger amounts than could be produced in the laboratory. It proved impossible to persuade any of the large chemical manufacturers to make meprobamate at an affordable price, but I was fortunate in having Bob Milano, president of a small chemical plant in New Jersey, assume the risk involved in setting up manufacturing facilities for a new drug. Meprobamate soon became available, and Selling was able to start the clinical evaluation of the drug in January 1953. He quickly recognized its value in the treatment of anxiety and tension states. His findings were published in the *Journal of the American Medical Association* in April 1955 (10). They were confirmed by Borrus (11) and others, and the drug was approved by the FDA in July 1955.

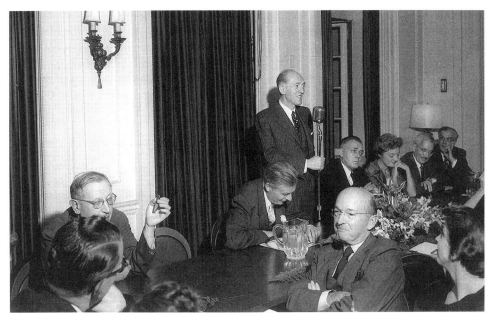

Aldous Huxley (left of speaker), Frank M. Berger (speaking), Laura Huxley (right of speaker), and Julian Huxley (far right)

Meprobamate soon became very popular. In October the following year, a conference on it and other agents used in mental disturbances was held in New York City under the auspices of the New York Academy of Sciences (12). At the conference, leaders in the fields of medicine, psychiatry, and psychology reported on their experiences with the drug. The meeting was introduced by Aldous Huxley, who welcomed the arrival of new tranquilizing drugs which would, as he put it, be less costly from the physiological and psychological point of view than the agents that humankind had turned to in the past in search of self-transcendence and relief from tension. Meprobamate soon became the most widely used prescription drug in the United States and in many other countries. By the end of 1965 the bibliography on the subject numbered more than 4,000 papers.

The clinical utility of meprobamate had been widely accepted by 1958, and I decided to focus my attention on questions relating to the vindication of its use (13). At that time most American psychiatrists considered Freudian psychoanalysis to be the only acceptable treatment of psychoneurotic conditions. I attempted to show that the chemotherapy of mental diseases is medically sound, morally acceptable, and scientifically justified. I did this by pointing out the neuropharmacological differences between meprobamate and the barbiturates. I also drew attention to the fact that anxiety is not a disease, but a symptom of a disease. As well, I tried to challenge the idea that, in limited amounts and under the proper circumstances, anxiety is necessary, and that without it we would lose our initiative and desire to work. I realize that I have not been completely successful in this respect, in spite of some incontrovertible evidence showing that anxiety is a maladaptive influence that invariably impairs performance and makes subjects unwilling to venture (14).

I am happy that I had the good fortune to participate in the introduction and acceptance of antianxiety agents which, together with the antipsychotics and antidepressants, demonstrated that mental disorders can be ameliorated by pharmacological agents. These agents have become the cornerstones of the new discipline of biological psychiatry. But let us not forget that this is not the end of the road. In many respects, our emotional life has not changed greatly since the dark ages. The future will reveal new ways, we hope, to liberate our minds from these primitive and outdated attitudes, so that we may clear them of prejudice and superstition and, in Spinoza's words, live according to the dictates of reason alone.

REFERENCES

1. Berger, F.M. (1944). Extraction and purification of penicillin. *Nature* (London), 154: 459-460.
2. Berger, F.M., and Bradley, W. (1946). The pharmacological properties of alpha:beta dihydroxy-gamma-(2-methylphenoxy) propane (Myanesin). *Brit. J. Pharmacol.*, 1: 265.
3. Berger, F.M. (1947). Mode of action of Myanesin. *Brit. J. Pharmacol.*, 2: 241.
4. Schlesinger, E.B., Drew, A.L., and Wood, B. (1948). Clinical studies in the use of Myanesin. *Am. J. Med.*, 4: 365-372.
5. Berger, F.M., and Schwartz, R.P. (1948). Oral Myanesin in treatment of spastic and hyperkinetic disorders. *J. Am. Med. Assoc.*, 137: 772.
6. Riley, R.F., and Berger, F.M. (1949). Metabolism of Myanesin. *Arch. Biochem.*, 20: 159.
7. Berger, F.M., and Riley, R.F. (1949). The preparation and pharmacological properties of the acid succinate of 3-(0-toloxy)-1,2-propanediol (Myanesin). *J. Pharmacol. exper. Therap.*, 96: 269.
8. Ludwig, B.J., and Piech, E.C. (1951). Some anticonvulsant agents derived from 1,3-propanediol. *J. Am. Chem. Soc.*, 73: 5779-5781.
9. Berger, F.M. (1952). The anticonvulsant activity of carbamate esters of certain 2,2-disubstituted-1,3-propanediols. *J. Pharmacol. Therap.*, 104: 229.
10. Selling, L.S. (1955). Clinical study of a new tranquilizing drug. *J. Am. Med. Assoc.*, 157: 1594-1596.
11. Borrus, J.C. Study of effect of Miltown (2-methyl-2-n-propyl-1,3-propanediol dicarbamate) on psychiatric states. *J. Am. Med. Assoc.* 159: 596-598.
12. Berger, F.M. (ed.). Meprobamate and other agents used in mental disorders. *Ann. N.Y. Acad. Sci.*, 67 (1957): 671-894.
13. Berger, F.M. (1964). The tranquilizer decade. *J. Neuropsychiat.*, 5: 403.
14. Cattell, R.B., and Scheier, I.H. (1958). The nature of anxiety. *Psychological Reports,* 4: 351-388.

FUNCTION AND DYSFUNCTION OF THE BASAL GANGLIA

Paul A.J. Janssen

QUESTION: At this moment, after more than fifty years of studying and research, I still wonder why you started out in research and continued to do it, instead of pursuing some other interesting career such as, for example, treating patients in a more rational way?

It was not that much of a choice. Whenever I am asked my profession, I say that I take care of patients. This has always been an important part of my life. However, my dissatisfaction with conventional treatments provided a strong motivation to look for change. I certainly did not agree with pharmacology as it was taught when I was a medical student. It was a blend of one part fact and three parts fantasy about how existing compounds worked. At the same time I was unhappy with the medicinal preparations my father was importing from Hungary. We frequently had discussions about their value until one day my father said, "If you think you can do better, go ahead."

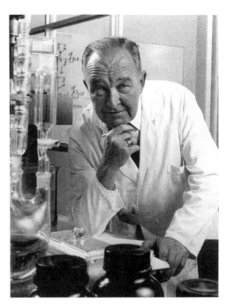

Paul A. J. Janssen

The result is that I am now better known for my research than as a physician.

At the beginning of my career in medicinal research in 1953, I was aware of two major conditions which had to be met in order to succeed. These conditions in my opinion are equally relevant today. The first is the synthesis of new organic molecules by simple reactions – to the extent that this is possible. The second is that one must be very familiar with the characteristic actions of existing drugs on inexpensive biological materials, such as intestinal segments, or centrally-acting drugs, tested directly on mice or rats. When both conditions are systematically

Paul A. J. Janssen completed medical training in Belgium in 1951. From 1953 until 1991 he was president and director of research of Janssen Pharmaceutica NV. He holds over one hundred patents as the inventor of drugs, has authored more than 828 scientific publications, and has received more than 70 scientific and professional awards. Currently he is the chairman of Janssen Research Foundation Worldwide.

Janssen is an Honorary Fellow of CINP. Elected fellow in 1964, he served as Councillor of the 7th, Treasurer of the 9th, 10th and 11th, President Elect of the 12th and President of the 13th Executive. He presented papers on "Recent advances in the butyrophenone series" and on the "Pharmacological aspects of neuroleptic drugs" at the 3rd and 4th Congresses respectively. He also presented the Moderators' Report on the 4th Working Group (Pharmacological and clinical aspects of neuroleptic drugs) at the 4th Congress.

pursued, structure-activity relations emerge and drive synthesis in the direction of improved activity.

QUESTION: This must have resulted in a substantial number of rules to guide your medicinal research. Can you tell me more about this, or are these rules top secret?

In fact, many so-called rules last only until the exception is found. The rule is adjusted so as to accommodate the exception and then the new rule is there until it is broken again. That is part of the reality in research. But every medicinal chemist will tell you that interatomic distances are important. In some series of chemical compounds a well-defined activity is dependent on the distances between readily identifiable atoms. This helps classification and guides creativity.

A further complication in structure-activity relationships may arise from drug metabolism in the organism; an observed activity can be the result of a metabolite rather than of the originally administered compound. Around 1955 Arnold Beckett of the Chelsea School of Pharmacy in London studied the metabolism of the analgesics morphine and pethidine and found, as others before him had, that these drugs penetrate the brain, where they are N-demethylated at the piperidine nitrogen. Beckett proposed that the resulting normorphine and norpethidine were the effective analgesics.

This hypothesis on the mode of action of morphine-like drugs was new but not well substantiated. Curiosity got the better of hesitation, and we decided to enter this field by synthesizing novel norpethidine derivatives by a relatively simple Mannich reaction. The first compound, R951, a propiophenone derivative of norpethidine, induced excitation, mydriasis and Straub tail in mice; R951 was unquestionably a morphine-like drug. Analgesia occurred with R951 at doses at least ten times lower than with morphine and pethidine.

QUESTION: So the new compound was metabolized more efficiently than morphine and pethidine, essentially proving that Beckett was right?

Arnold Beckett put us on the path to a problematic destiny, but it is generally admitted now that the original molecules themselves act as analgesics in accordance with their affinity for μ-opiate receptors. But the final scope of the program offered a greater surprise. A further compound, R1187, is the butyrophenone derivative of norpethidine. When injected into mice, R1187 again produced behavioural changes in line with the action of any morphine-like compound, but soon the animals became quiet and passive. This strange transition from excitation to quietness was observed every time and it puzzled us.

More butyrophenones were synthesized, with modifications of the norpethidine part. Among them in one, R1472, the early signs of morphine-like behaviour were absent, and quietness and passivity became dominant. These are prominent signs of a different central activity from morphine's. The bis-halogenated butyrophenone derivative, haloperidol (R1625), induced this specific behaviour to the point of catalepsy at low doses, over a long period of time.

On the basis of the early pharmacological investigation, therefore, it was concluded that haloperidol was a very potent and specific amphetamine antagonist in rats. Technically, as little as 0.02 mg/kg of haloperidol decreases the agitation of rats induced by a standard dose of amphetamine. The meaning of such observations is now masked by saying that "amphetamine is an indirect dopamine agonist." Forty years ago, however, when the neurotransmitter function of dopamine had not yet been established, the key observation was the identity of behaviour in two situations: amphetamine intoxication of cyclists and paranoid schizophrenia in patients. It is not surprising, then, that the unexpected observation of the potent amphetamine antagonism exhibited by haloperidol and other butyrophenones seemed to be promising.

QUESTION: But schizophrenia is a complex disorder. There is a lot of variation among patients and, in the same patient, there are marked changes over time. How can the value of treatment be assessed?

Psychiatrists from well-known European institutions were contacted to evaluate the effect of long-term oral administration of haloperidol to their patients. There was more than sufficient interest in haloperidol by the profession, and we organized an international symposium on haloperidol in September 1959. Psychiatrists from eight European countries representing fifteen clinical centres met in Beerse at the Janssen Research campus that had just been built. The proceedings of this symposium are a rich source of information on a wide variety of positive clinical evolutions that were reported with daily oral haloperidol, and on the quality of psychiatric practice at the time.

For example, Joseph Paquay reported on a group of seventy patients with chronic schizophrenia who were cared for at the Institut Saint-Martin in Dave, Belgium. Moderate daily doses of 2 to 7 mg of haloperidol were administered. After several months of treatment the status of the seventy patients was as follows: 11 patients had improved to the point where they could be discharged, 44 experienced clear relief from their hallucinations, delusions, affective flattening and disturbing ward behaviour, and 15 were considered poor responders. The observations and conclusions of other groups of psychiatrists, including Jean Delay's group in Paris, were essentially very similar, although the conclusions were reached in a very different way. In some cases treatment with haloperidol was initially grossly overdosed and some extrapyramidal side-effects were induced. It was unnecessary and might even have been counterproductive. It happened because, in the absence of prior experience with haloperidol in treatment, the potency of the substance was underestimated. Another reason for it was that the individual neuroleptic threshold, which determines the narrow therapeutic margin for optimal benefit in a particular individual, was not well established as yet.

QUESTION: At the third CINP Congress in Munich in 1962 you reported on the pharmacology of the butyrophenones. I assume that after the development of haloperidol a systematic study of similar molecules was made. Was a super-haloperidol found in these investigations?

When it was synthesized in 1958, the chemical structure of haloperidol was original and hence a fresh source of inspiration to chemists who wished to find out what kind of activity changes might appear as a result of various modifications. In a few years, hundreds of new butyrophenones were synthesized and studied in a series of pharmacological tests, of which two seem to be of particular relevance to clinical activity in schizophrenia. The first concerned amphetamine antagonism, which has already been mentioned as the core activity of haloperidol.

The details of how amphetamine acts on the brain have by now been worked out, and it is clear that the dopamine transporter at the nerve terminals is the main molecular site of its action. It is through the transporter, with its twelve transmembrane domains, that dopamine is driven out of the nerve terminal into the synapse, where the postsynaptic D2 receptors are stimulated. The direction of action in case of amphetamine is therefore the opposite to that of dopamine reuptake, and for some time now we have been considering the possibility of an endogenous amphetamine-like substance that is responsible for hyperactive dopaminergic neurotransmission in schizophrenia, or at least in paranoid schizophrenia.

A likely candidate is phenylethylamine, which is formed from phenylalanine by the action of aromatic amino acid decarboxylase. Our research is currently targeting the dopamine transporter and the amphetamine-like action of endogenous amines since it has been shown that amphetamine releases more dopamine in the brain of patients with schizophrenia than in the brain of normal volunteers; in addition, mice without the dopamine transporter as a result of selective genetic manipulation exhibit relentless running in their cages. Movement is one function supervised by dopamine in the basal ganglia, as is well-known from dopamine deficiency in Parkinson's disease. Planning and cognition however, appear also tightly coupled to dopaminergic neurotransmission.

The second test that has been very important explores serotonergic neurotransmission. It is the tryptamine test in rats. Even before the dopamine hypothesis of schizophrenia, Woolley had proposed that serotonin plays an important role in psychosis, in part because of the chemical relationship between serotonin and LSD-25, which is well known for its hallucinogenic properties. Tryptamine mimics serotonin, and a high intravenous dose in rats induces bilateral convulsions and tremors, which can be inhibited by central serotonin antagonists of the serotonin S2-receptor type.

In the study of newly synthesized butyrophenones, no relation was established between amphetamine and tryptamine antagonism; the potent amphetamine antagonism of haloperidol contrasted with very weak tryptamine antagonism. There was one compound with the opposite activity profile: pipamperone or dipiperone (R3345, synthesized in 1959) was markedly more potent as a tryptamine-antagonist than as an amphetamine one. Pipamperone is therefore a remote precursor of risperidone, and some early clinical observations with pipamperone raised expectations that were fulfilled many years later.

QUESTION: As you explained this I suddenly had an idea: pipamperone could have been called the first of the atypical neuroleptics and should have rivalled clozapine in the maintenance treatment of patients with schizophrenia.

The profile of clinical results obtained with pipamperone was much different from that with haloperidol. It was mainly Sugerman in the United States who described the improvement in sleep and reversal of affective flattening produced by treatment with pipamperone in the absence of extrapyramidal symptoms. That sounded very promising, but the so-called "experts" inside and outside the company did not recognize this profile for what it is: close to ideal for maintenance therapy. The same thing happened with clozapine, which had to be "rediscovered" in the United States ten years ago.

The use of the word "atypical," of course, makes no sense. For pipamperone, we simply say what it does: inhibition first of serotonin-S2 and then of dopamine-D2 receptors. When the word atypical is used for clozapine, one scientist thinks of "anticholinergic activity," a second of "mesolimbic selectivity," and a third and a fourth of "serotonin antagonism" and "dopamine-D4 antagonism." There is a tendency to link new neuroleptics through any arbitrary property to the "mystery" of clozapine.

QUESTION: In your chapter on antipsychotics in the Principles of Pharmacology *published in 1995, about 100 neuroleptics are classified according to chemical structure and pharmacological activities. The class of butyrophenones is followed by the class of diphenylbutylamines, which is headed by pimozide. What is important about pimozide and its analogs?*

Patients with schizophrenia who respond well to neuroleptic treatment may soon consider themselves cured. They tend to avoid further medication and run the risk of a psychotic relapse within a few weeks. In ambulant treatment, compliance is even more difficult to sustain with an oral medication that generally has to be taken several times daily. The chemical series of the diphenylbutylamines opened up the way for an alternative to injectable depot preparations. These amines have a lipophilic quality that results in a more gradual onset of action than that of the butyrophenones. Their duration of action is intrinsically long, up to one week for orally administered penfluridol. The concept of a weekend pill for ambulant treatment had arrived on the scene.

Penfluridol and the concept gave rise to considerable debate between the proponents of injection and those of oral treatment.

QUESTION: How did you resolve this?

Ultimately we developed both injectable haloperidol decanoate, which covers four weeks between injections, and the penfluridol or "weekend pill." Penfluridol is available in about thirty countries, though not in some major ones like the United States.

QUESTION: In the directory of members of the CINP for 1996 your name is on the short list of honorary fellows. During the two-year period of your presidency, the 10th Congress of the CINP was held in Jerusalem in 1982. You had presented a paper on the butyrophenones at the third congress in Munich in 1962. What stands out for you as being most important over all these years of close contact with the CINP?

Within a stable and qualified college like the CINP, the profession is present at all levels. Collaboration and exchange are facilitated and the friendships one makes last for life. There have been so many people with whom I had rewarding experiences that it is difficult to answer your question. That having been said, I have particularly fond memories of my relationship – fostered through the CINP – with Professor Hans-Joachim Haase of Düsseldorf, who died recently. When I first met him in the early days of haloperidol, the question of the optimal neuroleptic dose for psychotic patients was already his major concern. His approach was based on the study of alterations in fine motor control, which reveal the action of neuroleptics from very low doses on. His investigations resulted in the handwriting test and a practical definition of the optimal therapeutic dose for a given patient. Before medication the patient provides a first, reference sample by writing a standard text. Subsequently, handwritten samples of the same text make it possible to follow the patient's response to the neuroleptic. If the area of the post-medical sample is less than 12 percent smaller than in the pre-medication sample, the neuroleptic threshold has not been reached. If it is more than 30 percent smaller, the induction of extrapyramidal signs (EPS) is predicted. This empirical range, as established recently, corresponds to a range of 50 to 80 percent dopamine receptor occupancy in the striatum. [Private communication, to be published, Dr. U. Künstler, Leipzig.] As seen from the patient's perspective, the development by Haase of a simple method of initiating and maintaining appropriate neuroleptic treatment is a remarkable achievement.

QUESTION: Serotonin antagonism, specifically at 5-HT2A receptors, has dominated your research on centrally-acting drugs since about 1980. How fruitful has this approach been?

As I have already explained, serotonin and the potent hallucinogenic LSD were the substances Woolley related to schizophrenia several years before neuroleptic action was shown to be primarily based on dopamine antagonism. Hence, in the epoch of the first butyrophenones a double question arose: is serotonin antagonism important and is it safe? The fact that partial LSD-like activity was almost systematically reported for ergolines and other serotonin antagonists gave rise to doubts about safety. In 1978 it was shown that the tryptamine antagonism of pipamperone is linked to antagonism at the S2 receptor (later renamed the 5-HT2A receptor). Among the new compounds to come along in the following years, ritanserin and risperidone have taught us the most about the activity of serotonin at central S2 receptors.

Ritanserin by itself or added to haloperidol in the treatment regimen of patients with schizophrenia appears to improve mood through a robust effect on sleep; in normal subjects the time spent in deep-sleep phases doubles from two to four hours after a 5 mg dose of ritanserin.

In 1983 risperidone was synthesized. Within a large series of new benzisoxazole piperidine derivatives, risperidone, in experiments on receptor binding and behavioural responses in animals, was as close to the concept of a new type of neuroleptic as we could hope for. The activity of risperidone rests on those receptor interactions that have been known for quite some time, and the achievement of the right set of interactions in the right proportion makes a critical difference in the quality of treatment for a substantial number of patients. Risperidone is fully active at daily doses of 1 to 6 mg, which is again a traditional goal of our research as such low doses have the crucial advantage of a low incidence of general systemic side-effects. Within this dose range of 1 to 6 mg, the individual requirements and sensitivity of the patient must still be respected. Thanks to a somewhat larger therapeutic margin of about two-to-one, however, it is easier to obtain a side-effect-free, maximal therapeutic response with risperidone than with other neuroleptics.

QUESTION: Are there compelling reasons for avoiding extrapyramidal symptoms – I mean, in comparison with other possible consequences of neuroleptic treatment, such as tardive dyskinesia and malignant neuroleptic syndrome?

Even in the 'Pfalzklinik,' where Haase's handwriting test was systematically used to determine the optimal dosage, oral dyskinesias and tics were observed in about 5 percent of the patients with schizophrenia. That figure of 5 percent was also the mean prevalence of dyskinesia in unmedicated subjects, as reviewed by John Kane fifteen years ago. It is a general finding that aging alone is a major factor in the appearance of dyskinesia. In order to sort out all the contributing factors, Robin McCreadie conducted an additional important study in 1996. He observed four groups of older people in India: normal persons, relatives of the patients with schizophrenia, unmedicated and medicated patients with schizophrenia. Dyskinesia was relatively frequent (15 percent) in the first two groups; it was much higher in the last two groups (40 percent) but as common and as severe in the never-medicated as in the medicated patients. It follows that dyskinesia is associated with age and schizophrenic illness and not with antipsychotic medication.

QUESTION: After the development of neuroleptic drugs, from haloperidol to risperidone, where do you see further progress?

I am as interested as ever in the function and dysfunction of the basal ganglia.

THE DISCOVERY OF IMIPRAMINE FROM A PERSONAL VIEWPOINT

Alan D. Broadhurst

I joined Geigy in 1949 when I came out of the Services. The British branch of the Swiss pharmaceutical company was just starting its operations in Rhodes, a small mill town a few miles outside of Manchester. When I first arrived there I was surprised to find the new division at such an early stage of development. In fact, the main part of the operation at that time was to import finished pharmaceutical products from Basel and market them, almost entirely as ethical preparations, in the United Kingdom. One of the rooms in the small house, which served as our headquarters, was given over to packaging and another to an order department; there was a secretarial office, a few other rooms and a bathroom which in those early days was used as a makeshift laboratory. In day to day charge of the whole British operation was Leslie Robinson, an extremely competent man, a pharmacist with a business mind and a particular interest in drug research. During the first year of Geigy's life in Manchester, he had been trying to set up

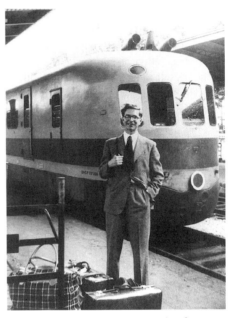

Alan D. Broadhurst commuting from Manchester to Basel, somewhere in France

out-of-house research projects, but these had been slow to get started, mainly because of the pressure of his heavy administrative load.

My job was to act as assistant to Robinson, especially within the scientific field. I should add that I was then only twenty-three years of age and uncomfortably aware of my pharmacological ignorance. Indeed, I wondered how I was going to fit into the organization. To add to my concern, I discovered within forty-eight hours of arriving that I was one of the senior members of the British company. The reason for this was, of course, that there was such a small staff. Very sadly, Leslie Robinson died within a year of my arrival, and for a while I had to take over his job, as well as continue with my own. I had to learn to cope very fast.

Alan Broadhurst is a consultant psychiatrist in private practice in Bury St Edmunds, England. He was formerly the senior consultant psychiatrist at the West Suffolk Hospital and a consultant physician at Addenbrooke's Hospital in Cambridge. For many years he lectured in psychopharmacology in the University of Cambridge. Before he became a psychiatrist, he worked as a clinical pharmacologist with Geigy Pharmaceuticals.

Right from the start there had been an intention to develop an in-house scientific base. This was to complement out-of-house research which was under way and to be expanded. Our parent company in Basel had quite a range of pharmaceuticals already on the market, some of which required further research, mainly in terms of setting up further clinical trials. Other drugs were in the process of early investigation. We hoped to try, as far as possible with our very limited resources, to begin parallel work in England. At about this point my job changed in another respect. It had been the original intention that I should spend most of my time in Rhodes and with British investigators. Now I found myself commuting to and from Basel and spending more and more time in Switzerland, working alongside the basic scientists.

My very first major task was to work within the field of anticoagulation. Clinical interest in this area was rapidly developing, and we were working with one of the early coumarin derivatives, ethyl biscoumacetate, known by the trade name Tromexan. Soon afterwards, I found myself in the antirheumatic field. After a long and exciting chase, our team developed phenylbutazone, the parent compound of many of the newer non-salicylic anti-inflammatory drugs. A variety of other projects followed and I realized how disadvantaged I was as a non-clinical scientist in setting up clinical trials. It was at this point that I made a major life decision to go off to medical school and train as a doctor. Clearly, I could not abandon my work at Geigy, and so I undertook my medical training in parallel with my research work. This was a fairly hectic undertaking, and it would have been easier to attend the medical school at the University of Manchester. I decided against doing so, however, because I had fairly recently put some screening work out to contract with the Department of Pharmacology at the university, and the professor of pharmacology was also Dean of the medical school. It therefore seemed to me that it would be undiplomatic to try for a place there. I did not want the Dean to feel uncomfortable about having to make a decision about whether or not to admit me as a student, and so I went to the next nearest university in Sheffield, from where I graduated in 1955.

Back at Geigy, we were working on antihistamines and already had a successful drug of this kind, halopyramine, on the market. We were, of course, aware of the exciting developments in France, where antihistamines were being used experimentally to reduce surgical shock and to potentiate anesthesia. Henri Laborit, an anesthetist working in Paris, had been collaborating with Charpentier, an organic chemist at Rhône-Poulenc, trying out different antihistamines emanating from the pharmaceutical company as they were made available. In 1947 Laborit tried out promethazine, the latest development from Rhône-Poulenc. This antihistamine was rather different since it was a phenothiazine. The drug had been created by grafting a side chain onto the -S position of the phenothiazine nucleus. Phenothiazine itself had been used for many years as a treatment for intestinal worms in horses. Laborit found promethazine to be more potent in anesthesia than the earlier drugs. His team began to use it in combination with pethidine. This was the birth of the so-called lytic cocktail.

Because of our own involvement with antihistamines, we followed this ongoing work in Paris with great interest. In 1949 Laborit was offered two more phenothiazines, promazine and chlorpromazine. These were even more powerful in their ability to potentiate anesthesia. Of even greater importance was the fact that they possessed a new property not found in earlier drugs: they were also thermolytic. They opposed the effect of the thermoregulatory mechanisms, whose function is to maintain a nearly constant core body temperature in warm-blooded animals. As a result, the technique of artificial hibernation was introduced. This allowed a patient to be pretreated with a thermolytic drug and then cooled with ice, thus making it possible for body tissues, including the brain, to be deprived of their blood supply for brief periods without sustaining serious damage.

Spurred on by Laborit's work, we felt that we ought to look again at halopyramine and our other, as yet unmarketed, drugs of this class. In fact, halopyramine and its close analogues had negligible thermolytic properties. It seemed likely that the effect on thermoregulation was mediated by the tricyclic phenothiazine ring structure. Our head of pharmacology, Professor Domenjoz, who incidentally was also professor of pharmacology at the University of the Saar, decided that there should be a new approach and that a search should be made for novel heterocyclic antihistamines, which might not only be thermolytic but also provide a starting point for the synthesis of compounds of potential value as sedatives, analgesics, and antiparkinsonian agents. It is interesting to note that, by this time, the phenothiazine derivatives were not only providing the possibility of major advances in cardiac surgery, but some remained as powerful antihistamines and others had useful anti-Parkinsonian effects. Domenjoz felt that we ought not to follow the phenothiazine route. He was keen to avoid accusations that Geigy was simply involved in "me too" drug development. The phenothiazine discovery had been the outcome of Rhône-Poulenc's work, and he wanted to leave it at that.

Accordingly, our chemistry and pharmacology departments put their heads together and thought about other possible heterocyclic compounds. Eventually, the spotlight fell upon iminodibenzyl, a tricyclic substance, at first glance rather similar to the molecular shape of chlorpromazine, but actually very different in chemical terms. Like phenothiazine, iminodibenzyl was not a new compound. It had been synthesized in 1898 and had been used briefly as an intermediate in the dyestuff, Sky Blue. It was then abandoned for more than half a century. This compound had very poor solubility and was therefore unlikely, in its unmodified form, to be of much therapeutic use.

Professor Domenjoz then asked two of Geigy's organic chemists, Schindler and Häfliger, to prepare derivatives of iminodibenzyl. A variety of side chains were added to the -N position on the central ring of the tricyclic nucleus by alkylation or acylation. Eventually, forty-two different substances were produced. Such is the enthusiasm of organic chemists! The compounds differed only in their side chains; the tricyclic nucleus remained unaltered. The side chains were of varying lengths, from two- to six-carbon atoms.

Pharmacological testing was then undertaken by Domenjoz, together with doctors Theobald, Herrmann, and Pulver. I was privileged and most fortunate to be able to work with Pulver, although I should add that I was, at that time, a very junior member of the Basel-based team. All forty-two of the new compounds were tested. The derivatives revealed the presence, in varying degree, of antihistaminic activity, together with sedative, analgesic, and spasmolytic properties. Some of the derivatives possessed a thermolytic component in their action. The properties of the derivatives varied according to the constitution of the side chain. The acyl derivatives with a -CO group next to the nitrogen atom on the central ring exhibited well-marked local anesthetic activity. In this respect, they were very similar to the analogous derivatives of phenothiazine. The presence of a quaternary carbon in the side chain enhanced existing analgesic activity in the alkylated compounds. Tissue distribution studies were then undertaken in a rabbit to measure the absorption levels in different organs and metabolic products of some of the most likely therapeutic agents.

Apart from fairly gross behavioural observations, such as the presence of sedation in treated animals, no specialized behavioural studies were carried out. Very few techniques of this type were in use, or even known, at that time. Moreover, even if such tests had been available, we were not looking specifically for the presence of any behavioural modification. In those early days, no particular guidelines were laid down for safety and toxicity testing. LDs on rat, mouse, and rabbit were undertaken. The next stage was to carry out pharmacokinetic studies of a few of the least toxic compounds in human volunteers. Inevitably, I found myself recruited into this study. Volunteering came with the job!

A few of the derivatives possessed pharmacological properties that were of interest and seemed worthy of further investigation. Although some of our compounds had been seen to possess thermolytic activity, we decided to delay trials in surgery. Rather, we thought it would be worthwhile to look more closely at those with a sedative effect, with a view to possibly developing them for clinical use as hypnotics. One of the least toxic of all the compounds in animal tests was the derivative given the Geigy code number G22150. Late in 1950 two of my colleagues, Paul Schmidlin and Otto Kym, both clinicians working in our pharmacology department, went to discuss G22150 with a psychiatrist, Roland Kuhn, at Münsterlingen Hospital on the shores of Lake Constance. They asked him if he would be prepared to try out this substance on some of his insomniac patients, and he agreed to help. The results were not startlingly good. Some patients slept well; others were barely touched by the potential hypnotic. Its sedative properties were, perhaps unusually, not uniform among the patient group. A decision was made to abandon this particular work with G22150.

After this disappointment, we decided that, after all, we ought to investigate the thermolytic properties of the compounds. One derivative with the code number G22355 looked interesting. It too had shown low toxicity in laboratory testing; it was not particularly sedating, it was an antihistamine, and it was thermolytic. Of particular importance was the fact that it was the iminodibenzyl analogue of promazine, which had been so successful in the French cardiac surgery units. We began to prepare a protocol for a clinical trial. But before we could get started, details of another major discovery emerged from France, a discovery which completely changed our plans.

Laborit had continued to use chlorpromazine in surgery with good effect. As he became more familiar with its action, he realized that it seemed to possess an additional, highly specific action. If given alone, it appeared to inhibit the response to stressful situations. Anxiety generated by the thought of impending major surgery was markedly reduced. Laborit noted in 1952 that, although the patients were in a state of full consciousness, they seemed to lack any interest in their surroundings. He believed that the drug might be of value in the treatment of psychiatric patients. He discussed this idea with two psychiatric colleagues, Jean Delay and Pierre Deniker at the Hôpital Sainte Anne, and they and other psychiatrists at the Hôpital Val de Grace tried the drug in a variety of psychiatric disorders. It was soon found to have a remarkable therapeutic effect in patients with schizophrenia. This was a most important advance, and back at Geigy we decided to investigate G22355, not in anaesthesia, but in schizophrenia. We wondered if it might share chlorpromazine's antipsychotic properties, for, of all the iminodibenzyl derivatives we had available, this drug was the directly analogous compound to promazine, with a straight side chain containing three -CH_2 groups.

The road to Münsterlingen was already well trodden, and soon we were retracing our steps to the psychiatric hospital there to ask Dr. Kuhn if he would try out our new drug in schizophrenia. I had initially thought that he might be reluctant to do so. He was a psychiatrist of the old school, an extremely perceptive clinical observer trained in the psychodynamic and psychoanalytic tradition. We had got to know him, of course, through the G22150 trial, and as far as I know, he had never been involved in clinical trials before. However, he had come to recognize that chlorpromazine was of great value in schizophrenia, and it was already in use at his hospital, though on a limited basis because of its cost. The idea of free supplies for clinical trials of what might turn out to be a successful substitute for the phenothiazine was attractive.

Those patients who were already being treated with chlorpromazine had it discontinued. Others had not received chlorpromazine at all. A group of these patients with schizophrenia were then started on the new experimental drug. Everybody thought that it would work in much the same way as chlorpromazine: perhaps more or less potent but, we hoped, with a definite antipsychotic effect. The clinical trial was, in modern terms, totally uncontrolled. In those days, double-blind comparative studies were virtually unknown. So any effect of the experimental drug would have to be of a high order for it to be regarded as significant.

In fact, such was the case. The whole team of workers medical and nursing staff at the hospital and scientists from Geigy waited with bated breath. At first, very little happened, but the excitement was intense. Then, within a period ranging from a few days to several weeks, certain very definite results began to appear. These were not only fascinating. They were, in some patients, quite alarming. Several previously quiet patients began to deteriorate with increasing agitation. Some developed hypomanic behaviour. One man, in such a state, managed to get hold of a bicycle and rode in his nightshirt to a nearby village singing lustily, much to the alarm of the local inhabitants. This was not a very good public-relations exercise for the hospital, and I cannot say that it improved relationships with Geigy either. Of course, not all the schizophrenic patients reacted in this way. Some even improved, especially if there was a major depressive component in their illness. Even so, it was clear that the effect of the drug was not particularly desirable in schizophrenia and that it was producing a very different effect from chlorpromazine.

Our disappointment was intense. The clinical trial was abandoned. We viewed the situation with dismay and had no real option but to go back to our drawing boards in Basel. However, it was certainly not the end of the story. Over the next few months we had a series of discussions with Dr. Kuhn, but these came to nothing. Schmidlin, Kym, and I spent many agonizing hours trying to find an explanation as to what might have happened to precipitate such a reaction in certain patients. We stumbled around, examining a number of unlikely hypotheses and mechanisms. During one of the brain-storming sessions in Schmidlin's office, an idea gradually crystalized. We stopped trying to elicit *why* the hypomanic reaction in the schizophrenic patients had occurred and began to allow our thoughts to wander in a different direction. Now, in retrospect, it all seems so naive, so preposterous, so mechanistic, and yet so simple, but we wondered if the apparent mood elevation seen in the schizo-

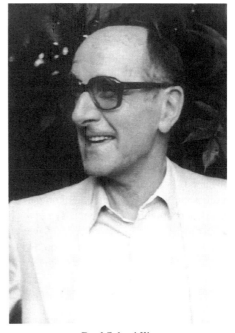

Paul Schmidlin

phrenic patients might also occur in depressed individuals, but in this case with beneficial outcome. I have no idea whose idea it was. Indeeed, I think it was not any one person's idea. It simply emerged.

Shortly after this, Schmidlin and I went to see Roland Kuhn again in order to talk things through. We sat on the harbour wall overlooking the lake – I think it was at Gottlieben – for our discussion. Paul and I felt somewhat diffident after the earlier unfortunate outcome, but we told Kuhn about our idea and asked him if he would be prepared to try G22355 in patients with depression. I well remember the look of suspicious disbelief on his face! He was clearly cautious about our proposal for a clinical trial, but he was persuaded.

The protocol was put together, final discussions took place, and the trial began in 1955. G22355 was given to a number of patients with major depressive illness. The drug was administered parenterally in the early patients and subsequently switched to oral therapy. At a later stage, all patients were treated throughout by means of tablets. Gradually ascending doses were used, and in most patients up to 150 mg was well tolerated. Occasionally, doses as high as 250 mg were used. This trial also was uncontrolled in the modern scientific sense.

The protocol required forty patients, in the first instance, to be included. Even the first three showed definite evidence of improvement after about three weeks on the drug. After forty patients had been treated, it was clear that G22355 was producing a dramatic, and this time beneficial, response. About two-thirds of the patients showed marked reduction in their depressive symptoms. Individuals with biological – or as Dr. Kuhn described them, "vegetative" – symptoms tended to do best.

This was a very exciting time for us all. In those days I had not received any postgraduate training in psychiatry. Indeed, my training in the field of mental illness as a student had been limited to being shown a few cases of paranoid schizophrenia. Nevertheless, during this trial I had seen some seriously depressed patients at Münsterlingen, and I was all too aware of what a merciless and devastating illness severe and unremitting depression could be. The fact that we might now, for the first time ever, have an effective treatment seemed incredible. If this therapeutic effect could be repeated in larger groups of patients, then G22355 represented a major advance in medicine.

Soon after this, the drug was given the generic name of imipramine and then the proprietary name Tofranil. Kuhn continued his work with imipramine and used it in several hundred patients with success. Schmidlin and Kym helped to get a number of other European drug trials started, but these were also uncontrolled.

Then things began to change. At some point in 1959, clinical trials started to be fully controlled, especially in the United Kingdom. Not only was the concept of comparison with placebo or standard drug introduced, but the development of rating scales provided a much more accurate means of making comparisons between groups where only small symptomatic differences might exist, especially in psychiatric disorders. One of the leading figures in this field was Max Hamilton in Leeds. I went to see him there, and he told me all about his new idea for a rating scale for depression. He was very excited to hear about imipramine and said that his rating scale might well be incorporated into future trials of the antidepressant.

My meeting with Max settled it. Important advances in clinical trials were being made in the United Kingdom, and we had to get some trials going. I went up to Newcastle and met Leslie Kiloh and John Ball. They too were very interested in imipramine and readily agreed to carry out a trial. Patients were given either imipramine or placebo, and the results were compared after four weeks of treatment. Among those patients considered to be suffering from endogenous depression, 74 percent responded well, as opposed to 22 percent of those receiving the placebo. This trial was published very quickly in 1959 and no doubt was a factor in stimulating other researchers. I was soon in touch with Linford Rees and his colleagues, Alexander Brown and Sylvio Benaim. They were keen to look at this drug in the treatment of very severely depressed patients, and theirs was a most carefully thought-out study. Imipramine was seen to have important antidepressant activity, even in these very ill patients.

An intriguing trial was that carried out by Hilda Abraham. She was a distinguished psychoanalyst, the daughter of Carl Abraham, and was the last person I would have expected to be interested in the drug treatment of depression. She contacted me out of the blue and asked if we could meet. She explained that she had read about imipramine and that it sounded remarkable. She had never really thought that medication could influence depression, but she was open-minded enough to want to see for herself. Abraham was not interested in simply trying imipramine in a few patients on a non-controlled basis, but insisted that she would have to do things properly. She joined forces with three colleagues, and one of them, Ismond Rosen, also a psychoanalyst, played a major part in the double-blind trial design. I remember how amazed Abraham was when nearly two-thirds of her depressed patients recovered with the drug.

There were other important clinical trials at that time, too numerous to mention here. During those years, some thirty-five further carefully controlled trials were carried out in the United Kingdom. By 1970 there were more than 4000 publications worldwide relating to imipramine. Beyond that point I lost count. The vast majority of these trials revealed imipramine to be an effective antidepressant.

From the time when I had started with Geigy, concerned with a broad range of pharmacological research, my field of interest had progressively narrowed until in 1959 I was involved more or less within the antidepressant area. From a therapeutic point of view, the introduction of imipramine into medicine had been of enormous significance, and it would have a major impact on the practice of psychiatry. The effect of the discovery upon me was no less. Indeed, it had been a remarkable experience, which changed the direction of my career. I wanted to be back in the clinical field, treating patients with medicines rather than researching them. I went off and became a psychiatrist, albeit one heavily involved in psychopharmacology. Like so many other discoveries in pharmacology, serendipity had played a major role. The antidepressant effect of imipramine was completely unexpected and was discovered entirely by accident. Luck was on my side too. I just happened to be working in the right place at the right time.

HISTORY AND FUTURE OF ANTIDEPRESSANTS

Roland Kuhn

Your invitation to contribute some of my auto-biographical memories of drug development to this volume impels me to ask myself these questions: by what means did I discover the antidepressant action of imipramine almost forty years ago, and what enabled me to offer CIBA Ltd. a modification of the chemical formula of a substance (later called maprotiline) which they could synthesize in their laboratories. My methods were entirely different from those which are nowadays applied in clinical research. I have never used "controlled double-blind studies" with "placebo," "standardized rating scales," or "statistical treatment of data based on a large number of patients." Neither have I ever looked for the "exact scientific validity" of my results.

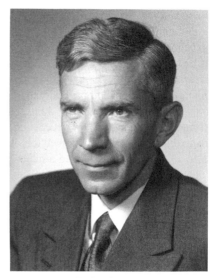

Roland Kuhn

Instead, I examined each patient individually, often every day, on several occasions, and questioned each patient again and again. The patients were attended to and observed in the hospital by doctors and the nursing staff under my personal supervision for years. I always took their proposals and criticisms seriously.

Thus, in 1957, I published the results of treating forty patients with imipramine for a minimum of one and a half years. Some years later, the outstanding Belgian psychiatrist Bobon told me: "The results of your research are surprising. Even more surprising, however, is the fact that in your first publication, you discussed 95 percent of everything there is to be said, in essence, about imipramine." Even today, at the most, only a small modification would have to be added to the original text.

The essential results of my first publication on imipramine can be expressed by the following quotation: "A particularly good effect is achieved with typically endogenous depressions... as far as they present symptoms of vital depression." Furthermore, at that time I also pointed out that reactive depressions may respond to treatment with antidepressants.

As it turned out, most psychiatrists did not know what is meant by the term "vital depression." For that reason, I provided the following definition: "Vital depression is a

Roland Kuhn was born in 1912 in Biel, Switzerland. After graduation from medical school he worked with Professors Klaesi, Wyrsch, Weber and Grünthal. Since 1939 he has worked in the Kantonal Psychiatric Klinik in Münsterlingen, becoming its director in 1970.
Kuhn was elected a fellow of the CINP in 1958. He presented "Gibt es heute schon Möglichkeiten, die störenden Nebenwirkungen der Antidepressiva beträchtlich zu mildern und ihre Wirksamkeit zu steigern?" at the 6th Congress and was a formal discussant of Working Group 5 (Pharmacological and clinical actions of antidepressants) at the 4th Congress.

syndrome which consists of tiredness that is often combined with disturbed sleep, psychomotor retardation, and difficulty in thinking, making decisions and acting. Furthermore, the patients have physical and psychological sensations of oppression and constriction, and they have lost their ability to experience joy. The most important feature is that all of these symptoms are much more marked in the morning than in the evening."

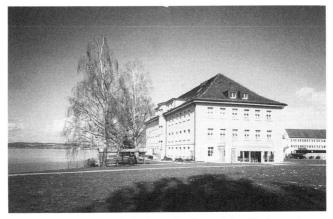

Münsterlingen Hospital where the first trials of imipramine in depression were undertaken

One needs to realize that the symptoms of vital depression are often not mentioned spontaneously by patients and cannot be discovered easily through questioning. They are often concealed by other symptoms which may seem to be more severe. They may not be recognised even by questioning with isolated questions in a structured interview. Patients may recognize and acknowledge the symptom only in the course of a free dialogue.

Nowadays we can read in the ICD-10 under F30-F39: "It is acknowledged that the symptoms referred to here as 'somatic' could also have been called 'melancholic,' 'vital,' 'biological,' or 'endogenomorphic,' and that the scientific status of this syndrome is in any case somewhat questionable... The classification is arranged so that this somatic syndrome can be recorded by those who so wish, but also can be ignored without loss of any other information." That is the exact opposite of what I wrote in 1957 and what I have stated again and again ever since! Vital depression is based on correct observation and while it is true that it may be associated with almost any kind of psychiatric disorder, it is a fundamental error to consider it as "nonspecific." In fact in any psychiatric disorder which includes vital depression, the vital depressive syndrome responds to treatment with an antidepressive medication, whatever the other psychopathological diagnosis may be. In a certain way the concept of vital depression has some resemblance to the state of depression that Guislain described about a hundred and fifty years ago as the first developmental stage of his unitary concept of psychosis. As I pointed out in 1964, some support for such a view comes from the generally acknowledged fact that many patients with obsessional disorders (perceived as a later developmental stage of the psychosis within Guislain's frame of reference) respond favorably to treament with antidepressants.

The problem facing us today is not only to find new medications, but to learn much more about how our present medications act and how could we use them optimally. We need to know, for example, if such substances as minerals, including iron and copper, vitamins and hormones are needed in order for antidepressants to exert their optimal effects.

I have never been urged to change my methods or the interpretation of my results. I have continued to practise and do research as I did before and have obtained significant results. However they have not received much notice!

THE STORY OF OPIPRAMOL AND CLOMIPRAMINE

George Beaumont

My career in psychopharmacology began in 1966. For six years previously I had worked in general practice. Although I found many aspects of primary care both interesting and rewarding, I had become sadly disillusioned with conditions in the British National Health Service (nothing changes!) and felt that I needed a fresh start. I answered an advertisement in the *British Medical Journal* by the then Geigy Pharmaceuticals Company, which was recruiting medical advisers. To cut a long story short, I was invited to join the company and began a long and happy association. Two positions were on offer, one in rheumatology and the other in psychiatry. On the strength of a six-month residency in my formative years, I accepted the latter.

It would not, I think, be an exaggeration to say that in the 1960s Geigy Pharmaceuticals was the foremost company in the United Kingdom in the field of psychopharmacology. Cyril Maxwell was

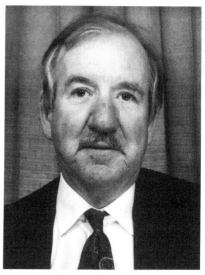

George Beaumont

already on staff. He was responsible for imipramine and desipramine, continuing the pioneering work that had been so ably begun by Alan Broadhurst. Cyril had more than enough to do. Someone had to take care of the other analogues in the series, hence my arrival on the scene. I was given the responsibility of evaluating opipramol (Insidon) and what we then called chlorimipramine (principally in the United Kingdom).

Opipramol had already been marketed, but was making little impact. It was, however, very successful in continental Europe, especially in Germany. The Swiss found it difficult to understand why the drug was not enjoying similar success in Britain. I discovered that the success was mainly achieved in primary care, but then came the difficulty. The principal indication was psychovegetative dystonia, and the compound was described as a psychic harmonizer. These concepts were totally alien to the British way of thinking. In fact, it was virtually impossible to explain them. The only apparently acceptable substitutes were mixed anxiety and depression and a variety of "psychosomatic" disorders. Some studies had already been done prior to my arrival which showed efficacy in mild to moderate depression.

George Beaumont is a founding member of the British Association for Psychopharmacology. He is currently visiting professor at the University of Surrey and editor of *Primary Care*.

Beaumont was elected a member of the CINP in 1976.

Of course, our ideas about nosology then were very different from what they are now. This was the heyday of the benzodiazepines, with chlordiazepoxide and later diazepam enjoying wide popularity and little awareness of any problems. My impression was that opipramol, because of its dual action in relieving both anxiety and depression, could do just as well, if not better, than the benzodiazepines. Combination products of anxiolytic and antidepressant were, in any event, popular in those days. A series of clinical trials succeeded in demonstrating efficacy in depression and anxiety, and also in the kind of psychosomatic disorders for which chlordiazepoxide was so widely prescribed. The portfolio of studies was extensive and comprehensive, and I thought that I had done well. However, the company believed that the moment had been missed, and that we were no longer capable of taking on the benzodiazepines in the market place. I myself felt that a great opportunity had been lost.

The imipramine (Tofranil) story is familiar to us all, a story that changed the face of psychiatry and one that contributed to the emergence of the relatively new science of psychopharmacology. Desipramine followed imipramine, and although the theory of its relative selectivity was quite impressive, it did not, in the United Kingdom at least, enjoy the kind of success that imipramine had. What then was the company to do with its third antidepressant, chlorimipramine?

When I arrived on the scene, a number of studies had already shown efficacy in what I suppose we would now call major depression (we preferred terms such as "endogenous" and "reactive" then), and there was a feeling abroad, based purely on anecdotal reports, that chlorimipramine was more "potent" than its forebears and might find a place in the treatment of more severe cases and those that had previously been resistant to treatment. I think that it would be fair to say that subsequent studies provided some confirmation of this impression. But the problem remained – how could we make our third antidepressant look a bit different? A search of the literature revealed a few anecdotal reports based on single cases of success in the treatment of obsessive-compulsive disorder. Back in the sixties there was a tendency to throw every newly introduced drug at all those conditions that had proved resistant to treatment or difficult to treat in the past. This "suck it and see" approach would be difficult or impossible to adopt in the present regulatory atmosphere. At the time, obsessive-compulsive disorder was regarded as a rare and bizarre condition. Nevertheless, it seemed a possibility worth pursuing.

The centre with the most experience was Professor López-Ibor's department in Madrid. So I took myself and a small party of potential investigators to see what was being done there. Fired with enthusiasm, we returned home and set up a series of studies. It was not easy. Initially, suitable cases were hard to find. There were no accepted methods of measuring severity or change, and we had to invent them or modify existing techniques. When I look back at what we did, it now seems crude. Nevertheless, the rest of the story is well known. Although the drug did not achieve the same publicity or success, I also began to feel that clomipramine (by this time the name had been changed) might have a place in the management of certain phobic disorders and in panic attacks. A number of what I can now only call primitive studies showed some success. Some of these were undertaken in primary care, with general practitioners as investigators. We also did a considerable amount of simple epidemiological research in family practice – regrettably, with the benefit of hindsight, never published – which indicated that fears, phobias, and obsessions were quite common.

When the program started, we really did not know why clomipramine should be effective in the management of obsessions, phobias, and panic. We were aware, however – thanks to the work of people such as Archie Todrick – that it was a very powerful inhibitor of the reuptake of serotonin. Gradually it began to dawn on us that perhaps there might be a connection. I like to think that this early work contributed to the subsequent interest in serotonin and the development of more specific and selective psychoactive agents.

The clomipramine story had some intriguing lateral developments. For example, we became very interested in the effect of tricyclic antidepressants on pain and in effects on sleep, and we were excited by the efficacy in cataplexy and effects on appetite, eating behaviour, and weight. All these formed part of the research program in the late sixties and the seventies.

In the light of current interest and concern, perhaps the observations and studies of the effect of clomipramine on sexual function were the most important. The first report of an effect on ejaculation came from a research chemist taking part in one of our studies of intravenous administration (that is another story which I do not have space to pursue here). Anorgasmia in the female was first reported by a general practitioner in Peterborough. Alerted by these incidents, we found that sexual side effects were common. We also realized that they could in some circumstances be turned to advantage. Small doses of clomipramine could be used to control ejaculation, and we were able to show that these could be very effective in premature ejaculation. Unfortunately, some of this work attracted the interest of the popular press. Geigy Pharmaceuticals had a Calvinistic background, and the management did not like what it regarded as "the wrong kind of publicity." Consequently, the sexual-function research was "put on the back burner." Given what we now know about the sexual side effects of commonly used psychotropic agents, and also considering the immense interest now in developing specific treatments for sexual disorders, here was perhaps another opportunity missed.

Quite apart from the psychopharmacological aspects, my association with the pharmaceutical industry has been very rewarding. I have been heavily involved in endeavouring to establish the specialist status of the pharmaceutical physician. I organized the first course in pharmaceutical medicine; I was subsequently involved in the development of a diploma in the subject; I served as the first external examiner for the diploma in clinical science, and more recently, I have been involved in devising the psychopharmacological content of an MSc in pharmaceutical medicine.

But I never lost sight of my initial interest in primary care. My belief was that the management of many common psychiatric disorders was most appropriately provided for in general practice, and that this was the best place to conduct clinical trials. To do so, we needed well-informed and well-trained general practitioners. At Geigy Pharmaceuticals, through our GP research group, we were among the first to take this approach. (I think it is fair to say that David Wheatley was the first.) My interest in organizing general practitioner research continues to this day. My more than thirty years in psychopharmacology have been a wonderful experience. I have made many good friends, travelled far and wide, had exciting experiences, and, I hope, contributed in a modest way to our knowledge of psychoactive agents and their value in the management of mental illness.

THE 1960S: MY EARLY YEARS WITH TRICYCLICS

Fridolin Sulser

Little was known in the early 1960s about central mechanisms of drug action. Understanding of the role of G-protein coupled receptor cascades would have to wait for at least another twenty years. Yet those were exciting times for psychopharmacology. Ironically, it was during that era of an almost total "mechanistic vacuum" that all the prototypes of psychotropic drugs were discovered, mostly as a consequence of the astuteness of clinical investigators. If serendipity played a role in the discovery of the therapeutic properties of psychotropic drugs, the "imipramine story" demonstrates that it favours the prepared mind.

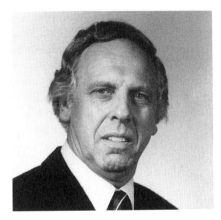

Fridolin Sulser

Soon after Ronald Kuhn discovered the therapeutic effect of imipramine as an antidepressant, I joined Bernard B. Brodie's group at the National Institutes of Health in 1959 as a young research associate. It was there that my love affair with tricyclics as both therapeutic agents and scientific tools to dissect mechanisms of brain function started. Although my main research interests in psychopharmacology have always been the use of psychotropic drugs as tools to understand mechanisms at the neurochemical, behavioural, and, more recently, molecular level, I was nonetheless able to contribute in a small way to the development of new prototypes of psychotropic drugs, such as the secondary amines of tricyclic antidepressants. I associated with colleagues who complemented my own scientific background: Donald Bogdanski, who patiently taught me about the ergotropic/trophotropic concept of W.R. Hess; Jim Gillette and Jim Dingell, who introduced me to microsomal enzymes and the power of solvent extraction procedures; Park Shore, the late Ken Finger, and Ronald Kuntzman, who made me aware of the principles and application of the fluorescence assay; and Marcel Bickel, with whom I explored the early antireserpine actions of desmethylimipramine (DMI). We needed to distinguish the antidepressant drug imipramine from the structurally related, phenothiazine-like antipsychotic agents. In this context, we became aware of the potential of reserpine, at that time used as an antihypertensive drug, to precipitate

Fridolin Sulser received his MD in 1955 from the University of Basel, Switzerland. Between 1958 and 1963 he worked in Dr B.B. Brodie's Laboratory of Chemical Pharmacology at the National Institutes of Health. After a short detour into the pharmaceutical industry from 1963-65, he joined the faculty at Vanderbilt University School of Medicine as professor of pharmacology (1965) and professor of psychiatry (1986).

Sulser was elected a fellow of CINP in 1970.

depressive reactions necessitating hospitalization in a number of patients. Consequently, we decided to take advantage of the reserpine-like syndrome elicited also by synthetic benzo-quinolizines (e.g. tetrabenazine and RO-41284) as a model depression to uncover antidepressant activity that could not be detected in normal animals. To my surprise, imipramine, particularly when administered chronically, inhibited both peripheral and central symptoms elicited by the reserpine-like drugs, a pharmacological property not shared with the structurally related chlorpromazine. Thus, in animals given imipramine, the effect of tetrabenazine or Ro-41284 was to elicit exophthalmos instead of blepharospasm, mydriasis instead of miosis, hyperthermia instead of hypothermia, and increased exploratory and compulsive motor activity instead of the almost complete loss of motor activity observed after the reserpine-like drugs alone. Importantly, these antagonistic effects of imipramine occurred without inhibition of the monoamine oxidase enzyme. The increase in parasympathetic activity following reserpine administration (lacrimation, salivation, diarrhea) was also blocked, but this was not surprising since imipramine displays considerable anticholinergic activity.

I wondered why chronic administration of imipramine was more potent in antagonizing the reserpine-like syndrome than a single dose of the drug. Could it be that the drug accumulated in brain tissue and took time to reach a "therapeutic" level? It so happened that Jim Dingell, for his PhD thesis, had developed a fluorometric method to measure imipramine quantitatively. Thus we naturally joined forces and worked to discover the suspected accumulation of imipramine in brain tissue. To our surprise, there was no accumulation of imipramine in brain tissue after chronic administration of the drug, but a significant increase in fluorescence was noted in the buffer phase, identified in due course as being the result of the demethylated secondary amine of imipramine, desmethylimipramine (DMI) (1). Jim and I were excited when we could show that DMI, formed from imipramine by oxidative N-demethylation in vivo, yielded a drug with stronger antireserpine activity and with a considerably longer biological half-life than the parent substance. The demonstration that DMI was an effective antidepressant in humans added to our satisfaction. In due course, a large number of secondary amines were synthesized as potential antidepressants by the pharmaceutical industry, for example, desipramine, nortriptyline, protriptyline, maprotiline, and others, which were all active in the reserpine model and useful as therapeutic agents in major depression in humans.

In addition to reserpine's value in "model depression" in animals, Marcel Bickel and I took advantage of the reserpine model to study the mechanism of action of tricyclic antidepressants. We investigated the biogenic amines in the antireserpine actions of DMI in animals whose brains had been selectively depleted of catecholamines by means of alpha-methyl-metatyrosine. These studies revealed that DMI failed to antagonize or "reverse" the reserpine-like syndrome during the period of maximal depletion of brain catecholamines, but the antireserpine activity of DMI returned gradually as the levels of catecholamines in the brain returned to normal (2, 3), thus clearly establishing the pivotal role of catecholamines in the antireserpine action of DMI-like drugs. These findings coincided with pioneer discoveries by Julie Axelrod and his collaborators (also at the NIH), who found that tricyclic antidepressants blocked the neuronal reuptake of norepinephrine (NE) in peripheral and central noradrenergic neurons (4), thus providing a rational basis for the enhancement of peripheral noradrenergic activity observed many years earlier by Ernest Sigg (5) and for the absence of the drug's antireserpine effect observed by us in NE-depleted animals.

In retrospect, DMI was the first selective NE reuptake inhibitor, discovered in the brain of Sprague-Dawley rats after the administration of imipramine, and it paved the way for other selective amine uptake inhibitors. Soon after the discovery of the action of tricyclic antide-pressants on the uptake of NE, Arvid Carlsson, who preceded me as a visiting scientist in Brodie's laboratory, demonstrated in Göteborg that tricyclic antidepressants also inhibit the uptake of serotonin into central serotonergic neurons and that the tertiary amines are more potent than the corresponding secondary amines in inhibiting the transport of serotonin, while secondary amines are more potent in inhibiting the uptake of NE than the corresponding tertiary amines (6). These findings have profoundly affected the further development of selective amine uptake inhibitors as antidepressant drugs.

It is hard to convey the excitement that permeated the NIH campus in the early 1960s. The laboratories of Bernard Brodie and Julie Axelrod were truly Meccas of psychopharmacology. They facilitated the development of new psychotropic drugs and of sound methodology to measure drugs and their metabolites in plasma, brain, and other tissues as well as the synthesis, release, and metabolism of biogenic amines. Data generated in these laboratories in the early 1960s catalyzed the concepts of the clinically relevant catechol and indoleamine hypotheses of affective disorders – hypotheses that have dominated research strategies in biological psychiatry for the last thirty years. The evolution of these theories has reflected changes in our understanding of the mode of action of antidepressant drugs. The research focus has shifted over the last three decades from acute presynaptic events to delayed adaptive changes in receptor sensitivities, and more recently to the convergence of aminergic signals beyond the receptors, leading ultimately to changes in programs of gene expression. Today's molecular psychopharmacology, with its sophisticated methodologies, is, however, firmly based on the findings and progress made in the 1960s, the decade responsible for the "golden era in neuropsychopharmacology" and for the evolution that is still in progress in molecular psycho-pharmacology and molecular psychiatry at the dawn of the third millennium. I make no apologies for the rather crude tools we had at our disposal in the 1960s.

REFERENCES

1. Gillette, J.R., Dingell, J.V., Sulser, F., Kuntzman, R., and Brodie, B.B. (1961). Isolation from rat brain of a metabolic product, desmethylimipramine, that mediates the antidepressant activity of imipramine. *Experientia* 17 : 417-420.
2. Sulser, F., Watts, J., and Brodie, B.B. (1962). On the mechanism of antidepressant action of imipramine-like drugs. *Ann. N.Y. Acad. Sci.* 96: 279-286.
3. Sulser, F., Bickel, M.H., and Brodie, B.B. (1964). The action of desmethylimipramine in counteracting sedation and cholinergic effects of reserpine-like drugs. *J. Pharmacol. Exp. Ther.* 144: 321-330.
4. Axelrod, J., Whitby, L.B., and Hertting, G. (1961). Effect of psychotropic drugs on the uptake of 3H-norepinephrine by tissues. *Science* 133: 383-384.
5. Sigg, E.B. (1959). Pharmacological studies with Tofranil. *Can. Psychiatric Assoc.* J. 4: S75-S85.
6. Carlsson, A., Corrodi, H., Fuxe, K., and Hökfelt, T. (1969). Effect of antidepressant drugs on the depletion of intraneuronal brain 5-hydroxytryptamine stores caused by 4-alpha-ethyl- meta-tyramine. *Eur. J. Pharmacol.* 5: 357-366.

FROM IMIPRAMINE TO DESIPRAMINE

Marcel H. Bickel

When imipramine (Tofranil) appeared in the final years of the 1950s, it soon revolutionized the treatment of depression. This was clearly a new type of drug. The observation that it counteracted clinical depression but did not produce excitation in "normal animals" or humans was baffling at that time. Surprisingly, imipramine even had a weak chlorpromazine-like action. Neither the people at the Geigy company nor the discoverer of imipramine's antidepressant action, Roland Kuhn, nor the pharmacologists were able to make an educated guess about its mechanism of action. But this was precisely the type of challenge enjoyed by Bernard B. Brodie, who had just around that time switched his research interest from drug metabolism to neuropsychopharmacology. By 1960 he and Fridolin

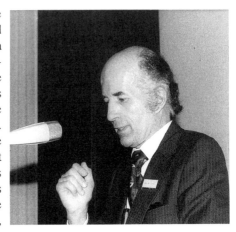

Marcel H. Bickel

Sulser had started a project aimed at elucidating the mechanism of action of imipramine. The following year I joined the Brodie group at the National Institutes of Health as a postdoctoral student from Switzerland, and since Geigy, Kuhn, and Sulser were all Swiss, I became part of the Swiss "imipramine mafia."

I knew little about neuropsychopharmacology at that time and next to nothing about imipramine. I learned that Brodie and Sulser had just shown that it prevented and even reversed the sedative action of reserpine in rats, which was an important finding in light of the fact that patients under reserpine therapy occasionally experienced clinical depression. It was the finding which led to the use of reserpine (and reserpine-like compounds) as tools for producing a "model depression" in animals. The observed imipramine-induced "reserpine reversal," I further learned, begins slowly and is mediated through desmethylimipramine (DMI), a metabolite of imipramine, identified in Brodie's laboratory by J.R. Gillette and J.V. Dingell in 1961.

Marcel H. Bickel obtained his PhD at the University of Basel in Switzerland in 1959 and did postdoctoral studies with D. Bovet in Rome and with B.B. Brodie at the National Institutes of Health in Bethesda, Maryland, between 1961 and 1964. He then joined the University of Bern Medical School, where he was professor of biochemistry in the years 1967-76 and of pharmacology from 1977 to 1993. He is now a member of the Department of the History of Medicine in the medical school.

Bickel was elected a fellow of the CINP in 1968. He presented a paper on "Pharmacokinetic studies in animals as a model system for human therapy" and on "True and apparent non-penetration of the blood-brain-barrier by psychotropic drugs" at the 6th and 7th Congresses, respectively.

All this was intriguing for me, to be sure. It was also sufficiently stimulating to trigger research directed at the pharmacology of DMI. In the course of these studies it was learned that unlike imipramine, DMI, even in large doses, caused no obvious sedation in rats. On the other hand, it blocked or reversed the action of reserpine much more quickly and effectively than did imipramine. It also counteracted the whole range and not only some of the reserpine-induced symptoms, such as sedation, muscular rigidity, diarrhea, blepharospasm, and miosis. (It was noted that the administration of imipramine or chlorpromazine delayed or prevented these effects of DMI.) However, the most striking effect of DMI was that reserpine-induced sedation was not only prevented but also "reversed" into a singular type of coordinated hyperactivity.

In order to get a better understanding about this new type of hyperactivity, we switched to behavioural studies. The results were described in 1964 by Brodie, Sulser, and myself as follows: "Control rats, placed on top of the cage, moved around, exploring the environment for a few minutes, after which they usually huddled together and groomed themselves. Rats given RO-41284 [a reserpine-like compound] and placed on the cage-top remained motionless and isolated from each other, in a hunched-back position, for about three hours."

In contrast, the rats given DMI together with RO-41284 showed the following behaviour patterns:

(a) The animals ceaselessly circled the perimeter of the cage-top, peering over the sides and frequently leaping from cage-top to floor, where they continued their avid exploratory behaviour. Rats placed inside the cage almost invariably scrambled over the sides. In contrast, animals treated with d-amphetamine (5 mg/kg) dashed about erratically, not only around the perimeter, but over the entire cage-top.

(b) In a treadmill, the rats treated with DMI and RO-41284 turned the wheel much more frequently than normal animals. The animals plodded on like automatons, rarely changing direction, walking but never running. In contrast, amphetamine-treated animals displayed erratic haste .

(c) Apparently compulsive behaviour was [also] shown by the rats placed on a platform near the ceiling. The animals moved around, repeatedly looking over the edge, each time stretching outwards a little more, until finally many tried an impossible descent, which resulted in their toppling to the floor. Replaced on the platform, they would repeat the performance despite the previous hard fall. By contrast, animals treated with d-amphetamine (10 mg/kg) or methylphenidate (15 mg/kg) did not attempt the descent.

The performance of our rats on the "jumping board" near the ceiling of our lab became an attraction. Our colleagues came from the neighbouring labs and from remote NIH locations; Brodie brought in guests, and all wanted to watch our "suicide rats." I should add that we always spared the poor little fellows a hard fall by gently catching them in mid-air in the palms of our hands. At one point we thought that it would excite our boss if we made the "crucial experiment" by offering the rats a jump from the top (fourteenth) floor of the Clinical Center; however, Brodie could not be provoked.

The findings that higher doses of DMI could prevent and even reverse sedation into a unique hyperactivity, proved to be useful in developing a test for the screening of the potential antidepressant activity of compounds.

Furthermore, the findings in our pharmacological studies were indicative of DMI's potent antidepressant effects. They also suggested that DMI was an active antidepressant, whereas imipramine was an inactive precursor. Thus, we believed that once again a prominent action of a drug was due to the formation of an active metabolite, in this case by N-demethylation of a tertiary to a secondary amine. It was on the basis of this discovery that the possibility was raised that secondary, and perhaps primary, amines exert central effects which are different from those produced by their tertiary analogues.

An important question was whether the anti-reserpine action of DMI was in any way a reflection of its clinical action in depressed patients. It was important to find out whether this was the case not only with respect to the mechanism of action of the drug, but also with respect to the possibility that the neuronal pathways disturbed by reserpine might be similar to those disturbed in clinical depression. In the midst of these laboratory investigations, we heard of the exciting news from Nathan Kline's psychiatric clinic that DMI was more effective and more rapid in its action than imipramine in the treatment of endogenous depression. Shortly after, the Geigy company launched DMI as an antidepressant under the generic name desipramine and the optimistic trade name Pertofrane. A new antidepressant drug was born!

All this sounds like a success story. It looked as though desipramine would replace imipramine, as the "real" prototype antidepressant. Hopes were high that its use in animal experimentation would result in the elucidation of its mechanism of action and thus provide a clue to the better understanding of depression. It was also hoped that its clinical use would accelerate the onset of antidepressant action and improve therapeutic performance. Indeed, in the following years we saw intensive studies of desipramine in many laboratories. In the course of these studies much was learned about how desipramine interacted with the various neurotransmitters; about the metabolism and metabolites of desipramine; and about the difference between the pharmacological profiles of desipramine and imipramine. However, after many years and much work, no serious pharmacologist would pretend to understand desipramine's mechanism of action. Equally unfortunate, it became clear that the drug's performance in clinical therapy was somewhat disappointing; as a whole it was not superior and may even be inferior to imipramine. As a result, desipramine became a second-choice drug antidepressant in treament and imipramine was re-established as the prototype antidepressant.

Thus in the long run, ours was not a success story, but we were not frustrated. Since the 1960s several theories about the mechanism of action of the antidepressants have been advanced. I remember telling my students a slightly different story or hypothesis almost every year. Furthermore, many new antidepressant drugs have appeared, some with fewer side effects than the older ones. However, it seems doubtful whether old imipramine has lost its role as the prototype antidepressant.

The fact remains that we still have too little knowledge about depression. It is unlikely that even with the sophisticated technology we have today its secrets will be unravelled. Nevertheless, there is no reason for discouragement because it is more important that we are able to help depressed patients than that we know exactly how our drugs work.

THE CHEESE STORY

Barry Blackwell

When I graduated from high school in Canterbury, England, in 1952, chlorpromazine had been "discovered" as an antipsychotic. By 1957, when I graduated from Cambridge University, iproniazid was known to be an antidepressant, and as I completed my medical school training at Guy's Hospital in 1961, imipramine also became available. So, by the time I arrived at the Maudsley Hospital in London in the fall of 1962 to begin residency training in psychiatry, our specialty had the basic tools to deal with all the major "biochemical disorders."

The Maudsley was in its heyday. Aubrey Lewis had consummated his vision of a multidisciplinary Institute of Psychiatry that included all the basic and clinical sciences. The staff and faculty were among the leaders in European descriptive and biological psychiatry, and the Institute attracted many of the best graduates from medical schools around the world. Sir Aubrey had a knack of selecting trainees

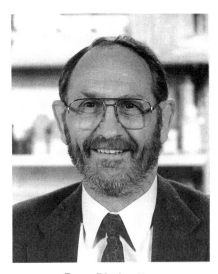

Barry Blackwell

with diverse abilities and a capacity for divergent thinking. If you had not already obtained board certification in general medicine, you had to at least show some unusual talent – perhaps an Antarctic expedition, a musical or literary skill, or even athletic ability. I had a talent for playing rugby and had published my first article in *The Lancet* (Why patients come to a casualty department) while still an intern. Even so, I only made it to the B team. The brightest began at the Maudsley, while the remainder were posted to the Bethlem Hospital in the suburbs.

Within three months, at the age of twenty-nine, I stumbled upon the discovery that would give me worldwide recognition. The "cheese story" has been told in two ways, as a scientific inquiry (1) and as a personal saga (2). Like almost all the early discoveries in biological psychiatry, mine was a blend of serendipity and preparedness. While I was an intern in neurology, my chief resident constantly reminded me that patients treated with tranylcypromine sometimes suffered a hypertensive crisis and more rarely a subarachnoid hemorrhage.

Barry Blackwell served as professor and chairman of Psychiatry at the Milwaukee Clinical Campus of the University of Wisconsin School of Medicine from June 1980 to 1992. He retired from medicine in July 1998 to pursue numerous other interests and hobbies.

Blackwell was elected a fellow of the CINP in 1972. He presented a paper on "Hypertensive interaction between MAOI and foodstuff" (Blackwell and Marley) and on "The use of MAOI and specific response to them" (Blackwell and Taylor) at the 5th Congress.

Although I took assiduous drug histories, I never witnessed or talked to anyone who witnessed the connection – until I was eating lunch in the cafeteria at the Bethlem Hospital one day and heard some fellow residents discussing a young woman who had experienced an unexpected stroke.

There had been six independent letters to *The Lancet* about this side effect over the preceding twenty months. Eager for a publication, I wrote my own report, which was also published as a letter. Shortly afterwards a reply arrived from a hospital pharmacist, G.E.F. Rowe, who had read *The Lancet* report in the local library and wrote that his wife had experienced sudden, excruciating headaches while taking tranylcypromine, both times after eating cheese, and asked "could there be a link between the effects and the amino acids of the cheese?" I shared this letter with my fellow residents as a joke, but later that week a pharmaceutical company representative, Gerald Samuels, told me that his company, Smith, Kline and French had received similar reports. Although he suggested that I check the amino acid content of cheese only, I also did a retrospective review of the hospital menus. Cheese is full of protein, and the Bethlem patient my fellow residents discussed had eaten a cheese pie on the day of her subarachnoid hemorrhage.

Fulfilling an ancient tradition of self-experimentation, another resident and I now took tranylcypromine and sat down to eat a breakfast of Cheddar cheese. Nothing happened. Deterred by this outcome and the growing ridicule of my fellow residents, I temporarily dropped the idea. Shortly afterwards, I was moonlighting for a local family practitioner when a request to make a house call came from a man whose wife, who was taking tranylcypromine, was suffering an intense headache. She had just eaten a cheese sandwich for lunch, and when I took her blood pressure, she was in the midst of a hypertensive crisis.

I now found a patient on tranylcypromine who was willing to undertake the experiment that had failed on myself. After she ate the cheese, my bedside vigil on her blood pressure went unrewarded for two hours. I left, only to be called back almost immediately by the nurses for permission to give "aspirin for headache." When I returned, I found the patient in the throes of a hypertensive crisis. The blood pressure records on this patient became part of the article that was published in *The Lancet* in October 1963. Within nine months I had been able to assemble twelve patients, of whom eight had eaten cheese shortly before their hypertensive episode. Coincidence had continued to play a part. Walking down a Maudsley corridor one evening, I was overtaken by the on-call resident en route to a ward where two patients were simultaneously complaining of sudden, severe headache. Both were taking a MAO inhibitor and both had just returned from the hospital cafeteria after eating cheese.

My *Lancet* article was met with considerable scepticism: one critic found the concept "unscientific and premature," while another noted that "everyone eats cheese," and that people who had experienced one episode often ate cheese again with impunity. These criticisms were silenced when the research workers at another London hospital ate Gorgonzola cheese and demonstrated that tyramine appeared in the chromatograms of their body fluids.

By now I had been elevated to Aubrey Lewis's own professorial unit, where he kept a close eye on me. Observing my predilection for complex psychosocial assessments, he expressed a concern that I might be flirting with psychoanalysis, and he recommended that I take time out to study the mechanism of this side effect further and obtain special training in psychopharmacology.

For the next two years I worked under Ted Marley in a Second World War Nissen hut and learned to perform smoked-drum experiments on cats and rats which explained the mechanisms of the interaction between tyramine contained in foodstuffs and the MAO-A inhibitors. What we learned in animals was confirmed in a series of human experiments on Gerald Russell's metabolic unit. We also collaborated with the National Institute for Research in Dairying to study the composition and tyramine content of different cheeses. Along the way Professor Marley and I published articles in *The Lancet, The British Journal of Pharmacology, Nature,* and *The Journal of Food Science.* Ultimately in 1967 the entire scientific story was published in *The British Journal of Psychiatry* (1) and documented the many variables in the patient, the medication, and the composition of cheese that determined the sporadic occurrence and severity of the interaction.

This was an experience with personal lessons of its own. First, I found that much of what I had "discovered" was already known. Sir Aubrey, who was a Greek scholar, recalled that Hippocrates had said something about cheese. Consulting a biography, I discovered what he has said: "It is not enough to know that cheese is a bad article of food in that it gives pain to anyone eating it in excess, but what sort of pain, and why, and with what principle in man it disagrees." The amino acid tyrosine was first isolated from cheese by a German chemist in 1846 and named after *tyros,* the Greek word for cheese. Tyramine was also first identified in cheese and discovered to be a hypertensive agent by Sir Henry Dale in 1909. Two years later, Findlay used tyramine in experiments to calibrate the first sphygmomanometer and was sufficiently alarmed at its pressor potential that he warned that sudden tyramine-induced rises in blood pressure might cause cerebral hemorrhage. I also found that monoamine oxidase was originally named tyramine oxidase after its first known substrate. The role of the enzyme in the gut and liver were thought by Blashko in 1952 to include the prevention of access to the circulation of amines in foodstuffs.

Not only were all the mechanisms known that would predict this side effect when MAO-A inhibitors were given to humans, but the side effect itself was clearly described before these drugs were used for depression. In 1955 Ogilvie conducted a trial of iproniazid in patients with tuberculosis and noted severe throbbing headache and hypertension in four out of forty-two patients. At least another forty cases, including several deaths, were reported before I began my own research in 1963, and tyramine was incriminated.

A second personal lesson that I learned was that I was not cut out to be a basic scientist. This was a bitter disappointment to Ted Marley, who had hoped I might become a disciple and follow in his footsteps. But I was a klutz and could no more become a pharmacologist than a surgeon. My experiments were littered with broken syringes and smudged smoked drums. For a while I remained involved and interested in psychopharmacology. After completing my residency training, I took a postdoctoral fellowship to work with Michael Shepherd. Together we reanalysed the claims made by P.C. Baastrup and M. Schou that lithium was a prophylactic agent in the long-term management of depression. This critique was accompanied by data to suggest that tricyclic antidepressants might be equally effective if analysed in the same flawed manner. Our paper, published by *The Lancet* in 1968, questioned whether lithium was truly prophylactic or simply another panacea. It was a typical product of another aspect of the Maudsley environment – a critical, but sceptical appraisal that others viewed as sterile and nihilistic.

Despite all the training that I now had and the attention I had attracted, I still doubted my choice of career specialty and decided to take time out from psychiatry to try my hand at family medicine. Here I worked with David Goldberg to develop one of the first validated screening instruments for psychological disorders in a primary care setting (General Health Questionnaire). Although I returned to psychiatry and emigrated to the United States a year later, it was this experience in primary care that reaffirmed Sir Aubrey Lewis's suspicions – I was really far more interested in the psychosocial aspects of medicine than in psychopharmacology. Although I continued throughout my career to teach and write, my focus has been at the interface of psychiatry and medicine within what Engel called the biopsychosocial model. My latest task (and perhaps my last) has been to edit a book entitled *Treatment Compliance and the Therapeutic Alliance* (3). This is a close examination of the ways in which people with severe and persistent mental illness can obtain the benefits of treatment through a broader understanding of the relationship between consumers and providers.

As I write this memoir, I am acutely aware of how ephemeral are knowledge and fame. Not only was what I "discovered" already known and forgotten, but the same fate now confronts me. The last edition of *The Comprehensive Textbook of Psychiatry* mentions that the cheese discovery was made by "an American psychiatrist" whose date of birth was 1903 (thirty-one years before I was born). If you look up the cheese reaction in the official APA text on psychopharmacology, you will not find any of the original articles or authors, only a secondary citation. But a quarter-century has passed. We now have newer antidepressant medications that are virtually free of serious side effects, and our patients are better served. It is a trivial scientific matter if the gods reward youthful hubris with obscurity.

REFERENCES
1. Blackwell, B., Marley, E., Price, J., and Taylor, D. (1967). Hypertensive interactions between monoamine oxidase inhibitors and foodstuffs. *British Journal of Psychiatry,* 113: 349-365.
2. Blackwell, B. (1984). The process of discovery. In J.Frank. Ayd and B. Blackwell (eds.), *Discoveries in Biological Psychiatry.* Baltimore: Ayd Medical Communications.
3. Blackwell, B. (ed.) (1997). *Treatment Compliance and the Therapeutic Alliance.* Toronto: Harwood Academic Publishers.

DEPRENYL, THE FIRST CATECHOLAMINERGIC ACTIVITY ENHANCER

Joseph Knoll

My work during the 1960s was focused on the development of deprenyl (selegiline) and after receiving your invitation to contribute some of my memories of drug development from the 1960s, I decided to give a brief account of the history of research with the drug.

Deprenyl, developed in the early 1960s, is a peculiar stimulant of the catecholaminergic system in the brain, possessing a still unique, complex pharmacological spectrum, one component of which, the selective inhibition of monoamine oxidase type B (MAO-B), made the drug famous in the 1970s.

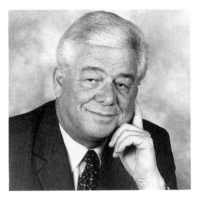

Joseph Knoll

SELECTIVE MAO-B INHIBITOR

In 1968 Johnston described clorgyline, a new MAO inhibitor which preferentially inhibited the deamination of serotonin. He proposed the existence of two isoforms of MAO: one, type A, highly sensitive to clorgyline and one, type B, relatively insensitive to it. Further studies with clorgyline focused attention on the need for a new pharmacological tool, a highly selective inhibitor of MAO-B, for the final verification and detailed in vivo mapping of the two forms of MAO. I was lucky to discover in 1970 that deprenyl is the highly selective inhibitor of MAO-B. I presented the finding in my lecture at the 1st International Symposium on MAO in Cagliari (Italy). Our paper, published in 1972, demonstrating that deprenyl is a selective MAO-B inhibitor became on January 15, 1982, a "citation classic."

From another aspect, deprenyl also proved to be a unique MAO-inhibitor. In 1963, B. Blackwell published the finding that the inhibition of the metabolism of tyramine in foodstuffs

Joseph Knoll, born in 1925, entered the medical faculty (now Semmelweis University of Medicine) of Pázmány Péter University in Budapest in 1946 and received his MD in 1951. He began his research career in the department of pharmacology of the university in 1949 and he has remained with this institute, of which he has been professor since 1963, and head from 1962 until 1992. He developed deprenyl (selegiline) and discovered the satientins, an endogenous family of anorectics. He is currently vice-president of Semmelweis University.

Knoll presented papers on "Methods for evaluation of tranquilizers" and on "The deconditioning effect of some beta-aminoketones, a new group of tranquilizers" at the 1st and 2nd Congresses, respectively.

– for example, cheese – can lead to the serious, sometimes fatal, hypertensive reactions in patients treated with MAO inhibitors. The "cheese effect" cast a shadow on the MAO inhibitors, one of the first significant family of antidepressants, which had achieved a resounding success in the late 1950s. I had observed that deprenyl, in contrast to other potent MAO inhibitors, inhibits the noradrenaline-releasing effect of tyramine, and in 1965 asked a good friend of mine, the psychiatrist Ervin Varga, to check this in volunteers. He studied the consequences of the concurrent administration of deprenyl with tyramine and found that deprenyl did not potentiate the effect of tyramine; but he did not publish his results. Considering the practical importance of this finding, when summarizing the results of our research with deprenyl during the 1960s (in our paper published in 1968) we wrote: "As the so-called cheese reaction, namely clinical symptoms after cheese consumption, similar to a paroxysm induced by pheochromocytoma, is absent, this tyramine inhibiting property of deprenyl may be highly valuable for human therapy." Regrettably, the proposal did not attract attention at the time, although the first clinical trial with racemic deprenyl was performed in depression, with encouraging results by Varga and his co-workers in the late sixties. A potent MAO inhibitor free of the "cheese effect" would have filled the need for a MAOI antidepressant which can be used without dietary and other considerations such as drug interactions. The possibility of introducing deprenyl as an antidepressant has remained unexploited to this day.

Interestingly, deprenyl found its first clinical application in Parkinson's disease, precisely because it was an MAO inhibitor free of the cheese effect. After Hornykiewitz discovered in 1960 the striking dopamine deficiency in the striatum of patients who died from Parkinson's disease, and Birkmayer and Hornykiewitz demonstrated in 1961 the dramatic therapeutic effect of dopamine substitution by levodopa in patients suffering from Parkinson's disease, they tried immediately to lessen the serious side effects of treatment by the concurrent administration of a MAO inhibitor. This was, however, unworkable because of the potentiation of the catecholamine-releasing effect of levodopa by MAO inhibitors. As deprenyl was the first MAO inhibitor free of catecholamine releasing property, Birkmayer combined it with levodopa in Parkinson's disease. The combination worked and by now the value of deprenyl in the treatment of Parkinson's disease has been established.

ENHANCEMENT OF CATECHOLAMINERGIC ACTIVITY

My further studies with deprenyl also revealed that the substance is an exceptionally fortuitous chemical modification of phenylethylamine (PEA), an endogenous substance in the mammalian brain. Deprenyl, unlike PEA, has no catecholamine releasing effect. It only became clear with these findings how fortunate it was to select deprenyl in the early sixties for further research and possible clinical development. Apparently by introducing the propargyl group intentionally into methamphetamine to change the molecule to a strong, irreversible MAO inhibitor (pargyline was our model), we unintentionally created a selective inhibitor of MAO-B; and by attaching the bulky substitution of the propargyl group to the nitrogen in methamphetamine, for the first time the catecholamine-releasing property of an indirectly-acting sympathomimetic amine was eliminated, while its effect of enhancing catecholaminergic activity, or CAE effect, was maintained.

According to our present knowledge, the nigrostriatal dopaminergic neurons are the most rapidly aging neurons in the human brain. The dopamine content of the human caudate nucleus decreases steeply, at a rate of about 13 percent per decade over age forty-five. We know that symptoms of Parkinson's disease appear if the dopamine content of the caudate nucleus sinks below 30 percent of the normal level. The age-related decline of the nigrostriatal dopaminergic brain mechanism plays a significant role in the decline of performance with the passing of time. Safe and effective prophylactic medication is needed to slow these changes, and I proposed in 1982 to use deprenyl for this purpose. Pursuing this line of research further, first we found that maintaining rats on 0.25 mg/kg of deprenyl, three times a week, prolonged their life significantly. Later on we also revealed that deprenyl-treated rats lived not only longer than saline-treated rats, but also that deprenyl-treated males maintained their ability to ejaculate for a significantly longer period and remained better performers in the shuttle box than their saline-treated peers. The prolongation of life in deprenyl-treated animals was attributed to the peculiar CAE effect of the drug. Deprenyl keeps the catecholaminergic, mainly the dopaminergic, neurons in the brain on a higher activity level.

There is solely a quantitative difference between the physiological age-related decline of the dopaminergic input and that observed in Parkinson's disease. In the healthy population, the calculated loss of striatal dopamine is about 40 percent at the age of seventy-five, which is the average lifetime. The loss of dopamine in Parkinson's disease is about 70 percent at diagnosis and over 90 percent at death. That deprenyl is capable of slowing the rate of the functional deterioration of the nigrostriatal dopaminergic neurons was shown not only in rats, but also in patients with early, untreated Parkinson's disease. Age-related deterioration of the striatal machinery is a continuum and any precisely determined short segment of it is sufficient to measure the rate of decline in the presence or absence of deprenyl. As a matter of fact, a segment of this continuum – the time elapsing from diagnosis of Parkinson's disease until levodopa was needed – was studied, and it was found that deprenyl delayed the need for levodopa therapy. The patients selected for the study with early, untreated Parkinson's disease still had a sufficient number of dopaminergic neurons whose activity could be enhanced by deprenyl; thus, the need for levodopa therapy was delayed. As drug effects in Parkinson's disease are necessarily transient in nature, it is obvious that, parallel with further decay of the striatal dopaminergic system, the responsiveness of the patients to deprenyl decreased with the passing of time.

Deprenyl, though still not used for this purpose, is primarily destined to serve as a prophylactic agent in the healthy population for slowing the physiological age-related decline of the striatal dopaminergic neurons. It is reasonable to assume that if the patients selected for our studies had the opportunity to take just two to three tablets of deprenyl weekly during the whole postdevelopmental period of their life preceding the precipitation of the symptoms of Parkinson's disease, they would have either avoided reaching the low level of striatal dopamine within their life time, or at least would have crossed the critical threshold substantially later.

FUTURE ASPECTS

The real challenge for future pharmacological and clinical research is to take up the fight against the physiological age-related activity decline of the catecholaminergic system in the healthy brain, via long term, small-dose administration of a proper catecholaminergic-activity enhancer-substance, like deprenyl, during the postdevelopmental phase of life. It is reasonable to expect that preventive medication with a safe, small dose of a catecholaminergic activity enhancer substance will slow the age-related decline of behavioural performance, delay natural death, and decrease susceptibility to Parkinson's and perhaps even Alzheimer's disease.

THE RISE OF LITHIUM TREATMENT IN THE 1960s

Mogens Schou

To test an observation made by others is gratifying; to test an observation made by oneself is exciting. The 1950s were a decade when, together with Juel-Nielsen, Strömgren, and Voldby, I tested and confirmed in a partially double-blind trial John Cade's observation of an antimanic action of lithium. That was gratifying because until then only strongly sedative barbiturates and electroconvulsive treatment had been available for treatment of manic episodes. The neuroleptics came on the scene a little later.

The 1960s were a decade when, together with Poul Christian Baastrup and G. P. Hartigan, I observed, and together with Baastrup tested and confirmed, a prophylactic action of long-term treatment with lithium. That was exciting because until then maintenance ECT had been the only agent available, and its effect was dubious. Prophylactic lithium treatment was found effective in both bipolar and unipolar disorder, and it brought new hope to those suffering from these devastating and dangerous disorders.

Baastrup's and my first study of prophylactic lithium treatment was prospective and non-blind. It involved eighty-eight patients and lasted six years. The treatment produced a marked and long-lasting change in the disease course of patients who, prior to the lithium treatment, had had an average of five manic or depressive episodes. The change coincided with the start of the lithium treatment and was unlikely to have been fortuitous. Most of the patients were discharged after the start of the treatment, and it was accordingly the general practitioners, ignorant of the ongoing trial and therefore not biased, who decided when a recurrence had taken place.

I had personal reasons for being satisfied with the outcome, but not because I myself was manic and in lithium treatment as I later learned, Michael Shepherd thought at the time I was not. But from the age of twenty-five my brother had had yearly episodes of depression. In spite of ECT, drug treatment, and hospitalization, the depressive attacks came again and again, inexorably. Lithium treatment completely changed his life and the lives of his wife and children. When at a meeting in Göttingen, where Shepherd was present, I reported our findings and mentioned my brother. For Shepherd this was apparently testimony of my bias and folly,

Mogens Schou was born in Copenhagen in 1918 and graduated from Copenhagen University in 1944. He trained in clinical psychiatry and experimental biology in Denmark, Norway, and the United States. He was appointed head of the Psychopharmacology Unit at the Psychiatric Hospital in Risskov, Denmark, in 1951. He became professor of biological psychiatry in 1971 and retired in 1988.

Schou is an honorary fellow of the CINP. Elected in 1962, he was a councillor on the 9th and 10th executives, and presented papers on "Therapeutic and toxic properties of lithium," on "Lithium: relation between clinical effects of the drug and its absorption, distribution and excretion," and on "Concerning the evidence for a prophylactic action of lithium" at the 1st, 6th, and 7th Congresses respectively. He also contributed to the general discussion of the Third Symposium (Ten years of psychopharmacology) and a discussion of Opitz's presentation (Studien über den Einfluss psychotroper Substanzen auf den Glucosegehalt des Blutes) in the General Communications session, at the 3rd Congress.

and it seemed to convince him that lithium must be ineffective. It was in this spirit that he and Barry Blackwell criticized the study undertaken by Baastrup and myself. Shepherd did not understand that my personal involvement motivated me even more to put the efficacy of the treatment on the firmest possible ground.

The first move was to check whether others could find the same results as we had, so we joined forces with Paul Grof in Czechoslovakia and Angst and Weis in Switzerland. Data from 244 lithium-treated patients at the three clinics in Glostrup, Prague, and Zurich were pooled. Regression analyses showed that in bipolar and unipolar patients the frequency of recurrences fell to about one-third of what it had been before the treatment; in schizoaffective patients it fell to about one-half. This decrease in frequency was in marked contrast to the grad-

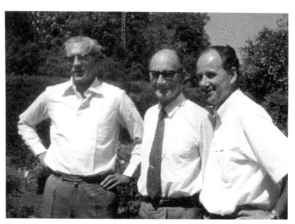

From left: Poul Christian Baastrup, John Cade, and Mogens Schou

ual increase of recurrence frequency, which Angst and Weis had previously found in manic-depressive patients not given prophylactic treatment.

In the summer of 1968 the situation was as follows: prophylactic treatment with lithium had become widespread in Scandinavia and a large part of continental Europe, and the results were good. The usage in England and the United States was more uneven. Many psychiatrists in those countries used lithium prophylactically and found it efficacious, but the debate with Blackwell and Shepherd had left a feeling of uncertainty in others, and they hesitated. Baastrup and I could not help being worried about manic-depressive patients in the English-speaking countries who were deprived of a valuable treatment. It was tempting to carry out a double-blind, placebo-controlled trial, but we were held back by the fear of exposing patients allocated to a placebo to suffering and risk of suicide when we had seen so many of them become stabilized on lithium after years of ravaging mood swings.

In the end we decided to do such a trial, but only after we had devised a protocol of a special design. A total of about 100 patients who had been in lithium treatment for a year or more were switched double-blind to a placebo or continued lithium treatment, the two treatments being allocated randomly. Sequential analysis was used, involving a pairing of lithium-treated with placebo-treated patients and the termination of the trial as soon as a predetermined degree of statistical significance ($p<0.01$) had been reached. When a recurrence developed, the trial was terminated for that member of the pair, antimanic or antidepressant treatment was immediately instituted, and the patient was transferred to open lithium treatment. In this way the number of recurrences and of patients put at risk was minimized, as was the ethical problem involved in withdrawing a putatively effective treatment from patients apparently benefiting from it.

The trial was terminated by the sequential analysis within half a year. It showed lithium to be significantly superior to·a placebo. But those six months were strained. We worried incessantly about each patient's health and life. At that time there were no ethical committees and no requests for informed consent, but Baastrup and I felt deeply our double obligations to the patients who participated in the trial and to the manic-depressive individuals around the world who were not given a chance with prophylactic lithium treatment. If the treatment was as good as our observations indicated, we were morally obliged to demonstrate this fact in such a way that psychiatrists everywhere would start using it. If, on the other hand, our interpretation of the observations was wrong, then we were obliged to establish this fact and spare our own patients treatment with an ineffective drug associated with side effects and possible risk. Yes, the excitement of scientific endeavour was there, but it was an excitement with heavy responsibility rather than one of triumph.

The term "enthusiastic advocate" has clung to me ever since Shepherd first used it, and I gladly accept the first word. Rather than sheer ambition, engagement should be the driving force of research, and who would not be enthused when his or her research led to effective treatment of a long-lasting and serious illness? But the designation "advocate" I refuse to acknowledge. Advocates collect data and arguments that speak for or against a particular point of view or person. Scientists, on the other hand, gather and weigh all available evidence concerning a question or problem, and then on the basis of their assessment of the evidence, they draw a conclusion, often a tentative one with reservations. The conclusion is not a judgment in any legal sense, but rather a working hypothesis, which the true scientists are ready, even eager, to reject if new data or arguments speak convincingly against it. Baastrup and I drew our conclusion about a prophylactic action of lithium because we found this interpretation more likely than any other. Numerous controlled studies have later confirmed its validity.

The CINP and lithium have had little to do with each other during the early years of the organization. The proceedings of the first congress in Rome in 1958 do not show a single paper with the word "lithium" in the title. The very last presentation of the book appears under the heading "General discussion." It was a cry of despair and defiance, and yet it contained elements of prophetic truth: "On the chemotherapeutic firmament lithium is one of the smaller stars, and until now it may not even have been noticed by all psychiatrists. But its light appears unmistakable, and it may turn out to be more steady than that of several other of the celestial bodies which now shine so brightly." (Schou 1958).

This was the nadir. By 1970 the situation had changed. At the seventh CINP congress in Prague the very first symposium was titled "Clinical and pharmacological aspects of lithium therapy," and it included contributions from Belgium, Canada, Czechoslovakia, Denmark, Ireland, and the United States. The possibility of prophylactic protection against recurrences of mania and depression had caught the attention of the psychiatrists. The following decade brought a deluge of publications about lithium, but it was the 1960s that saw the breakthrough in psychiatric lithium treatment.

LITHIUM IN CANADA

Edward Kingstone

It is an honour to be asked to recall some of the events surrounding drug developments in the 1960s, especially as they related to my own career. In writing this memoir, I have consulted a slender, but important volume entitled *Psychopharmacology in Perspective,* a personal account by the founders of the Collegium Internationale Neuro-Psychopharmacologicum (1). One of those founders was D. Ewen Cameron, for many years the director of the Allan Memorial Institute in Montreal and chairman of the Department of Psychiatry at McGill University. I contributed a biographical sketch of Dr. Cameron, who died in 1967, some three or four years after he left the Allan and McGill. That activity – both the writing of the article and its rereading – gave me an opportunity to recall those early days of psychopharmacology. On an earlier occasion, at a symposium on

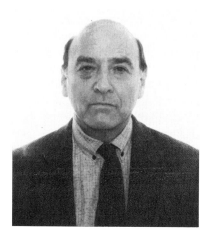

Edward Kingstone

lithium in 1974 (2), I had been able to record that that year was the fifteenth anniversary of my association with the lithium ion. This memoir is based on those two publications.

However, it might be of interest to establish the scene in 1959, particularly in Montreal. In the first place, McGill University held a pre-eminent position in psychiatry in Canada. At that time the Allan Memorial Institute was probably unique in the country. Its director, Cameron, had been there since 1944. I have always felt that the organization as it existed then was a historical accident which could probably not be repeated. Because of the financial support available, many of the psychiatrists on staff were primarily resource people and had little to do with the day-to-day running of the institute. Today, of course, it is almost impossible to find the same level of financial support, so that most people attached to academic institutions have, of necessity, to be heavily involved in patient care.

The era itself was one of excitement, optimism, and a belief that all psychiatric problems would and could be solved by the use of organic or psychological therapies. It was a time when new compounds were being introduced almost monthly in the therapeutic field. The major

Edward Kingstone, after a productive decade at the Allan Memorial and at McGill University in Montreal, became head of the Department of Psychiatry at Sunnybrook Medical Centre and eventually professor at the University of Toronto. Later he spent two terms as Chair of Psychiatry at McMaster University in Hamilton. He was a founder of the Canadian College of Neuropsychopharmacologists and also editor of the Canadian Journal of Psychiatry from 1977 to 1995. Currently he is applying psychopharmacological knowledge on medical and surgical wards of St. Michael's Hospital in Toronto, while practising consultation-liaison psychiatry.

Kingstone was elected a fellow of the CINP in 1970.

psychopharmacological agents were already available and were widely used; these included chlorpromazine, imipramine, and the MAO-inhibitors, as well as some minor tranquilizers. Only a few years earlier in 1954 Heinz Lehmann had introduced chlorpromazine in North America, and an international conference on imipramine had been convened at the Allan Memorial Institute in 1959.

With regard to lithium, I recall, during ward rounds one day in the latter part of 1959, the team was discussing the treatment of patients in one of the wards at the institute. Ward rounds then consisted of the same routine, by and large, as they do today: that is to say, a group of doctors, nurses, and other staff sat in an office surrounded by charts and went over the reports of the various staff interactions with a particular patient. During these rounds the service chief, who was Cameron himself, and I as the senior resident would make suggestions that sent one of us residents scurrying off to the literature, which usually opened up a completely new area of endeavour about a particular problem. The day in question was no exception; during what seemed to be the usual discussion about the treatment and progress of a patient suffering from a manic disorder, Cameron turned to me and suggested that we try lithium. He casually mentioned a reference to the drug in the *Journal of Mental Science* (now called the *British Journal of Psychiatry*). At first this suggestion seemed likely to be another wild idea, though one that might improve our knowledge and capabilities. But given an entrée into the literature on the subject and a commission to investigate the usefulness of the drug, I soon discovered the other sources of information that existed at that time.

It also became evident that there was a considerable literature about the toxic effects of lithium, particularly when used in the relative absence of sodium, as had occurred in the past when lithium salts were tried out as a substitute for sodium in low-salt diets in the treatment of hypertensive and other cardiovascular conditions. Despite the clarity in the literature that lithium toxicity and poisoning took place only when it was administered in large doses or in the relative absence of sodium, considerable apprehension existed about the use of this ion.

Perhaps something should also be said about the research climate with regard to new drugs at that time. This was the era before the thalidomide tragedies, and each investigator acted as his or her own "ethics committee." Since there was no manufacturer distributing lithium carbonate for use in any specific condition, we had to appeal to the hospital's pharmacy to obtain and put up the medication in usable form. As it turned out, this was not a difficult thing to do since a biological grade of lithium carbonate was all that was needed, and it was readily available. The pharmacy arranged with a small pharmaceutical manufacturer to provide the medication. As I remember, because of the small cost involved, the pharmacy was able to obtain it without charge. The biochemistry technicians at the institute quickly set up a method for detecting lithium in the blood, and we were able to proceed.

Initially, we felt considerable apprehension about our venture into the unknown, but within a few months some seventeen cases had been treated, with those admitted to the study at the beginning maintained on lithium until the end, which was about three or four months later. Treatment proceeded relatively smoothly. Despite the fact that in some cases fairly high doses were used, no untoward incidents occurred. The literature on toxicity at that time was particularly full and useful. The concept of adjusting doses on the basis of clinical effects stood us in good stead and prevented any unfortunate occurrences.

At some point it was decided to terminate the project, even though new patients continued to be treated with lithium. The results indicated that the majority of cases recovered or improved from their attacks of mania as a result of treatment with the drug. The results were written up with the inclusion of some case histories to represent the variety of situations we had seen: a case that responded, one that did not respond, and another whose response was somewhat ambiguous. All this material was sent off to the *American Journal of Psychiatry,* whose editor at that time resided in Toronto. In short order, a letter came back stating, if I remember correctly, that the data and contents of the article would not be of interest to readers of the journal. This response was difficult to understand, especially since we believed that this would be the first publication on the use of lithium in mania in North America.

It was decided to submit the article to another journal that had just come on the scene, *Comprehensive Psychiatry,* of which Cameron was an editor. He suggested that the cases reported should be our most successful ones, not any failures. His view was that the readership would understand that the worse cases were probably not being reported. The article was accepted by this journal (3), and it was the first publication on lithium use in Canada. I was suitably gratified, and at the end of that academic year I went on a fellowship to the Maudsley Hospital in London, England, where I discovered that lithium carbonate was not used or even considered.

After my return to Canada, some attempts were made by other institutions in the Montreal area to investigate the possible use of lithium. However, for many years concern about its toxic effects, particularly fears about its nephro-toxicity, caused many people to be extremely cautious. Nevertheless, as time went on, further evidence was garnered about its value as a prophylactic agent in the treatment of recurrent mania and its possible use in preventing the depressive phase as well, which created an interest in this drug that has of course continued until this day.

After I joined the staff of the Allan Memorial Institute and the Department of Psychiatry at McGill, I received a fellowship from the Canadian Pharmaceutical Manufacturers Association that allowed me to become conversant with the issues of drug development and testing. It also permitted me to pursue interest in this burgeoning field at the Allan. My clinical responsibilities were centred on ambulatory care, including day care, outpatient care, and ultimately follow-up care, and we began to set up specialty clinics that provided very fertile ground for further clinical drug testing. Methodological practice was still in its infancy, and most of the emphasis was on obtaining adequate numbers of patients to produce valid statistical results.

We were able to use the specialty clinics for drug testing and I recall that at the time we were testing a newly introduced long-acting injectable formulation of an antipsychotic there was a treatment-refractory patient included in the clinical trial. Not only did the patient benefit, but an improvement in relations with family members was observed. The trial contributed to lowering the emotional tension in the household.

My early and intimate introduction to psychopharmacology cemented its relationship with the clinical, psychological and social aspects of my work. Becoming a biopsychosocial psychiatrist was an easy and logical development, a fact that allowed me to have a rich and rewarding career in psychiatry.

REFERENCES

1. Kingstone, E., and Cameron, D.E. (1992). In T.A. Ban and H. Hippius (eds.), *Psychopharmacology in Perspective.* Berlin: Springer-Verlag.
2. Kingstone, E. (1976). The history and current status of lithium in Canada. In A.Villeneuve (ed.), *Lithium in Psychiatry: A Synopsis.* Québec: Les Presses de l'Université Laval.
3. Kingstone, E. (1960). The lithium treatment of hypomanic and manic states. *Compr. Psychiat.,* 1: 317-320.

FIGHTING THE RECURRENCE OF AFFECTIVE DISORDERS

Paul Grof

If you compare the state of affairs thirty years ago and today you will realize how profoundly psycho-pharmacology has changed during this relatively short period of time, and appreciate how much of what we do today with strong conviction will likely become outdated within three decades.

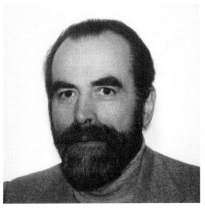

Paul Grof

There have been striking changes in the process of approving new drugs for testing. In the 1960s, in my native country (Czechoslovakia), we could start with the clinical investigation of a potentially psychoactive substance (with the necessary pre-clinical data) about two weeks after its arrival at our clinic. Currently (in Canada) I have been working on a new protocol for well over two years, and we still do not know when – and whether at all – the signatures needed for starting the study will arrive.

During those years in Czechoslovakia we had an outstanding team of researchers to synthesize new psychotropics and pharmacologists to perform efficiently, without delay, the necessary preclinical screening and safety evaluations with the new drugs. A review of this information by a few preclinical and clinical experts – roughly a half day session at the Ministry of Health – was all that was needed to proceed further. Then, in the "old tradition" of the great Bohemian scientist, J.E. Purkyne (1787-1869), we might have popped a couple of capsules into our mouths to get a feel about tolerability, and if everything was fine, we received the green light to go ahead with the drug. Subsequently, in a couple of weeks, after a verbal explanation from the investigator and verbal consent from patients, the first cases were enrolled in the clinical trial at the psychopharmacology research unit of the Psychiatric Research Institute in Bohnice, near Prague; and after the administration of the substance to thirty to forty patients for a few weeks, the first pilot (open) study was completed with the new drug. One might argue that the kind of approach I just described contributed to the thalidomide tragedy. Considering the current situation, however, when it takes over ten years and easily $300 million to bring a new drug to the market, one can't help wondering if there should be a more rational "middle way" between the two extremes.

Paul Grof is a psychopharmacologist and a clinical and research psychiatrist trained in Czechoslovakia. He has practised in Germany, the United States and Canada. Currently he is Professor of Psychiatry at the University of Ottawa. He has published two books and over 250 articles.

Grof was elected a fellow of the CINP in 1968.

For those who entered psychiatry after the 1970s, it is hard to believe that in the early 1960s virtually all mood disorders were treated with medication just for the duration of the episode, without any consideration of the recurrent nature of depressive illness. The psychoanalysts employed the only continous, long-term treatment approach to depression and manic-depressive disorder. In the early 1960s, thanks primarily to Julius Axelrod, an early version of the norepinephrine (NE) hypothesis emerged, stimulating new hopes. It had a strong impact on us in Prague since, at that time, we still believed whatever was published in the English, or more precisely in the American literature. For me, the association of depression with NE deficiency implied that keeping a patient on a maintenance dose of the medication that would elevate his brain NE levels, as the tricyclic antidepressants do, should prevent the recurrence of depressive episodes. Given that until then the dominant theories of depression were psychological or social, and the course of affective disorders was considered to be capricious and unpredictable, that idea of mine was considered to be heretical.

I feel that I should mention here that I became a psychopharmacologist against my best intentions. It was Freud, thanks to his "wonderful" performance as a novelist, who attracted me to a career in psychiatry very early. The fact that his birthplace and mine were just a few kilometres apart also possibly helped. His books were prohibited in Communist Czechoslovakia, but I happened to have a friend whose cousin worked in the university library. There, in the same place where in medieval times the Jesuits had locked away heretical writings, Freud's volumes dwelled in peace – except on weekends, when they travelled to our apartment, to be returned before Monday morning. Inspired by my readings, I obtained clandestine psychoanalytic training in the 1950s and, while still a medical student, began studying child psychiatry. It seemed to me at that time that the source of all emotional trouble must lie in childhood. Today my views are somewhat broader.

I thought that it was necessary to provide you with this account in order to make it possible to understand why I was hired to help develop research in child psychiatry in 1960 at the Psychiatric Research Institute, which had just opened. My appointment in child psychiatry, however, did not last long. As I understand it, my boss gave his support to the "wrong Communist" as director of the Institute, and my unit was disbanded. I was given a choice between working far away in the countryside or at the front line with a fellowship in psychopharmacology. The latter choice had important personal ramifications, and I selected that option. My stipend was about half what the nurses were paid.

By that time I had already had some involvement with psychotropic drugs by using them as a clinician (since 1959) and by participating in some of the early clinical trials with antidepressants and antipsychotics in Czechoslovakia. I had the opportunity of working with Professor Milos Vojtechovsky, who was involved at the time in developing a pharmacological model for mood disorders by the intravenous administration of psychostimulants. We tried to augment the therapeutic effect of imipramine by fever treatment, using pyrifer. I was also assisting my brother, Dr. Stan Grof, with modelling acute psychosis by hallucinogens and developing psycholytic therapy with LSD. Given what occurred in subsequent years, it is now probably hard to believe that one could work extensively with LSD for nearly ten years without seeing any evidence of abuse. The explanation simply is that in a totalitarian state it is impossible to operate an underground private laboratory to produce LSD.

During the early 1960s there was a dramatic shift from a psychosocial to a biological orientation in psychiatry in Czechoslovakia. The department became obsessed with double-blind trials. All the psychotropic drugs on the ward were in numbered bottles, with the exception of a few for emergency use. I was learning a great deal about drug trials methodology, but little about individual patients. Further, I was frustrated with not being able to find out for two years or so what I treated my patients with. Fortunately, I succeeded as early as 1962 in setting up an affective disorders clinic where I could treat discharged patients according to their needs without the binds of the double-blind, but with the option of readmitting them to the psychopharmacology department if they relapsed. I suppose that today many people would prefer to use the term "mood disorders" clinic than "affective disorders" clinic. But the term "mood disorders" only became popular during the 1980s. I believe the English term "affective disorders" was a literal translation of "affektive Störungen" in the textbooks of the German psychiatric pioneers.

As the expression "long-term treatment" indicates, it takes a long time to generate the necessary data in such a study that can be meaningfully analyzed. In view of this, it was critical to develop a suitable methodology for completing a long-term study within a reasonable period of time. Inspired by the work of Chassan, I designed a system of interindividual comparison that included periods of active drug, placebo, and no treatment. We completed several investigations with this method between 1966 and 1969 and described it in several papers. We adapted, later on, the method of interindividual comparison to acute treatment as well. In combination with sequential analyses, our method of interindividual comparisons speeded up greatly the evaluation of drug studies to the extent that we were able to complete our studies in less than half of the usual time.

On the basis of findings in our long-term studies we were able to conclude that reduced maintenance doses of tricyclics, such as 75-100 mg of imipramine a day, were effective for continuation treatment, but ineffective in the prevention of recurrences. In bipolar patients, however, the maintenance dose of antidepressants shortened the symptom-free interval. I also made the serendipitous observation that urea provided some prophylactic action against recurrences, but I dropped my work with urea when I came across the concept, more developed by then, of lithium prophylaxis.

When I met Jules Angst and told him about my work, he urged me to get in touch with Mogens Schou. I knew of Schou's research with lithium from the literature, but the negative results of our own systematic work had made me sceptical that any medication could prevent the fateful pace of recurrences. It did not help that he used neologisms like "normothymotics" in the titles of his papers. But Angst knew Schou well, and he insisted that his work was solid. The drive to Denmark was long, and as we arrived in Aarhus very late at night, the clutch in my old car burned out. It was no fun having to call upon a senior colleague whom I had never met for help in the middle of the night. But Schou came immediately and rescued us, as he would so many times in different situations on subsequent occasions. I had come to see him in order to bring to his attention that his findings about prophylactic efficacy of lithium must be wrong. But in the course of our meeting the strength of his data convinced me that his conclusions were valid. I was also impressed by his dedication and knowledge of his patients, by his tremendous grasp of the topic, and by his eloquence and personal charm. I returned to Prague determined that instead of fighting him, I would collaborate with him.

As I had a large number of patients in Prague with recurrent episodes in follow-up, finding suitable candidates for our research was easy. What was difficult was everything else. To measure serum lithium levels, my old friend Petr Zvolsky had to rescue a thirty-year-old flame photometer from the basement of the psychiatric hospital at the university, and patients had to travel all the way across Prague to have their lithium concentrations measured. The director of the institute, Professor Hanzlicek, responded in his characteristic way. A courageous experimenter himself, he had had a couple of tragic experiences with lithium in acutely overactive patients before the necessary precautions became known. It was not in his nature to stop me, but he made it crystal clear that if I ran into any toxicity, I would be dismissed immediately from the Institute. As is often the case with new treatments, the first two years were quite stressful and lithium treatment gave me some sleepless nights. But the prophylactic effects seen in patients, and especially in those I had seen relapse repeatedly over the years, were greatly satisfying. In the next three years, my efforts were directed at polishing the methodology of long-term trials and helping to demonstrate that lithium indeed has remarkable prophylactic efficacy.

Given how difficult it was to convince others of the efficacy and safety of lithium treatment, it was fascinating to see over the years how the attitudes of my colleagues in the profession changed; how something "undesirable" could become the fashion, and how lithium could be used in such indiscriminate fashion , far beyond what was originally intended. Indeed, lithium, which was considered too toxic to be given to a single person, is now used widely and wildly. Long-term treatments given to virtually no one thirty years ago are now prescribed for nearly everyone with recurrent affective disorders, to the point that the natural course of illness is not known anymore. With the use of lithium, the concept affective disorder has dramatically broadened and mood symptoms, rather than comprehensively assessed psychopathology, have become the centre of psychiatric assessment. Having observed these changes, I have a deep appreciation of how many similar cycles psychiatry must have undergone in the past, and how much more in psychiatry we still have to clarify and to learn.

Neurochemical Underpinnings

THE IMPACT OF LABORATORY TECHNOLOGY ON ADVANCES IN NEUROPSYCHOPHARMACOLOGY

Theodore L. Sourkes

Neuropsychopharmacology and biological psychiatry are fields that take advantage of techniques in many different disciplines while transcending the boundaries of those disciplines. The methods of biochemistry play an especially prominent role in these investigations. During the last four decades photometric and chromatographic techniques, in a variety of modes, have undergone developments that now provide very high sensitivities, permitting measurements to be made on minuscule samples of tissue or body fluid. Thus, the increased physical sensitivity provides greater anatomical, even histological, specificity. In what follows I describe how these developments applied in my laboratory.

After coming to the Department of Psychiatry at McGill University, I continued work that I had been carrying on at the Merck Institute of Therapeutic Research in Rahway, New Jersey, research that dealt with means of inhibiting the biological synthesis of the catecholamines. I justified this research

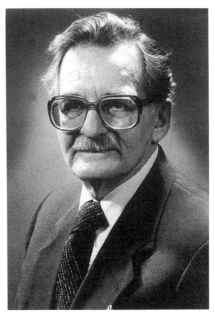

Theodore L. Sourkes

in my new environment on the grounds that the catecholamines, bioactive substances functioning in so many physiological processes, probably served some mental functions as well. I was encouraged in this direction by my chief, Robert A. Cleghorn, the director of the Laboratory of Experimental Therapies at the Allan Memorial Institute. Much of my previous work had dealt with the search for inhibitors of dopa decarboxylase, and out of that came alpha-methyldopa, which within a few years had undergone clinical trials and become the first specific drug for the treatment of essential hypertension.

In Montreal, monoamine oxidase was soon added to the roster of enzymes that my group studied. At the time (in the 1950s), we made use of the Warburg manometric apparatus and

Theodore L. Sourkes is Professor Emeritus in the Department of Psychiatry at McGill University in Montreal. In researching the metabolism and functions of biogenic amines since the early 1950s, he has contributed significantly to the drug treatment of essential hypertension and Parkinson's disease. In recent years he has been writing on the history of neurochemistry and neuropharmacology.

Sourkes was elected a fellow of the CINP in 1976.

the Beckman DU spectrophotometer, then honourable tools of the biochemical trade, although the Warburg has now been relegated to history. Methods with these instruments were applied successfully to the purification of monoamine oxidase and dopa decarboxylase.

As the work progressed, the need to measure the catecholamines became imperative, and we were able to secure an Evelyn fluorometer, then the state-of-the-art instrument for a technique that is intrinsically more sensitive than photometry. My students and postdoctoral fellows established standardized

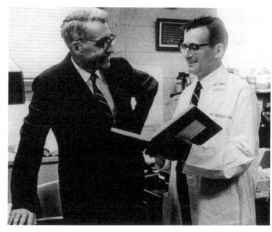

Robert Cleghorn and Theodore L. Sourkes (right)

methods for measuring norepinephrine and epinephrine, and soon we had studies going on catecholamine metabolism in various clinical states. The coloured filters employed in this instrument, though providing band-pass selectivity, restricted measurements to the visible range of excited fluorescence. Within a few years we were able to obtain a spectrophotofluorimeter, the second one in Canada. It had been pioneered in England by Gregorio Weber and in the United States by Robert Bowman, and featured quartz optics and diffraction gratings instead of filters for wave-length selection. These innovations extended the range of fluorometric studies to the ultraviolet region, so that many substances fluorescing below the visible range could be estimated. In fact, it made measurements even in the visible range more specific and provided greater sensitivity than ever before. We witnessed a turning point in the development of psychopharmacological research, as now serotonin and dopamine were measured with facility, and the actions of drugs on a host of monoamines in the brain and other organs could be studied.

As evidence piled up from laboratories in Japan and Sweden in the late 1950s about the high concentrations of dopamine in the basal ganglia, we began to investigate the metabolism of catecholamines in diseases related to those nuclei. The only abnormality we detected was the significantly subnormal excretion of dopamine in Parkinson's disease. This was also true of the excretion of homovanillic acid, the terminal metabolic product of dopamine. Knowing from our animal work that L-dopa reaches the brain and yields much dopamine there, we administered the amino acid to Parkinson's-disease patients and found an amelioration of their condition. This result was matched by the simultaneous trial undertaken independently in Vienna by W. Birkmayer and O. Hornykiewicz. It marked the start of L-dopa treatment for Parkinson's disease and these studies soon became the model for the study of extrapyramidal syndromes generally, as well as other disorders potentially associated with a neurotransmitter deficiency. Dopamine, which had been the Cinderella of the catecholamines, soon became the subject of one symposium after another at neuroscience, neurological, and psychiatric meetings.

We regularly monitored the catecholamines, dopa, their metabolic derivatives, and enzymes acting on them, and in collaboration with L.J. Poirier, a neuroanatomist and experimental neurologist, we were soon able to establish the existence of the hitherto unknown dopaminergic

nigrostriatal tract, a finding that contributed decisively to the physiopathological understanding of Parkinson's disease.

In clinical-chemical studies of Parkinson's and other diseases, we used the cerebrospinal
fluid obtained from patients at the time of neurosurgical operations. The acids stemming from
monoamine metabolism were at first determined quantitatively by a tedious, but sensitive
method of thin-layer chromatography and then by fluorometry. The results matched the brain
studies.

Radioactive techniques with ^{14}C-labelled amino acids and other compounds played an
important role in much of our laboratory research, but an unusual opportunity arose from our
work on the metabolism of tryptophan and its synthetic alpha-methyl analogue. We found that
administration of the latter compound yields alpha-methylserotonin in the brain, with replacement of serotonin itself from that organ. The fact that alpha-methylserotonin is not a substrate
for monoamine oxidase meant that, once formed, it has a long residence there. My colleague
M. Diksic at the Montreal Neurological Institute has been able to develop, by positron labelling
of alpha-methyltryptophan, a method for assessing the rate of synthesis of serotonin in the
brain, and we have demonstrated its physiological validity. The method is being applied now
to studies of depression and other clinical entities. In recent years this work has made much
use of the very sensitive high-performance liquid chromatography (HPLC) technique for
monitoring the concentrations of indolic compounds.

Alpha-methylserotonin appears to have the same type of action as serotonin, so that its
amino acid precursor could prove useful in conditions where a sustained level of neurotransmitter is deemed important therapeutically.

The work described above from our laboratory – concerned with the aromatic amino acids
and their derivatives in metabolism and function – illustrates how methodology and instrumentation have made possible advances in neuropsychopharmacology and biological psychiatry during the last four decades. Ancillary tools have also undergone development. For
example, at one time we used a programmable calculator in our catecholamine work, as a great
labour- and time-saving device. Now computers are built into instruments for programming
and controlling analytical procedures, as in HPLC, and can automatically transform dial
readings directly into desired units of quantity.

We now have a plethora of advanced physicochemical techniques for studies of the nervous
system in vivo and in vitro. Among them are autoradiography, GC/MS (gas chromato-
graphy/mass spectroscopy), magnetic resonance spectroscopy, in vivo microdialysis of the
brain, voltammetry, immunochemical techniques, and the methods of molecular biochemistry.
These techniques find their application in measurement of neurotransmitters and their transporters, evaluation and quantification of receptors and ionic channels, signalling pathways,
and other functions, so that the innermost activities of the neuron are being revealed.

We may well ask: What awaits the neurochemist in the next four decades?

ON THE EVE OF THE NEUROTRANSMITTER ERA IN BIOLOGICAL PSYCHIATRY

Alfred Pletscher

In the mid-1950s, at the beginning of the developments described in this paper, only three biogenic amines – acetylcholine, noradrenaline, and
5-hydroxytryptamine (5-HT, serotonin) – were
known to occur in the brain, and monoamine receptors existed only as hypothetical constructs. Although the role of biogenic amines in brain function, including their involvement in the action of
neuropsychotropic drugs, was virtually unknown,
there was already a considerable amount of information about the biosynthesis and metabolism of
these substances. At the National Heart Institute of
the National Institutes of Health (NIH) in Bethesda,
Maryland, alone there were two research groups,
one led by J. Axelrod and the other by S. Udenfriend, carrying out pioneering biochemical work
on biogenic amines, i.e., catecholamines and 5-HT.
In addition, Bernard B. Brodie (then head of the laboratory of biochemical pharmacology at

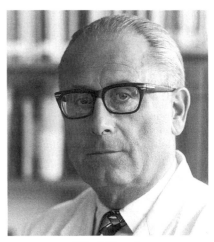

Alfred Pletscher

Alfred Pletscher was born in Switzerland in 1917 and holds both an MD and a PhD in chemistry. After
eight years of clinical training, he was a member of the research department of F. Hoffmann La Roche
Inc. between 1955 and 1978. He spent the greatest part of 1955 as a visiting scientist at the National Heart
Institute in Bethesda, Maryland (USA), and he acted as research director of Hoffmann-La Roche in
Nutley, New Jersey (USA), in 1957, and in Basle (Switzerland), from 1967 to 1978. As well, Pletscher
has been professor of psychophysiology at the University of Basle, chairman of the department of research
of the university clinics, and president of the Council of the Swiss National Science Foundation and the
Swiss Academy of Medical Sciences.

Pletscher was elected a fellow of CINP in 1958. He presented papers on "Biogenic Amines," on
"Pharmacologic and biochemical basis of some somatic side effects of psychotropic drugs," on "Diffe-
rences between neuroleptics and tranquilizers regarding metabolism and biochmical effects" (Pletscher,
de Prada and Foglar), on "Mechanism of action of neuroleptics" (Pletscher and de Prada), and on
"Alterations of cerebral monoamines by aromatic amino acids and effect of decarboxylase inhibitors"
(Pletscher and Bartholini) at the 4th, 5th and 7th Congresses respectively. He coauthored a paper on
"Metabolism of C14-L-3,4-dihydroxyphenylalanine after inhibition of extracerebral decaboxylase in rats
and man" (Bartholini, Pletscher, and Tissot), at the 6th Congress. He gave Moderator's report on Working
Group 1 (Experimental and clinical biochemistry) at the 4th Congress, and was a formal discussant
(Pletscher, Steiner and Voelkel) in the Third Symposium (Comparison of abnormal behavioural states
of animals and man) at the 1st Congress.

the NIH) and his associates had just presented their interesting pharmacological findings with 5-HT. These led our group later on to formulate the hypothesis that reserpine might exert its action by the liberation of endogenous 5-HT.

I joined Brodie's laboratory in early March 1955 as a visiting scientist from F. Hoffmann-La Roche of Switzerland, a pharmaceutical firm that had just hired me. I felt fortunate that I could work in a laboratory with the leading experts in transmitter research of the time and learn directly from Drs. Brodie and Parkhurst A. Shore about their findings:

- that reserpine and 5-HT potentiated the action of hypnotics,
- that there was an antagonism not only between 5-HT-,

Parkhurst A. Shore

but also between reserpine-induced potentiation of hypnotics and lysergic acid diethylamide (LSD, a 5-HT-antagonist), and
- that reserpine administration produced an enhancement of the urinary excretion of 5-hydroxyindolacetic acid (a major metabolite of 5-HT) in dogs.

Reserpine, an alkaloid of the *Rauwolfia serpentina* plant which was used in Indian folk medicine as a tranquilizing agent, had just been isolated, synthesized, and pharmacologically characterized by researchers at CIBA S.A. in those days. Clinically, the drug had beneficial effects in arterial hypertension, and initially it showed promise for psychiatry as one of the first neuroleptics in the treatment of schizophrenia.

RESERPINE AFFECTS BRAIN SEROTONIN

When I started my work in Brodie's group, I was assigned the task of proving that reserpine affected endogenous 5-HT stores in animal tissues. Brodie and Shore's findings with reserpine in dogs indicated that reserpine had an effect on endogenous 5-HT stores, but with the methodology used – which measured the concentration of a 5-HT-metabolite in the urine – they could provide only indirect evidence for reserpine's 5-HT-liberating effect. Therefore, experiments with animal tissues had to be performed. We decided to look first at the gastrointestinal tract, which contains relatively large amounts of 5-HT, and to carry out the experiments on rabbits, a species of animal with particularly high gastrointestinal 5-HT concentrations. A colorimetric method for the detection of 5-HT, which proved to be better than the previously used biological assays, had just become available from Udenfriend's laboratory. However, I had to modify it for use in intestinal tissue because there were interfering substances in the tissue extracts. By employing the modified method, we found to our great delight that reserpine in doses between 0.25 and 5 mg/kg caused a profound, dose-dependent decrease of serotonin (1). Thus, the hypothesis of a 5-HT-releasing action of reserpine was confirmed.

However, it was still uncertain whether reserpine also acted in the same way on brain 5-HT stores as on the 5-HT stores of the gastrointestinal tract, because intestinal 5-HT is in the enterochromaffine cells, i.e., in non-neuronal cells. The colorimetric method I used for measuring 5-HT in the gut was not sensitive enough for this research because in the rabbit, the concentration of 5-HT in the brain is more than an order lower than in the gastrointestinal tract. Fortunately by that time, in a laboratory close to ours, R.L. Bowman, in collaboration with Udenfriend, had constructed a new type of instrument which was to become known as the spectrophotofluorimeter. With this new device, which had a higher sensitivity than the colorimetric method, it became possible to identify specific biological compounds and measure them quantitatively. The spectrophotofluorimeter that was available for us in Bowman's laboratory was an early model, an open prototype that needed careful manipulation to avoid getting electric shocks. (Later on, safe spectrofluorimeters became commercially available). Nevertheless, the device enabled us to design a method for the specific estimation of the small amounts of 5-HT present in the brain (2). Already the first injection of 5 mg/kg reserpine I gave to the rabbits caused a practically complete depletion of 5-HT in the hypothalamus (3), together with marked behavioural sedation. Even more, the reserpine effect on brain 5-HT proved to be dose-dependent. Thus, in 1956 it was demonstrated for the first time directly that a psychotropic drug, reserpine, had an effect on the concentration of a neurotransmitter in the brain. It became a cornerstone of the hypothesis that 5-HT has a role in brain function (4) and that the liberation of 5-HT in the brain is responsible for the psychotropic action of reserpine. The findings that only those Rauwolfia alkaloids that had a sedative action decreased cerebral 5-HT (5) provided further substantiation for the role of serotonin in psychotropic effects.

NEUROBIOLOGICAL EFFECTS OF A MODERN ANTIDEPRESSANT

During my stay at the NIH, while working with reserpine, another drug, developed by F. Hoffmann-La Roche in the course of the company's anti-tuberculosis program, came to our attention. By the time it came to us, the compound, iproniazid (Marsilid), was reported to have psychotropic effects, and there was even some evidence from Nathan S. Kline and his colleagues that it had a beneficial action on depressed mood. But even before iproniazid's psychotropic effects were noted, E.A. Zeller's group had shown that the drug is a specific inhibitor of monoamine oxidase (MAO), one of the main metabolizing enzymes of monoamines such as 5-HT in the brain. Prompted by these findings we decided to perform experiments with iproniazid as well. In the course of this research we found that, after the injection of iproniazid into rabbits (and later in Basel, into mice and rats also), cerebral

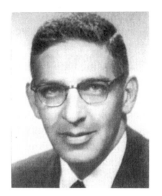

Nathan S. Kline

5-HT content increased, and that pretreatment with the drug not only attenuated the reserpine-induced decrease of 5-HT in the brain, but was associated with behavioural stimulation by reserpine. The attenuation of reserpine-induced changes in brain 5-HT was for me an expected finding, but the associated behavioural changes came as a surprise because iproniazid alone did not produce overt behavioural changes. Reserpine alone caused deep sedation, and the administration of iproniazid after reserpine treatment (when the 5-HT stores were already depleted) did not influence reserpine-induced sedation at all (6, 7, 8). Later on, we encountered similar findings with the combined administration of the monoamine oxidase inhibitor, iproniazid and tetrabenazine. It was on the basis of these observations that we assumed that the reserpine-induced sedation was not due to a decrease of the stored, functionally inactive 5-HT, as previously believed, but rather to the decrease in the availability of free (active) 5-HT, in the synaptic cleft, as a result of the rapid breakdown of released 5-HT; and that the reserpine-induced behavioural stimulation after pre-treatment with iproniazid was due to the excess of free 5-HT at the synaptic cleft resulting from the interference with the breakdown of the reserpine-released neurotransmitter by the monoamine oxidase inhibitor (6, 7, 8).

The experiments with iproniazid and with the iproniazid-reserpine combination also supported the hypothesis that the action of psychotropic drugs is mediated by biogenic amines and that biogenic amines play a role in the functioning of the brain. I remember how interested Kline was when I demonstrated to him, on the occasion of his visit to our laboratory, that the sedative effect of reserpine was "reversed" by pretreatment with iproniazid. As he told me later, this experiment reassured him that his clinical findings regarding the antidepressant effect of iproniazid were on solid ground. The MAO-inhibitors were initially quite successful as antidepressants, but their triumph was of relatively short duration, mainly because of adverse effects (e.g., hypertensive crises resulting from the inhibition of the breakdown of tyramine contained in food). The original MAO-inhibitors have to a great extent been replaced by the tricyclic and other antidepressant drugs, but some of the early inhibitors are still used as antidepressants. Also, in recent years the MAO-inhibitors have seen a certain revival in the treatment of depression, at least outside of the United States, with the discovery of isoforms of MAO (MAO-A and B) and the availability of reversible MAO inhibitors with a relatively specific action on MAO.

A NEW CLASS OF RESERPINE-LIKE COMPOUNDS

Back in Switzerland towards the end of 1955, we started a screening program at F. Hoffmann-La Roche for 5-HT-releasing synthetic compounds, in order to substantiate the "monoamine hypothesis" of psychotropic effects and detect new neuroleptics of the reserpine type. We soon found a class of substances, the benzo(a)quinolizines, which attracted our interest. Some of these drugs, for example tetrabenazine, caused a marked decrease of cerebral 5-HT (also noradrenaline and dopamine) in animals, which could be attenuated by pretreatment with iproniazid. Tetrabenazine also displayed reserpine-like sedation, which was "reversed" by pretreatment with iproniazid (9, 10). Although the benzoquinolizines seemed to be more selective for the brain than reserpine, they had a shorter duration of action with regards to both 5-HT-release and behavioural effects. Nevertheless, our findings with these first groups of synthetic 5-HT-releasing agents reassured us that we were on the right track with our monoamine hypothesis. Today, tetrabenazine is still used occasionally in the treatment of Huntington's chorea, and the radiolabelled compound and some of its derivatives (e.g. dihydrotetrabenazine) serve as specific ligands for the vesicular monoamine transporter, especially VMAT-2.

THE USE OF BLOOD PLATELETS AS PERIPHERAL MARKERS IN PSYCHIATRY

The spectrofluorimetric method of 5-HT determination allowed us to perform experiments with blood platelets, which had been shown to contain 5-HT. In the platelet, as in the brain, reserpine causes a profound, long-lasting depletion of 5-HT (11). Also, repeated administration of iproniazid to humans was found to lead to a marked increase of platelet 5-HT content. The detection of the 5-HT-storage organelles (dense bodies) in platelets of animals (12) and humans (13), and the description of some of their pharmacological properties (14), revealed other similarities between platelets and monoaminergic neurons as well. These and other findings (such as those regarding the 5-HT transporter at the plasma membrane) led psychiatrists to use platelets as peripheral markers of mental disorders. Such investigations seem to be of interest for determining the in vivo activity (e.g., on 5-HT-uptake and MAO-B activity) of neuro-psychotropic drugs in humans. However, regarding the use of platelets as markers of psychiatric disorders, the results have been controversial, and further investigations using accurate, standardized methodology are needed in order to reach definitive conclusions.

FUTURE DEVELOPMENTS

Our results in Brodie's laboratory had an impact on research at F. Hoffmann-La Roche. They contributed to our decision to concentrate our efforts on the new field of neuropsychopharmacology, in which Roche had not been active before. This, in turn, led not only to the discovery of the 5-HT-releasing benzoquinolizines but also to the discovery of the benzodiazepines (15, 16), such as chlordiazepoxide and diazepam, which became important tools for elucidating the role of the GABA-ergic system in the brain. In collaboration with Birkmayer, Vienna, another advance was made in the improvement of levodopa treatment by combining the substance with an extracerebral decarboxylase inhibitor (benserazide). The rationale for this combination was based on the discovery that the decarboxylase inhibitor enhanced the levodopa-induced rise of cerebral dopamine, whereas it decreased the level of dopamine in the extracerebral tissues (17, 18). Levodopa, combined with a decarboxylase inhibitor, such as Roche's Madopar and Sinemet, are still being used as the standards in the drug treatment of Parkinson's disease. Our original 5-HT hypothesis has been further elaborated by many investigators, leading to the monoamine hypothesis of mental disorders and psychotropic drug action. The demonstration that reserpine, benzoquinolizines, and MAO-inhibitors interfere with cerebral neurotransmitters other than 5-HT, e.g., noradrenaline and dopamine, and the elucidation of the action mechanism of reserpine-like compounds (interference with the vesicular monoamine transporters), were essential contributions which opened up progress in the field. The discovery of antidepressants other than the MAOIs (e.g., the tricyclics in the late fifties) which act on brain monoamines by mechanisms different from those of reserpine and MAO-inhibitors (e.g., by interference with the uptake of monoamines at the cytoplasmic membrane), added evidence for the validity of the monoamine hypothesis.

Our knowledge about the significance of monoamines in brain function and drug action has been considerably refined by the discovery of a wealth of monoamine receptors and subtypes, the elucidation of their molecular structure, signalling pathways, and functional role, and so on. In the light of these and other developments, our original 5-HT hypothesis looks quite primitive. Nevertheless, it contributed to the birth of biological psychiatry, which has now been widely accepted, even by many of those psychiatrists who initially had difficulty adopting the new paradigm.

REFERENCES
1. Pletscher, A., Shore, P.A., and Brodie, B.B. (1955). Serotonin release as a possible mechanism of reserpine action. *Science, 122:* 374.
2. Bogdansky, D.F., Pletscher, A., Brodie, B.B., and Udenfriend, S. (1956). Identification and assay of serotonin in brain. *J. Pharmacol. exp. Ther.,* 117: 82-88.
3. Pletscher, A., Shore, P.A., and Brodie, B.B. (1956). Serotonin as a mediator of reserpine action in brain. *J. Pharmacol. Exp. Ther.,* 116: 84-89.
4. Brodie, B.B., Pletscher, A., and Shore, P.A. (1955). Evidence that serotonin has a role in brain function. *Science,* 122: 968.
5. Brodie, B.B., Shore, P.A., and Pletscher, A. (1956). Limitation of serotonin-releasing activity to those Rauwolfia alkaloids possessing tranquilizing action. *Science,* 123, 992-993.
6. Brodie, B.B., Pletscher, A., and Shore, P.A.. (1956). Possible role of serotonin in brain function and in reserpine action. *J. Pharmacol. exp. Ther.,* 116: 9.
7. Pletscher, A. (1956). Wirkung von Isonicotinsäurehydraziden auf den 5-Hydyrdoxytryptamin-stoffwechsel in vivo. *Helv. Physiol. Acta,* 14: C76-C79.
8. Besendorf, H., and Pletscher, A. (1956). Beeinflussung zentraler Wirkungen von Reserpin und 5-Hydroxytryptamin durch Isonicotinsäurehydrazide. *Helv. Physiol. Acta,* 14: 383-390.
9. Pletscher, A. (1957). Release of 5-hydroxytryptamine by benzoquinolizine derivatives with sedative action. *Science,* 126: 507.
10. Pletscher, A., Brossi, A., and Gey, K.F. (1962). Benzoquinolizine derivatives: A new class of monoamine-decreasing drugs with psychotropic action. *Int. Rev. Neurobiol.,* 4: 275-306. New York: Academic Press Inc.
11. Shore, P.A., Pletscher, A., Tomich, E.G., Kuntzman, R., and Brodie, B.B. (1956). Release of blood platelet serotonin by reserpine and lack of effect on bleeding time. *J. Pharmacol. exp. Ther.,* 117: 232-236.
12. Tranzer, J.P., da Prada, M., and Pletscher, A. (1966). Ultrastructural localisation of 5-hydroxytryptamine in blood platelets. *Nature,* 212: 1574-1575.
13. Da Prada, M., Tranzer, J.P., and Pletscher, A. (1972). Storage of 5-hydroxytryptamine in human blood platelets. *Experientia,* 28: 1328-1329.
14. Da Prada, M., and Pletscher A. (1968). Isolated 5-hydroxytryptamine organelles of rabbit blood platelets: Physiological properties and drug-induced changes. *Brit. J. Pharmacol.,* 34: 591-597.
15. Sternbach, L.H., and Reeder, E. (1961). Quinazolines and 1,4-benzodiazepines. II. The rearrangement of 6-chloro-2-chloromethyl-4-phenylquinazoline 3-oxide into 2-amino derivatives of 7-chloro-5-phenyl-3H-1,4-benzodiazepine 4-oxide. *J. org. Chem.,* 26: 1111-1118.
16. Randall, L.O. (1961). Pharmacology of methaminodiazepoxide. *Dis. Nerv. Syst.* 21 (see 2, supp): 7-10.
17. Bartholini, G., Burkard, W.P., Pletscher, A., and Bates, H.M. (1967). Increase of cerebral catecholamines caused by 3,4-dihydroxyphenylanine after inhibition of peripheral decarboxylase. *Nature,* 215: 852-853.
18. Bartholini, G., and Pletscher, A. (1968). Cerebral accumulation and metabolism of C14-dopa after selective inhibition of peripheral decarboxylase. *J. Pharmacol. exp. Ther.,* 161, 14-20.

THE UPTAKE OF NEUROTRANSMITTERS AND PSYCHOACTIVE DRUGS

Julius Axelrod

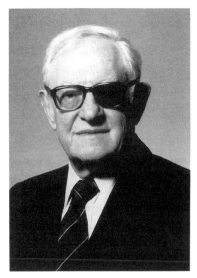

Julius Axelrod

When I joined the National Institute of Mental Health in 1955, I knew very little about neuroscience or mental illness. My impression of neuroscience was that it mainly involved electrophysiology, brain anatomy, and behaviour. But I was aware that a revolution was taking place in psychiatry with the introduction of drugs to treat manic-depressive illness (lithium), schizophrenia (chlorpromazine), depression (tricyclics), and anxiety (diazepam). Before I joined the NIMH, I had described the metabolism of amphetamine and ephedrine while working at the National Heart Institute.

The philosophy of Seymour Kety, then director of the intramural program at NIMH, was to allow investigators to carry out research on any problem that they thought potentially important and solvable. Instead of working on a problem related to mental health, I thought I would work on one with which I was familiar and that would be appropriate to the mission of the NIMH. I first worked on the metabolism and physiological disposition of LSD, which was then a fashionable tool for studying the nature of schizophrenia. I also studied the metabolism of narcotic drugs and proposed a mechanism responsible for the development of tolerance.

In the late 1950s two Canadian psychiatrists, Humphrey Osmond and Abram Hoffer, reported that schizophrenia might be caused by abnormal metabolism of adrenaline to adrenochrome in the body. In searching the literature I was surprised to find that hardly anything was known about the metabolism of adrenaline and its chemical relatives, noradrenaline (NA) and dopamine in the body at that time. I had hoped that a study of the metabolism of adrenaline might give a clue regarding a biological abnormality in schizophrenia.

Julius Axelrod was born in New York City in 1912. He received a PhD at George Washington University in 1955 and soon after was appointed to a research position at the National Institute of Mental Health. He formally retired in 1984, but continues his work as a Guest Researcher.

Axelrod, a Nobel Laureate, is an Honorary Fellow of the CINP. He was elected fellow in 1958. He presented a paper on "The effect of antidepressant drugs on the uptake and metabolism of catecholamines in the brain" at the 5th Congress and delivered a brief contribution to the third plenary session (The present state of neurochemistry) at the 1st Congress.

In the late 1950s, adrenaline was believed to be metabolized and inactivated by deamination by monoamine oxidase (MAO). However, it seemed that after the administration of MAO-inhibitors (MAOI) the physiological actions of administered adrenaline and noradrenaline were rapidly terminated. This indicated that enzymes other than MAO are involved in the metabolism of adrenaline.

A possible alternative route of adrenaline metabolism, I thought, might be via oxidation. I spent many frustrating months searching for the oxidative enzymes of adrenaline without success. Just then Armstrong and co-workers reported that patients with pheochromocytoma – tumours that secreted large amounts of adrenaline and NA – also excreted large quantities of the O-methylated product, 3-methoxy-4-hydroxymandelic acid, referred to as vanilmandelic acid (VMA). This indicated to me that VMA could be formed by the O-methylation and deamination of adrenaline and NA.

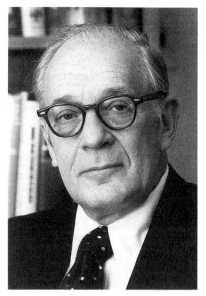

Seymour Kety

The enzymatic O-methylation of the catecholamines, adrenaline, NA, and dopamine was an intriguing possibility that could be experimentally tested by using a methyldonor, such as S-adenosylmethionine. I soon discovered an enzyme, to be named catechol-O-methyltransferase (COMT), that O-methylated catecholamines and other catechols in the presence of a methyl donor. COMT was found to be present in the brain and many other tissues. My colleague, Irv Kopin and I subsequently identified the many metabolic products of the catecholamines in the body, such as metanephrine, normetanephrine, 3-methoxy tyramine, and 3-methoxy-4-hydroxyphenylglycol (MHPG). Thus, catecholamines were metabolized by O-methylation, deamination, glycol formation, and conjugation with glucuronide and sulphate. In view of my research on catecholamine metabolism I felt justified in considering myself a neuroscientist.

The description of the various metabolic products of adrenaline and NA made it possible to test whether there was an abnormal metabolism of adrenaline in patients with schizophrenia. However, when Kety and co-workers compared the metabolic products of adrenaline in patients with the disease, they found no difference from those of normal subjects. Nevertheless, the metabolites of catecholamines, and especially MHPG, have been used as a marker in many studies in psychiatry.

By the 1960s, it became apparent that drugs which relieved depression, schizophrenia, and anxiety interfered with the actions of neurotransmitters such as NA, dopamine, serotonin, and gamma-amino butyric acid (GABA). One important characteristic of a neurotransmitter is that its actions must be rapidly terminated, because otherwise its persistence might cause problems. In the late 1950s, when I began my work on catecholamines, there were only two established neurotransmitters – acetylcholine and NA – and a few putative ones, such as dopamine, serotonin, and GABA. Since the actions of acetylcholine were were found to be ended by the enzyme acetylcholinesterase, I assumed that the actions of NA would be inactivated by the enzymes MAO or COMT. However, when these enzymes were inhibited by specific enzyme blockers and NA was injected into cats, NA's blood-pressure-elevating actions were rapidly abolished. These findings indicated that there were other mechanisms than MAO and COMT for terminating the actions of NA. I thought that a study examining the distribution of injected NA might give me a clue. To do such a study it was necessary to use a tracer ^{3}H NA, of high specific activity. When the labeled NA was injected into cats, it was found to be highly localized after two minutes in tissues rich in sympathetic nerves, such as the heart and the spleen. Little ^{3}H NA was detected in the brain, indicating that it did not cross the blood-brain barrier. An unusual observation was that the ^{3}H NA persisted in tissues long after its blood-pressure-elevating action had ended. This suggested that it was taken up in sympathetic nerves and held there, providing an effective way for terminating the actions of NA.

George Hertting, a visiting scientist then in my laboratory, and I thought of a simple experiment to find out whether NA was taken up in nerves. We removed the superior cervical ganglia of cats unilaterally, a procedure that resulted in the degeneration of sympathetic nerves on one side after a week. When we injected ^{3}H NA, large amounts of the unchanged radioactive catecholamine were found in tissues on the innervated side, but hardly any on the denervated side. This finding indicated that NA was taken up in sympathetic nerves and held there. Such a phenomenon, which we named reuptake, was novel and could serve as a mechanism for inactivating neurotransmitters. Because of the potential importance of reuptake in nerve function, we then carried out other kinds of experiments to confirm our findings. In one of these experiments ^{3}H NA was injected into a dog's skeletal muscle. We found that when the sympathetic nerves to the skeletal muscle were stimulated, there was a marked increase of ^{3}H NA released into the blood stream. A compelling proof of re-uptake was the demonstration by visualized autoradiography that after the injection of labeled NA, the substance was highly localized in sympathetic nerves.

My postdoctoral students later demonstrated that dopamine, serotonin, and GABA were also taken up by nerves. These observations, as well as subsequent findings, established re-uptake as a major mechanism for the inactivation of neurotransmitters. In the early 1990s the transporter molecule responsible for the uptake of several neurotransmitters was cloned and sequenced.

As soon as it was found that catecholamines could be taken up and inactivated by re-uptake into sympathetic nerve terminals, my students and I turned our attention to the effect of drugs on this process. We designed relatively simple experiments for this study, injecting the drug into animals and then measuring the uptake of injected ^{3}H NA in certain tissues. Cocaine was the first drug we examined. It had been previously postulated that cocaine causes supersensitivity to NA by interfering with its inactivation. After we pretreated cats with cocaine, there was a marked reduction of ^{3}H NA in tissues that were innervated by sympathetic nerves after the injection of the radioactive catecholamine. The findings of this experiment indicated that cocaine blocked the reuptake of NA in nerves, and thus allowed larger amounts of the catecholamine to remain in the synaptic cleft and act on the postsynaptic receptors more intensely and for a longer period of time. Using a similar approach, we observed that tricyclic antidepressant drugs, amphetamine, and other sympathomimetic amines also block the uptake of NA.

Most of our initial work on catecholamines was done on the peripheral nervous system because catecholamines could not cross the blood-brain barrier. My postdoctoral student Jacques Glowinski and I circumvented this problem by devising a technique to introduce ^{3}H NA directly into the brain by injection into the lateral ventricle. Subsequent experiments showed that ^{3}H NA can mix with the endogenous catecholamine. As in the peripheral nervous system, ^{3}H NA was found to be metabolized in the brain by O-methylation and deamination.

After labelling brain noradrenergic neurons, Glowinski and I examined the effect of psychoactive drugs on brain NA. We found that only clinically effective tricyclic antidepressants block the re-uptake of ^{3}H NA in nerve terminals. We also discovered that amphetamines blocked the re-uptake, as well as the release, of ^{3}H NA in the brain. The finding that antidepressant drugs blocked the reuptake of neurotransmitters made it possible for pharmaceutical companies to rapidly evaluate the effectiveness of numerous synthetic compounds for their antidepressant activity. A result of this was the introduction of the specific serotonin re-uptake inhibitor fluoxetine (Prozac), as well as many other types of drugs to treat depression.

INITIAL INVESTIGATIONS OF THE CENTRAL METABOLISM OF RADIOACTIVE CATECHOLAMINES

Jacques Glowinski

My interest in neuropharmacology started almost forty years ago when, in 1960, I spent a stimulating year at the Institute of Pharmacology in the Faculty of Pharmacy in Paris, where a few selected young pharmacists received a specialized training in pharmacology. The field of central monoamines was just emerging, and I was asked to write a small review of MAO-inhibitors (MAOIs) and their properties as antidepressants. At that time, I was particularly impressed by three series of observations: first, the articles of M. Vogt, A. Pletscher, and others, who described the effects of drugs such as amphetamine, reserpine, and MAOIs on brain monoamine levels, and who attempted to correlate changes in monoamine levels and the behavioural effects induced by the drugs; second, the study of A. Carlsson and his colleagues from Sweden demonstrating for the first time the occurrence of high dopamine levels in the rat striatum, findings which suggested that dopamine was not only the precursor of noradrenaline in nor-

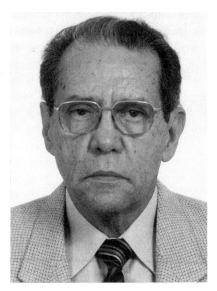

Jacques Glowinski

adrenergic neurons but also a central neurotransmitter; and third, the elegant metabolic studies on the fate of radioactive noradrenaline by J. Axelrod, I. Kopin, and G. Hertting, at the National Institute of Mental Health (NIMH) in Bethesda, Maryland. The NIMH researchers described how injected labelled noradrenaline was taken up into peripheral noradrenergic neurons, then released from nerve terminals under nerve stimulation, and finally inactivated by re-uptake and catabolism through the actions of catechol-O-methyltransferase (COMT) and monoamine oxidase (MAO).

Fascinated by these studies and highly stimulated by Professor D. Albe Fessard, my supervisor at the Faculty of Sciences, I decided to prepare my dissertation in neuropharmacology. D. Albe Fessard and her husband, A. Fessard, were directors of the Marey Institute in

Jacques Glowinski was a postdoctoral fellow under Dr Julius Axelrod from 1963 to 1966. He is presently professor and vice-president of the Collège de France and Directeur of an INSERM Unit (U114) in Paris, France.

Glowinski was elected a fellow of the CINP in 1968. He co-authored a paper on "The effect of antidepressant drugs on the uptake and metabolism of catecholamines in the brain" (Iversen, Axelrod and Glowinski) presented at the 5th Congress.

Paris, the prestigious centre of French neurophysiology where a large number of French and foreign neurobiologists were trained. D. Albe Fessard was particularly interested in the mechanisms of action of anesthetics and suggested that I train in neurochemistry, a new field still poorly developed in our country. After long discussions, I succeeded in convincing her that I should work on central dopamine using a strategy similar to that chosen by Axelrod and his colleagues in their investigations of the peripheral metabolism of noradrenaline. My scientific career, however, began with two serious difficulties. First, radioactive dopamine was not available; second, even if it were, I had to find a procedure through which it could cross the blood-brain barrier.

Working first at the Marey Institute, I developed a stereotaxic method that allowed me to introduce glass cannulae into the lateral ventricles of the rat brain and inject compounds into the CSF. Then, I joined the Laboratory of Radioisotopes at Pasteur Institute directed by G. Milhaud, J.P. Albert, and J.P. Aubert. This laboratory was interested in bacterial sporulation and in calcium metabolism in humans. It was also the only place in France where labelled ^{14}C amino acids were synthesized. Fortunately, our lab was near J. Monod's laboratory, a very attractive place in which several foreign scientists were working during this exciting period of molecular biology. In spite of this remarkable scientific environment, I felt completely isolated, because nobody was interested in dopamine and neurobiology. I was asked several times to work on something more interesting. Nevertheless, with the help and advice of Aubert, an outstanding biochemist, I started to synthesize labelled ^{14}C dopamine from ^{14}C tyrosine. This was achieved by using a mushroom polyphenol oxidase as a first step, and then a dopa-decarboxylase from the rat kidney to obtain ^{14}C dopa and ^{14}C dopamine, as the second. The process was not easy since ^{14}C dopa was contaminated by several compounds, but after a relatively brief period of six months, I was able to obtain 16 µCi of purified ^{14}C dopamine. Everything was in place for the crucial experiments, but then I had to join the army.

I was lucky enough to be asked to join the Navy Laboratory of H. Laborit, a scientist who impressed me by his great enthusiasm and imagination. As is well known, he was responsible for the discovery of the central effects of chlorpromazine. Laborit helped me to return to the Pasteur Institute, where I injected ^{14}C dopamine into the rat brain. After tedious separations by ion-exchange chromatography and bidimensional paper chromatography, the several labelled dopamine metabolites formed through the actions of COMT and MAO (already described in peripheral tissues) could be shown in the brain, indicating that ^{14}C dopamine was rapidly taken up into brain tissue. Several unknown radioactive metabolites were also present, but to be able to proceed further, cold dopamine metabolites, particularly the alcohol derivatives of homovanillic and dihydroxyphenylacetic acids, had to be synthesized. As expected, ^{14}C dopamine metabolism was extensively modified when ani-

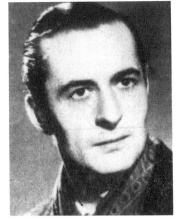

H.-M. Laborit

mals were previously injected with either MAO or COMT inhibitors. Since ^{3}H noradrenaline had just become available, similar studies were then performed with this ^{3}H catecholamine. Although these initial studies on the metabolism of catecholamines in the brain were published in 1962 and 1963 in the *Compte-Rendus de l'Académie des Sciences,* their impact was unfortunately very limited.

In the course of this work, I wrote to Axelrod partly asking him for advice and partly in order to acquire some dopamine and noradrenaline metabolites, which were not easy to find. In the spring of 1963, I received a letter from Julie: he was passing through Paris and wanted to meet me. I remember very well the day of his visit. We went to the flea market and then discussed several topics extensively. I was absolutely delighted. It was quickly decided that I should join his laboratory. Soon after, I obtained a National Institutes of Health (NIH) postdoctoral grant, and two months later my wife, my three-year-old son, and I were in Washington. This was the beginning of a wonderful adventure that changed my life. In mid-1963 Dick Wurtman and Sol Snyder were working with Julie in a section of the prestigious Laboratory of Clinical Sciences. Seymour Kety was the chief of the laboratory, and outstanding scientists such as L. Sokoloff and I. Kopin were acting as section chiefs. Besides Wurtman and Snyder, several young postdoctoral fellows were also there. I particularly remember J. Musacchio, J. Fisher, R. Baldessarini, and M. Reivitch. It was a very pleasant and stimulating group. It was particularly enjoyable to work with Julie, who was always positive about new ideas. A year later, Les Iversen joined us, and he and I immediately started to work together. E. Costa was working with B. Brodie in the same building. There was a noble competition between the two groups. It was an exciting time.

During my thirty-month stay in Washington, I extended the work I had done in Paris, and several questions were resolved in studies I mostly performed with Iversen and Axelrod. I also collaborated with Kopin, Snyder, and Reivitch. As a result of employing several complementary approaches, we were able to demonstrate that labelled, exogenous catecholamines injected into the cerebrospinal fluid (CSF) were rapidly taken up and stored in large amounts in nerve endings. Tricyclic antidepressant drugs were shown to act as inhibitors of noradrenaline uptake into noradrenergic neurons. The blockade of catecholamine storage by reserpine was confirmed, and evidence for a releasing effect of amphetamine obtained. As in peripheral tissues, COMT was shown to play a prominent role in the extracellular inactivation of released catecholamines in the brain. An autoradiographic study indicated that the brain distribution of ^{14}C noradrenaline was closely similar to the distribution of the ascending noradrenergic neurons just described at the time in the first superb histochemical studies by K. Fuxe and A. Dalhström. Turnover studies on ^{3}H dopamine or ^{3}H noradrenaline in different parts of the brain were carried out, and these experiments were rounded out by research on dopamine and noradrenaline synthesis from their labelled precursors. The turnover rates of these amines were found to be similar to those obtained in the first studies performed with alpha-methylpara-tyrosine, the potent inhibitor of catecholamine synthesis. Differences in the rate of noradrenaline turnover between brain structures could be demonstrated, and thanks to the radioactive tracer technique employed, the heterogeneous storage of noradrenaline and dopamine in their respective nerve terminals could be shown. The time spent at the NIH was a very productive scientific period for me. But even more important, I established excellent relationships with a number of other scientists, and we have remained close friends. It was indeed a privilege to have been part of the Axelrod and Kety scientific family.

I very soon benefited from this privilege after my return to Paris. Indeed, thanks to Axelrod and Kety, I obtained an important NIH grant to set up a small laboratory at the Collège de France. My first collaborators were Anne-Marie Thierry and André Chéramy, who are still working with me. In 1966 Ross Baldessarini came to Paris for a few months to write a review with me on the metabolism of central noradrenaline for the *Pharmacological Review.* Soon after, I received a letter from Seymour Kety asking if he could spend a sabbatical year with us. It was like a dream come true; we could not believe it. We all benefited from Seymour's extraordinary personality. Using the tracing techniques developed at the NIH to estimate noradrenaline and dopamine turnover in brain areas, we carried out a series of investigations which indicated that stressful situations, electric shocks, and amphetamine accelerated noradrenaline turnover in the rat brain.

After Kety left, a collaboration with M. Jouvet and J.F. Pujol enabled us to show that central noradrenaline turnover was also markedly enhanced during the rebound of paradoxical sleep induced by prolonged sleep deprivation. Tracing techniques were also used to study the central metabolism of labelled serotonin. At the same time, several approaches were used to demonstrate that, in their respective nerve terminals, newly synthesized noradrenaline and dopamine were located in a functional pool preferentially involved in the release process and that older labelled amines were located in a main storage compartment from which they could be used in emergency situations. In 1971, M.J. Besson, A. Chéramy, P. Feltz and I published our first release study on the cat caudate nucleus, performed by the employment of a cup technique which made it possible to measure the release of ^{3}H dopamine continuously synthesized from ^{3}H tyrosine. This procedure also allowed us to demonstrate directly the effects of amphetamine and neuroleptics on dopamine release. However, it took us several years to apply the push-pull cannula method for measuring simultaneously the release of ^{3}H dopamine from nerve terminals and dendrites of the nigrostriatal dopaminergic neurons, and for demonstrating with Chéramy and A. Nieoullon, the effects of sensory stimuli on these processes. The year 1973 was also important for us because, with Thierry and other colleagues, we discovered the cortical dopaminergic innervation. This was the start of a new scientific adventure which provided further support for the dopamine hypothesis of schizophrenia.

These are some of my personal memories of this early period in modern neuropharmacology, during which several very active groups from different countries made major contributions to our present knowledge. Important new lines of research for the elucidation of the mechanism of action of psychotropic drugs were discovered. Now, like other scientists, I am confronted with the large number of articles that appear in our field every week, and it is difficult for me to believe that, when I started my research, only three publications on central dopamine existed.

NEUROPHARMACOLOGY

Arvid Carlsson

Forty years ago most neuroscientists probably believed that in the brain, in contrast to the peripheral system, the transmission between neurons was predominantly, if not entirely, electrical. It is interesting that, among the pioneers in the area of chemical transmission in the brain, we can actually quote, of all people, Sigmund Freud. In 1930, in a letter to Marie Bonaparte, he wrote: "The hope of the future here lies in organic chemistry or access to it through endocrinology." This comment was made not many years after Otto Loewi's discovery of chemical transmission in 1923. The term "chemical transmission" was probably not much used at that time, but Freud might very well have had that process in mind when he mentioned endocrinology because, after all, it is a related phenomenon. He continued, "This future is still far distant, but one should study analytically every case of psychosis because this knowledge will one day guide the chemical therapy." Here he uses the word "psychosis"; another term that he, of course, frequently employed was "neurosis." In that case, he had a very different story, as is well known. When he said that the future was far distant, he was right in a way, but we must remember that at about the same time, in India, two psychiatrists, Sen and Bose, described the antipsychotic action of *Rauwolfia serpentina*. It would take a couple of decades before Western psychiatrists rediscovered its action (1).

THE FIRST BREAKTHROUGH: BRIDGING THE GAP BETWEEN CLINICAL NEUROPSYCHOPHARMACOLOGY AND BRAIN NEUROCHEMISTRY

I am old enough to have seen a mental hospital before the advent of the modern psychoactive drugs. As a boy, I sneaked into a mental hospital, where on sunny days the patients were put outside in large cages, and one could see and listen to them. It was a shocking experience. Then in 1952 came chlorpromazine, and many schizophrenic patients responded with dramatic improvement in a few days. In fact, the responses tended to be more dramatic than can be seen nowadays in clinical trials, where one is not likely to have as many good responses.

Many people at that time were excited about these new findings, and one of them was Bernard B. Brodie. He was a very interesting personality. An organic chemist by training , he subsequently did pioneer work in the area of drug metabolism. Together with Sidney Uden-

Arvid Carlsson received his PhD in pharmacology from the University of Lund, Sweden, in 1951 and qualified as an MD the same year. After teaching at Lund for several years, he became professor of pharmacology and chairman of the department at the University of Göteborg, Sweden, in 1959. He has been professor emeritus since 1989. His research interests include neuropsychopharmacology, neurotransmitters, schizophrenia, Parkinson's disease, and other neuropsychiatric disorders.

Carlsson is an honorary fellow of the CINP. He was elected a member in 1958. Carlsson presented a paper on "Brain monoamines and psychotropic drugs" at the 2nd Congress and participated in Working Group 1 (Experimental and clinical biochemistry) as a formal discussant at the 4th Congress.

friend and Robert Bowman, he constructed the first spectrophotofluorimeter, which was a tremendous innovation in the 1950s. For the first time one could analyze by chemical methods, not only a number of drugs and their metabolites, but also several important compounds that occur in small amounts in the brain, such as the monoamines and their precursors and metabolites.

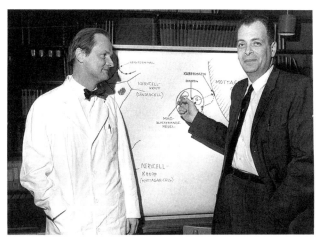

Arvid Carlsson (left) and Sidney Udenfriend

Brodie was not burdened by much knowledge about the brain, but he was a very courageous person. So when he heard about the spectacular improvement in the treatment of schizophrenia, he immediately started to work in that area. In this way, he became one of the great pioneers in psychopharmacology. One can understand that some of the established authorities in brain research witnessed his entrance onto this scene without enthusiasm.

Brodie's great discovery was that treatment of animals with reserpine caused the stores of serotonin to go down almost to zero. I was lucky that in 1955, only a few months after this discovery had been made, I could spend nearly half a year in Brodie's laboratory, where he and his colleague Parkhurst Shore generously introduced me to the new analytical methodology, as well as to the field of psychopharmacology generally. I suggested to them that we also look at how reserpine might act on the catecholamines, since they are closely related to serotonin. Brodie thought that this was not a good idea because he was so sure that serotonin was the really important factor. When I returned home to Lund, I got in touch with an extremely talented histochemist named Nils-Åke Hillarp. He had just made the important discovery that some intracellular organelles in the adrenal medulla store adrenaline. It occurred to me that these were perhaps the kind of organelles in the body that would be sensitive to reserpine. I proposed to Hillarp that we work together along these lines, and he agreed. We quickly found support for these speculations. When reserpine is given, the stores of not only serotonin but also the catecholamines are depleted. (A number of years later, we were able to localize the site of action of reserpine precisely in these intracellular granules, which in the nerve terminals are today usually called synaptic vesicles.)

DISCOVERY OF DOPAMINE IN THE BRAIN AND ITS ROLE IN IMPORTANT CENTRAL NERVOUS FUNCTIONS

We then found that the functional consequence of this depletion of amines was the opposite of what Brodie had predicted. He believed that reserpine caused an increased release of serotonin into receptors. But when we stimulated sympathetic nerves after reserpine treatment, we found that they no longer responded. That discovery led us to the next experiment. If there was a depletion of the amine stores, then we might be able to fill them up again. We therefore treated rabbits with reserpine and then with L-dopa, and they responded dramatically: all the sedation and immobility went away. That was how we stumbled on dopamine. When we analyzed the brains of these animals, we expected to see the norepinephrine stores filled up again because it was norepinephrine that we had found to be depleted in the brain. But the level of norepinephrine was still very low. To save face, we looked for the intermediate between L-dopa and norepinephrine, that is, dopamine, to see whether we could at least explain the action of L-dopa in terms of dopamine being formed. That hypothesis turned out to be true. We also found that dopamine normally occurred in much higher amounts in the brain than could be accounted for by a precursor. Thus we could report for the first time that dopamine occurs normally in the brain, where it seems not simply to play a role as a precursor, but rather as an agonist in its own right. This hypothesis was further supported by dopamine's depletion by reserpine and by the fact that L-dopa can fill up the store of dopamine again and thus reverse the action of reserpine.

Shortly afterwards, together with my students Bertler and Rosengren, I studied the distribution of dopamine in the brain. We then discovered the accumulation of dopamine in the basal ganglia. Since, at that time, reserpine was known to be able to mimic the symptoms of Parkinson's disease, we proposed a role for dopamine in that disorder and in extrapyramidal motor functions. Soon after our proposal, Ehringer and Hornykiewicz discovered, in 1960, that patients with Parkinson's disease have low levels of dopamine in the brain. This was followed one year later by the first successful attempt of Birkmayer and Hornykiewicz to use L-dopa in the treatment of Parkinson's disease. It was several years later, in 1967, that Cotzias and co-workers introduced their L-dopa treatment regime, which led to a breakthrough in the treatment of Parkinson's disease.

ENCOUNTERING DISBELIEF

In the late 1950s we were very excited by our findings, and we felt that we had good evidence that a compound such as dopamine could be an important agonist in the brain. Hillarp and I went to a CIBA Symposium on Adrenergic Mechanisms in London in 1960 (2), where we reported on our results. At this meeting nearly all the leading figures in the area of catecholamines were present. The most prominent was Sir Henry Dale, and around him was an impressive group of pharmacologists and biochemists.

At this time, Sir Henry was eighty-five years-old, but he was still strong and active, and it was interesting to see all his old pupils around him. They treated him much as schoolboys treat their teacher, even though they were themselves in their fifties or sixties. Dale was obviously still a very influential person. In 1936, together with Otto Loewi, he had received the Nobel Prize for his discovery of chemical transmission. Dale and his circle were not impressed by our findings, and he made this comment when we reported on L-dopa: "Is dopa a poison in the normal animal, which has not been treated with reserpine or anything else? It is rather extraordinary that there should be a poisonous amino acid, isn't it?" Following discussion, he concluded that dopa was a poison. Considerable skepticism was also expressed by Marthe Vogt and W.D.M. Paton. J.H. Gaddum finally observed: "The meeting was in a critical mood and no one ventured to speculate on the relation between the catecholamines and the function of the brain." But the paper I had presented had the title, "On the biochemistry and possible function of the catecholamines in the brain," and I had discussed this issue several times during the meeting. So obviously I was nobody!

EVIDENCE FOR A TRANSMITTER ROLE OF MONOAMINES

Hillarp and I were somewhat upset at our reception, but of course we were also stimulated. It was good for us to have this challenge. We decided that we must try to develop a method to demonstrate more directly that these amines were indeed in neurons and that they served the function of neurotransmitters. We tried several different methods, but finally Hillarp started out from an analytical approach that Udenfriend had published, in which formaldehyde was used to convert these amines into strongly fluorescent compounds. At this time Hillarp had joined me when I moved to the University of Göteborg to take over the chair in pharmacology. We had very good equipment and working conditions in the newly-built Department of Pharmacology. Together with Georg Thieme and Bengt Falck, he managed to work out a method by which one could convert the amines into strongly fluorescent compounds by treating tissue specimens with formaldehyde gas and visualizing them in the fluorescence microscope. Thus it became possible to map the pathways of the monoaminergic systems. The first one that we actually described was the nigrostriatal dopaminergic pathway. We could also, for the first time, outline the "synaptology." For example, we could demonstrate that there are two different uptake mechanisms, one located at the cell membrane where imipramine is inhibitory, and the other, as I have mentioned earlier, in the granules or vesicles where reserpine is an inhibitor. We then found a stimulating effect of chlorpromazine and haloperidol on the metabolism and turnover of catecholamines, most strongly for dopamine. On that basis we concluded that these drugs probably act by blocking receptors for dopamine and nor-epinephrine. A number of years later we could locate the amine-releasing action of ampheta-mine at the level of the cell membrane. It was in the early 1960s that we drew these first synaptology maps (3, 4).

There still continues to be considerable development in this field. The different transporters and receptors have been cloned, and the chain of events beyond the receptors is being elucidated.

EARLY NEUROPHARMACOLOGY OF ANTIDEPRESSANT DRUGS

The discovery in 1957 by Loomer, Kline, and their associates of the antidepressant action of the monoamine oxidase inhibitor iproniazid and the almost simultaneous discovery in 1957 by Kuhn of the antidepressant properties of imipramine mark important milestones in the evolution of modern psychopharmacology. While the first discovery had an immediate impact on neuropharmacology, the pharmacologists were at first puzzled by the latter because animal experiments with imipramine did not suggest a particular mechanism for its clinical effect. The first clue came in 1959 from Sigg, who observed a potentiation of sympathetic nerve stimulation and of norepinephrine's action on the nictitating membrane of the cat following imipramine treatment. Another important clue came from the discovery by Burn in 1960 of the uptake and storage of circulating noradrenaline by sympathetic nerves, as well as of the inhibition of this uptake/storage by cocaine and reserpine. The following year Axelrod confirmed Burn's observations, using elegant radioisotope techniques, and he demonstrated the important role of the uptake mechanism for the elimination of circulating catecholamines.

In the same year, 1961, Dengler and colleagues demonstrated the ability of imipramine to block the uptake of norepinephrine by brain slices. Subsequently the dual nature of the uptake/storage mechanism and its blockade by different drugs was elucidated, as described above.

During the 1960s the mechanism of action of imipramine and other tricyclic antidepressants was generally believed to be a blockade of norepinephrine reuptake. However, late in the decade this picture started to change somewhat. In 1968, working with K. Fuxe and U. Ungerstedt, both former students of Hillarp's, I found that imipramine blocked not only the reuptake of norepinephrine but also that of serotonin (5). We then studied a large number of tricyclic antidepressants. Among them, clomipramine had the strongest action on serotonin uptake, more so than did imipramine, which in turn was stronger in its action on serotonin than desipramine. For norepinephrine uptake, the ranking order was the opposite. From there we went on to study some antihistamines and discovered that they could also block the uptake of norepinephrine and serotonin, and that chlorpheniramine and brompheniramine were relatively strong on serotonin.

We then decided to try to develop a compound that was selective for serotonin reuptake. From brompheniramine, not much was needed to arrive at the first selective inhibitor of serotonin reuptake, zimelidine. In this context, I wish to mention Hans Corrodi, a very skilful organic chemist with whom I was working at the time. It was with him and Peder Berntsson, another talented organic chemist, that we synthesized and tested zimelidine and found it to be a selective serotonin uptake inhibitor. This research was carried out in the early 1970s, and the first zimelidine patent was published in 1972. Later, zimelidine was tested clinically, and in several well-controlled clinical studies, it was found to be a powerful antidepressant (6). Unfortunately, in a low frequency – something like 5 out of 10,000 patients – there was a fairly serious neurological side effect with paralysis. Even though this was a reversible phenomenon, the drug company Astra decided to withdraw the compound. Still, it was proven that a selective serotonin uptake inhibitor could indeed have very good antidepressant properties. Fortunately, after that, other drug companies developed similar SSRIs: fluoxetine, citalopram, and so forth.

I was somewhat surprised to read in a brief review in *Life Sciences* in 1995 that Prozac was the first SSRI, since Lilly started to work on the drug in 1972, shortly after the publication of the zimelidine patent. I recently managed to persuade Dr. David Wong at Lilly to co-author a correction in the same journal, in which it is clearly stated that zimelidine was the first selective serotonin reuptake inhibitor (7).

REFERENCES
1. Carlsson, A. (1988). Reflexions on the history of psychopharmacology. In D.E. Casey and A.V. Christensen (eds.), *Psychopharmacology: Current Trends* (pp.3-11). Berlin: Springer.
2. Vane, J.R., Wolstenholme, G.E.W.. and M. O'Connor (eds.). (1960). *Ciba Foundation Symposium On Adrenergic Mechanisms*. London: J. A. Churchill Ltd.
3. Carlsson, A. (1987). Perspectives on the discovery of central monoaminergic neurotransmission. *Ann. Rev. Neurol.*, 10: 19-40.
4. Dahlstrom, A., and Wong, D.T. (1986). Making visible the invisible (recollections of the first experiences with histochemical fluorescence method for visualization for tissue monoamines). In M.J. Parnham and J. Bruinvels (eds.) *Discoveries in Pharmacology*, vol. 3. Pharmacological Methods, Receptors & Chemotherapy (pp. 97-128). Amsterdam: Elsevier.
5. Carlsson, A., Fuxe, K., and Ungerstedt, U. (1968). The effect of imipramine on central 5-hydroxytryptamine neurons. *J. Pharm. Pharmacol.* 20:150-151.
6. Hope, K., and Attley, J. (eds.) (1982) Zimelidine (Zelmid). The First Antidepressant to Specifically Block 5-HT Re-Uptake. *Brit. J. Clin. Practice,* Symposium suppl., 19:1-125.
7. Carlsson, A., and Wong, D.T. (1997). A note on the discovery of selective serotonin reuptake inhibitors. *Life Sci.* 61, 1203.

Pharmacological Profile

BEHAVIOURAL PHARMACOLOGY

Pierre Simon

When my phone rang and I heard the sympathetic voice of Tom Ban asking me to write some pages about the behavioural pharmacology of psychotropic drugs in the 1960s, my first thought was that I was not the right man. After some discussion, it appeared that the reason for the choice was that the main actors were dead and my only advantage was that I was living...

The sixties! A wonderful time for a young chap interested in both psychiatry and pharmacology! After becoming a pharmacist and a medical doctor, I had a great opportunity to work with one of the leading pharmacologists of those times, Jacques-Robert Boissier. Following the discovery of the pharmacological properties of chlorpromazine by Suzanne Courvoisier, Louis Julou, and their co-workers – and of the therapeutic effects of the substance by Henri Laborit, Jean Delay, and Pierre Deniker – Boissier decided to create a specialist team in his laboratory in psychopharmacology. I had the honour and the responsibility of organizing this small team. At that time we were working at the Institut de Pharmacologie, part of the Faculté de Médecine de Paris.

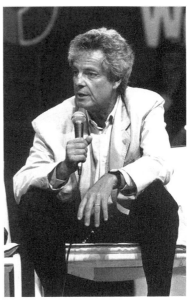

Pierre Simon

I vividly remember our first attempts in this field, carefully reading the scanty literature and especially dissecting the original paper of the Rhône-Poulenc team in the *Archives Internationales de Pharmacodynamie*. The tests that allowed for the discovery of chlorpromazine would certainly seem obsolete to young psychopharmacologists today! Our main goal was to

Pierre Simon was born in Caen, France, in 1934. He trained as a pharmacist and a medical doctor. From 1965 to 1985 he was professor of pharmacology at the Faculté de Médecine de Paris and head of the department of clinical pharmacology of the Hôpital Pitié-Salpêtrière. Then until his retirement in 1995, he was director of research and development for the pharmaceutical company SANOFI.

Simon was elected fellow of the CINP in 1966. He served as councillor on the 11th, 14th, and 15th Executives. He presented a paper on "Critères de sélection des antidépresseurs" (Simon et Lwoff) at the 6th Congress and coauthored papers on "Apport de la pharmacologie à la connaissance du mécanisme d'action des neuroleptiques" (Boissier et Simon), on "Etude pharmacologique prévisionnelle de deux neuroleptiques appartenant à une série chimique nouvelle" (Boissier et Simon), on "Activités psycholeptiques et psychoanaleptiques d'un dérivé du benzocycloheptathiophène (IB 503)" (Boissier, Simon et Breteau), and on "Histamine et cerveau: approches biochimiques et pharmacologiques" (Boissier, Tillement et Simon) at the 5th, 6th, and 7th Congresses respectively.

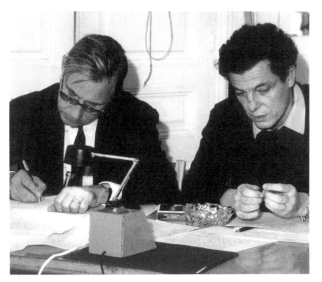

Jacques Boissier and Pierre Simon (right)

devise and validate new methods that would be more sensitive and specific in order to characterize first the psychotropic effects of chlorpromazine and its congeners, then the butyrophenone derivatives developed by Paul Janssen.

At the end of the fifties or early sixties, imipramine and iproniazid, representatives of a completely new class of psychotropic drugs – the antidepressants – appeared. Here again, the initial pharmacological studies were rather poor and non-discriminating, so much so that imipramine was proposed as a less-sedating substitute for chlorpromazine! During the same decade meprobamate and chlordiazepoxide appeared. They belonged to the new class of minor tranquilizers (the neuroleptics, like chlorpromazine, were then called major tranquilizers in the English-speaking world), now called anxiolytics. Of course, we also had amphetamine and its derivatives, caffeine (the subject of my medical thesis), barbiturates, and a few pharmaceutical plants.

To screen for new substances, it was necessary to profile the different pharmacological classes and invent new methods with the capability of detecting their differential characteristics. It was clear that one test would not suffice and that a battery of tests was needed – including the observation of the behaviour of animals, modification of conditioned reflexes, and antagonism or potentiation of "pharmacological reagents" – in order to do what we pompously called "previsional psychopharmacology."

In assessing the different kinds of tests, one must keep in mind what was asked from the experimental psychopharmacologists:

- Try to detect original new drugs, that is, substances with a profile different from the already existing ones.
- Propose "me-too drugs," neuroleptics with clear advantages in terms of potency, toxicity, side effects, and duration of action: for example, long-acting neuroleptics, neuroleptics without extrapyramidal side effects (regardless whether such a substance could be called a neuroleptic because induction of extrapyramidal side effects was part of the definition proposed by Delay and Deniker for a neuroleptic); antidepressants with fewer sedative, anticholinergic, and cardiovascular side effects; and antianxiety drugs without sedative effects.
- Help the clinicians find the best therapeutic regimen (which dose and how many times a day), but of course without having the necessary orientation points from pharmacokinetic studies, which were not yet in practical use.

The most important group of tests was based on the observation of animal behaviour. But which animals? Mainly rats and mice, for economic reasons. Of course, everybody dreamed about monkeys ... But quantitative studies with statistical validation were not possible! With preliminary observations, it was relatively easy to detect whether the substance induced sedation with or without catalepsy or motor incapacitation, or stimulation with or without stereotyped behaviour (in order to differentiate psychoanaleptics or amphetamine-like drugs from psychostimulants). We were of course also interested in the effects on aggressive behaviour and on convulsions.

In order to give relatively precise answers to the different questions, we needed quantification allowing dose-effect and time-effect curves and statistical analysis. For quantification of motor activity in rats and mice, many automated apparatuses were described, but as far as the experimental environments were different, it was always difficult to compare results. On the other hand, it was possible to quantify different patterns of behaviour in the rat for example by the open-field test, rearings, exploration, and emotional defecation. We initiated the hole-board test for mice in order to try to differentiate motor activity and curiosity (exploration of the holes in the board). As if it was yesterday, I remember the long afternoons in a very small, dark room without windows, the only place in the laboratory that was sufficiently sound-proof for testing.

All these tests could be performed in normal or anxiogenic conditions, on naive or previously trained animals. And the "repetition of passages" was sometimes used as a simple method for assessing memory. Motor incapacitation was quantified in mice by the rota-rod test, the traction test, or the chimney test. Catalepsy in rats was assessed by the four-rod test, the suspension test, or the ability to cross the homolateral legs.

The second group of tests was based on modifications of conditioned reflexes. American psychopharmacologists, with their background in psychophysiology, were very fond of these tests, but I have never been convinced that they were really useful. In any event, they were too sophisticated for screening and their interpretation was too doubtful to help understand the mechanism of action.

The third group of tests was based on the antagonism or potentiation of the different effects of "pharmacological reagents." The list of these reagents is long: apomorphine, amphetamine, reserpine, tetrabenazine, neuroleptics, oxotremorine, hypnotics, alcohol, convulsants, morphine, and so on.

All these methods allowed the researcher to determine the potency of the effect; to compare the effect by different routes of administration (giving a good idea of the absorption); to describe the kinetics of the effects (with a major advantage over the modern pharmacokinetic approach in that it provides information on the effect of the drug and of its possible active metabolites separarately); to study tolerance after chronic administration; and to detect possible withdrawal effects.

I personally regret that these simple, easy-to-perform and inexpensive tests are less and less used. Nowadays, you can find in the file for a new drug many sophisticated biochemical approaches, elegant neurophysiological methods, and quantitative EEG, usually without any description of the changes in the behaviour of the animals.

During these years I had the opportunity, especially during the CINP congresses, to meet all the people who were involved in the psychopharmacology revolution; and I will always remember the CINP meeting in Paris, organized by Jacques Boissier and our team. Great people, great times. Anyone who looks at the programs of the CINP meetings during the sixties

(Basel 1960, Munich 1962, Birmingham 1964, Washington 1966, Tarragona 1968), will find the names of the leaders in behavioural pharmacology:

L. Alexander, O. Benesova, G. Bignami, J.-R. Boissier, R. W. Brimblecombe, L. Cook, E.F. Domino, G. Everett, G.L. Gatti, C. Giurgea, A. Herz, W.R. Hess, S. Irwin, J. Jacob, E. Jacobsen, P.A.J. Janssen, M.E. Jarvik, C.B. Joyce, D. Joyce, L. Julou, R.T. Kelleher, J. Knoll, V.G. Laties, D. Loew, D.L. Margules, J. Metysova, I. Munkvad, H. Nakajima, C.J.E. Niemegeers, L. Otis, C. Radouco-Thomas, A. Randrup, O.S. Ray, R. Rushton, L. Stein, H. Steinberg, A.P. Silverman, M. Taeschler, D.H. Tedeschi, J. Thuillier, L. Valzelli, Z. Votava. My apologies to those whom I may have forgotten.

I cannot resist finishing this paper with a true story. I was, with much more distinguished scientists than myself, a member of the program committee of one of the CINP meetings. We met in a large European town, and one of the items on the agenda was to select a very distinguished speaker for the inaugural lecture – a Nobel prizewinner or someone like that – and we had difficulty finding the *oiseau rare*. Finally, I suggested the name of Czardash, a great speaker who had just recently emigrated from the east with completely

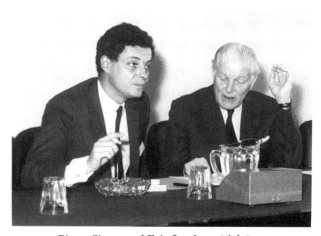

Pierre Simon and Eric Jacobsen (right)

new approaches and views. In fact, it was a pure invention, but no one dared to say that he did not know the man! And at the end of the meeting, I was in charge of trying to convince Czardash to accept the invitation! Moreover, that evening the committee was invited to the home of the local organizer. I was greeted by the host's wife: "Hello, Pierre! Nice to see you again. My husband told me that you know Czardash. Such a charming man! He dined here just two weeks ago ..." Unfortunately, Czardash was not free at the time of the meeting!

NEUROPHARMACOLOGY IN THE 1960s
From My Laboratory

David H. Tedeschi

Our neuropharmacology research program at Lederle Laboratories in the 1960s got started by exploring the possibility of using tryptamine potentiation as a means for measuring antidepressant activity. We had simply taken advantage of the fact that tryptamine was a convulsant and that a non-convulsant dose of it could be turned into a convulsant one by blocking the normal oxidative mechanisms (monoamine oxidase) responsible for its breakdown. As a result of our efforts we had developed a great test for the in vivo detection of monoamine oxidase inhibition.

In 1962 tranylcypromine was introduced as an antidepressant, based principally on its monoamine oxidase inhibitory activity. Subsequently, we had shown that monoamine oxidase inhibitors enhanced the pressor potency of orally-administered tyramine by preventing its oxidation in the gastrointestinal tract. Our findings contributed to the recognition of the need to avoid cheeses with high concentrations of tyramine. At last a really practical application for all our research effort!

In the mid-sixties we developed a test for measuring anxiolytic activity of "mild" tranquilizers (e.g., meprobamate, chlordiazepoxide) by their antagonism of foot-shock-induced aggressive behaviour. We also developed a novel approach for quantifying motor activity by the use of a confinement motor activity test. The confinement resulted in an exaggeration of the stimulant effects of drugs, such as caffeine, and thereby rendered quantifiable that which had previously not been easy to quantify.

An entirely different line of research in our laboratories was based on findings that tryptamine and serotonin share similar receptors in the brain. In the course of this research a fair degreee of correlation was found between the blocking activity of neuroleptics on these receptors and their activity as neuroleptics. Our findings indicated that all serotonin antagonists are neuroleptics, whereas not all neuroleptics are serotonin antagonists.

Finally, we had shown a good correlation between the potency of neuroleptics in causing (a readily reversible) ptosis and their potency as neuroleptics per se. We found that neuroleptics induced ptosis via the activation of branches of the facial nerve by a centrally induced decrease in the activity of the superior cervical sympathetics. We therefore proposed that the antipsychotic activity of neuroleptics was mediated by a selective inhibitory effect on central sympathetic outflow.

David H. Tedeschi received his BSc in Pharmacy at Rutgers University and a PhD in Pharmacology at the University of Utah with Swinyard and Goodman. He started his career in neuropharmacology at Smith Kline and French where he developed trifluoperazine and tranylcypromine and a number of test procedures in his field. He later went to Geigy and subsequently to Lederle as Director of Pharmacology. In 1978 he joined Minnesota Mining and Manufacturing (3M) as Director of Biosciences. He retired in 1996.

Tedeschi was elected fellow of the CINP in 1968. He presented a paper on "Comparative effects of neuroleptics on central and peripheral autonomic outflow," and one on "Criteria for the selection of pharmacological test procedures useful in the evaluation of neuroleptic drugs" at the 5th and 6th Congresses respectively.

BEHAVIOURAL PHARMACOLOGY AND THE RISE OF PSYCHOPHARMACOLOGY

Peter B. Dews

Psychopharmacology is the study of drugs in the clinic for the treatment of psychiatric disorders. As the title of this volume indicates, it originated in the 1950s and 1960s. I have been an observer of the rise of psychopharmacology, but essentially a bystander. My direct knowledge is in the basic science underlying psychopharmacology. This science is behavioural pharmacology, the systematic study of the effects of drugs on the behaviour of more or less intact subjects, from humans to rodents, and even members of other phyla. As a basic science, behavioural pharmacology must deal only with objectively defined phenomena, that is, phenomena that can be seen and confirmed by anyone competent to make the observations or carry out the experiments. Psychopharmacology, in contrast, is not limited to objectively defined phenomena. It can and must use any means that will optimize the efficacy of drugs in treating psychiatric disorders. For example, if the expectations of a patient can be changed to help the therapeutic efficacy of a drug, then psychopharmacology must take account of such factors, even when they are not susceptible to objective assessment.

My involvement with behavioural pharmacology began on my first day as a pharmacologist (as I hoped to be) in the laboratory of W.A. Bain in Leeds in May 1945, though the term "behavioural pharmacology" had not yet been invented at the time. Bain was working with the chemists Bergel (of Roche) and Todd (of Cambridge), with a psychiatrist, Stockings (of Oxfordshire), and with others, on agents with marijuana-like activity: distillates of *cannabis indicus,* a sticky "red oil," semi-synthetic and synthetic n-amyl, and n-hexyl tetrahydrocannabinols (THCs). My job was to make qualitative and quantitative comparisons between the compounds, and bioassays were needed. The principles of bioassay had been developed already by Trevan, Burn, Gaddum, and Schildt, and we were familiar with them from comparing adrenaline with noradrenaline, and measuring histamine, insulin, posterior pituitary extract, and even digitalis. The assays were demanding of skill and time, but yielded results of useful accuracy.

The best assays permitted repeated comparisons in different doses over time with a constant recording in real time: for example, a continuous recording of the arterial blood pressure of a dog or a cat. Dose-response curves could be drawn and relative potencies estimated. Even clues of qualitative differences emerged. A desirable feature of most bioassays is that the effect measured be an important effect of the agent.

Peter B. Dews was born in the United Kingdom in 1922. After attending medical school in Leeds, he moved to the United States in 1948. He subsequently spent two years with the former Wellcome Research Laboratories in Tuckahoe, New York, and three years at the Mayo Clinic. In 1953 he joined the Harvard Medical School, with which he has been associated ever since.

Dews was elected a fellow of the CINP in 1962. He was a formal discussant in the first symposium (Methods and Analysis of Drug-Induced Behaviour in Animals) of the 1st Congress.

When the attempt was made to apply these principles to assays of marijuana-like activity, great difficulties were encountered. Marijuana had exclusively behavioural effects, and I found no relevant behavioural assays in common use that objectively and quantitatively recorded behaviour in real time. There were mazes and runways for rodents, but these were a far cry from objective, continuous, quantitative recording in real time.

There were other difficulties with THCs, so I moved on. In 1949 I made a device that cast a simple light beam onto a photocell device for measuring "spontaneous" activity in mice, which provided objective, continuous, quantitative recordings in real time and permitted the generation of nice dose-effect curves, but it seemed a dead-end approach. Different aspects of the activity could have been separately recorded (and were by others), but it did not promise insightful analysis of the behavioural effects of drugs. The simple device itself has proved useful over the years, but in a limited, non-analytical way. Independently, at the same time, C. Winter was developing a more elaborate system at Merck, and he was also working on a method, derived from David Macht, that proved to be far more important. It was the method adopted by S. Courvoisier and colleagues (1) at Rhône-Poulenc and it led to the epoch-making discovery of chlorpromazine, surely one of the most seminal finds in the whole history of pharmacology. The story of that discovery is well known (2), so it will not be repeated here, except for certain aspects relevant to behavioural pharmacology. Although there had been sporadic attempts to develop behavioural pharmacology as early as the first decade of the twentieth century, I think that the experiments leading to chlorpromazine launched the field as a science.

In 1960 we thought that behavioural pharmacology would quickly provide a coherent scientific base for much of psychopharmacology, but we were unrealistically optimistic. Behavioural pharmacology has made enormous progress and has been crucial in the discovery of many new drugs, but a coherent scientific basis for much of psychopharmacology is still lacking. Our expectations in 1960 were unrealistic in view of the history of medicine's encounter with basic science. An example is cardiology. Much of the basic physiology and pharmacology of the heart was already established early in this century, as a result of about fifty years of previous work, but it was not until after World War II – almost a half-century later – that clinical cardiology became based on scientific physiology and pharmacology (as well as on pathology).

The lead method used in the discovery of chlorpromazine was a test on rats. A rat was placed in a cage with a grid floor that could be electrified and a pole that reached down from the roof of the cage. A buzzer sounded, and then some seconds later the grid was electrified. When the rat jumped onto the pole, the result was escape from the shock. After a number of trials, the rat came to jump onto the pole when the buzzer sounded, before the grid was electrified. When chlorpromazine was given over a dose range, the rat ceased to jump onto the pole while the buzzer was sounding, but did so when the grid was electrified. (This simple description omits many details that had to be observed in order to make the test reliable and predictable, but it suffices for the present purpose.) Thus, chlorpromazine abolished a "conditioned response" – jumping onto the pole when the buzzer sounded – but left more or less intact an "unconditioned response": jumping onto the pole to escape the shock. It attenuated conditioned responses before unconditioned responses. This is a statement of a principle of behavioural pharmacology. Unfortunately, it is nonsense. The "unconditioned response" of a rat to an electric shock, what it does on initial exposure to the shock and for a number of consecutive exposures, is to bite – something, another rat if present, anything – but not to jump onto a pole. That is something that happens to occur in the course of many rapid movements during the shock. The jump is reinforced by immediate escape from the shock and rapidly comes to occur as soon as the shock starts. A conditioned response has been developed. With repetitions, this response – jumping onto the pole – comes to occur on the sounding of the buzzer. (Why does the rat wait for the buzzer? Why not jump onto the pole and stay there? The answer is a "detail" of how to make the experiment work, and it need not be described here.) The point is that chlorpromazine does not differentiate between conditioned and unconditioned responses: it is differentiative between a conditioned response to two stimuli, a buzzer and a shock. Once we realize that the differentiation is between the efficacy of two stimuli, two questions follow: first, what is the difference between the stimuli that leads to the differential effects of chlorpromazine? second, can this difference be generalized to other pairs of stimuli?

What are the differences between buzzer and shock? Surely, the first surmise is that shock may be a more pre-emptive stimulus than a buzzer. In the jargon, the shock exerts "stronger" stimulus control over the response than the buzzer. That brings us to the second question: does chlorpromazine have a similar differential effect on other pairs or series of stimuli, exerting stimulus control of differing strengths? I reported experiments that I believe supported this suggestion – hypothesis, if you will – at the first CINP scientific meeting in Rome in 1958 (3). McKearney (4) showed that simply varying the intensity of a single stimulus – the brightness of a light – could lead to differential effects of a drug even when control performances were unaffected by the different intensities. Do the differential effects of chlorpromazine tell us anything about schizophrenia? Maybe the self-generated "internal stimuli" of hallucinations and delusions exert weaker control than those arising in the physical world, and are then preferentially attenuated by chlorpromazine. Human behavioural pharmacologists (a difficult profession) have still not performed enough analytical experiments for us to know whether the conjecture has substance.

By the mid-1950s, several groups were using methods of so-called operant conditioning to study drug effects on behaviour. The methods were appealing to pharmacologists because they were homologous to methods that had proved helpful in elucidating cardiovascular, respiratory, renal, and other systemic effects of drugs. They provided a visual record of behaviour occurring in real time and also gave objective and quantitative summaries of the behaviour. The ability to make nice measurements does not, of course, guarantee that the results will be interesting. It was quickly found, however, that schedules of reinforcement profoundly influenced the effects of drugs. The delivery of electric shocks could maintain responses quite similar to the delivery of food to deprived subjects, while, of course, there were situations where shock delivery and food delivery had essentially opposite effects. Drug effects played on these varied performances in consistent ways, but not in ways that would have been predicted by conventional psychological precepts. Fear, anxiety, and motivation had no useful role in helping to make sense of the many new findings.

Two developments may have slowed progress in recent years. One is the resurgence of non-scientific, so-called cognitive factors in the discourse. Medieval mysticism can only impair progress in science, behavioural pharmacology included. A second factor may be the intense interest in the study of chemical factors in the brain. In contrast to the cognitive nonsense, the major part of the work on humours, transmitters, and the like is good science, yielding important information. The difficulty for behavioural pharmacology is not the existence of the ongoing work; it is that it has distracted people who would otherwise be worrying about behavioural pharmacology. There seems to be a tacit assumption that the step from a chemical finding to a psychiatric therapy can be made without the intermediate stages of the relevant behavioural pharmacology. On occasion, that may, indeed, be possible, but not on the broad front. Modern advances in cardiological therapy have not come directly from the molecular biology of cardiac and smooth muscle, but have depended on continuing systematic studies in cardiovascular physiology and pharmacology (and in immunology, etc.) that go from chemistry to clinic. I believe that the systematic study of behavioural pharmacology will play an essential role in a better understanding of the pathogenesis and treatment of psychiatric disorders. Little more is understood today of the cause, for example, of schizophrenia, than when I was a student. We must do better: scientific investigation is the only route, and behavioural pharmacology will contribute.

REFERENCES
1. Courvoisier, S., Fournel, J., Ducrot, R., Kolsky, M., and Koetschet, P. (1953). Propriétés pharmacodynamiques du chlorhydrate de chloro-3- (dimethylamino-3'-propyl) -10-phenothiazine (4,560 R.P.). Etude expérimentale d'un nouveau corps utilisée dans l'anesthesia potentialisée et dans l'hibernation artificielle. *Arch. Intern. Pharmacodynamie*, 92: 305-361.
2. Swayzey, J. P. (1974). *Chlorpromazine in Psychiatry.* Cambridge, MA: The MIT Press.
3. Dews, P.B. (1959). Methods and analysis of drug-induced behaviour in animals (Discussion). In P.B. Bradley, P. Deniker, and C. Radouco-Thomas (eds.). *Neuropsychopharmacology. Proceedings of the First International Congress of the Collegium Internationale Neuro-psychopharmacologicum* (pp. 34-37). Amsterdam: Elsevier.
4. McKearney, J.W. (1970). *J. Exp. Anal. Behav.,* 14, 167-175.

ACKNOWLEDGMENT
I thank my colleague Dr. W.H. Morse for his help with this essay, though I of course, take full responsibility for its final contents.

THE CINP AND ANIMAL CONDITIONING RESEARCH IN THE 1960s

Oakley S. Ray

The CINP has become one of my most interesting, enjoyable, and active avocations since I was elected a member in 1970. But my involvement began in the 1960s. I had given several papers based on my personal research at CINP meetings in the early years of my career. I was trained as a clinical psychologist and did a two-year post-doctorate with Larry Stein in Pittsburgh, Pennsylvania, where I learned to conduct animal research (1).

I was interested in the effects of the then-new "tranquilizers" on clinical conditions. One of my early interests was to use animal research to test out possible clinical and side effects of the drugs.

A talk I gave in Washington DC in March 1966 was titled, "Preclinical Approaches to Clinical Psychopharmacology." In that paper I said, "... There are two main ways in which the preclinical behavioural pharmacologist can

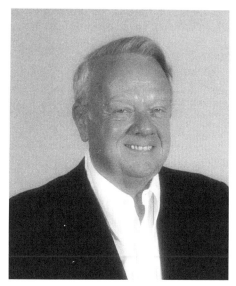

Oakley S. Ray

contribute to the clinical use of drugs: the first is by providing some rational basis to the obtained clinical effects and to the modes of actions of drugs; the second is by predicting clinical effects and clinical side effects without particular reference to the basis for the effects." I went on to say, "The appearance in the clinical literature of clearly differential effects of psychoactive compounds on sub-groupings within the classical diagnostic categories gives new life and new responsibilities to the preclinical worker. It has long been felt that the drugs

Oakley Ray received his PhD in Clinical Psychology from the University of Pittsburgh before spending two years as a postdoctoral student in the laboratory of Larry Stein. Stein's mentorship and friendship provided the momentum for a successful career in animal brain-behaviour drug research. Since 1970 Ray has been at Vanderbilt University where he is professor of psychology and psychiatry and associate professor of pharmacology.

Ray was elected a fellow of the CINP in 1970 and served as Councillor of the 17th, 18th, 19th and 20th Executives. He presented a paper on "Preclinical approaches to clinical psychopharmacology" at the 5th Congress and coauthored a paper on "Effects of electroconvulsive shock and strychnine sulphate on memory consolidation" (Bivens and Ray) at the same Congress.

used in the mental health field do not cure mental illness but in fact only suppress or control symptoms (2)." Someday I would like to update that statement!

In the 1960s and 1970s I attended meetings in Europe as often as I could afford to – we preclinical people did not typically have pharmaceutical company support – because my wife is a language teacher and she liked to use and hear languages other than English. (Even though it is true that "the language of science is English, spoken poorly," I regret that neither my ear nor my tongue ever mastered any language other than American.) My increasing friendships with researchers from around the world have developed in spite of my language shortcomings.

It's difficult today, in the late 1990s, to remember how different the research world was in the 1960s and 1970s. Everyone was grasping at ways of studying the effects of drugs on behaviour. We each came at the problem from our particular background. As a psychologist I tried to understand drug effects on the basis of what psychologists knew about controlling behaviour.

Many of my early papers – the one in Washington and one about five months earlier in Milan (3) –, looked at the relationships between drugs and behaviour in the context of the controlling characteristics of the behaviour. I concluded the Milan paper by saying, in part "... It is evident that the response, schedule, and reinforcement characteristics of a particular behaviour play as important a role in determining the effect of a drug on behaviour as does the dose, method, and time of administration of the drug." Pretty self-evident now, but thirty years ago it seemed to be a major revelation. What it said is that behaviour is not behaviour is not behaviour – any more than a drug is a drug is a drug!

During this period, groups and individuals were still trying to find optimal ways to exchange information. The CINP had not yet become the premier organization for staging congresses – that developed in the late 1980s. It was at a meeting in Liège, Belgium, in the mid 1960s that I first strongly pushed the idea that preclinical workers should spend as much time and effort in understanding and delineating their measures of behaviour as they put into the dose and mode of administration of the drug being studied.

Larry Stein and I had not worked together for about five years, and I still remember his amazement when I framed my presentation (including data) at the Liège Conference in terms of Clark Hall's theory of behaviour: the probability of a response being made was dependent on how many trials the animal had experienced, times the drive level of the animal (measured by deprivation), times the incentive value (magnitude) of the reward used. Those were the years of fun, fellowship, camaraderie, and arguments! Most papers had only one or two names on them – unlike the multi-authored papers of today. That's not good or bad, but it did mean that each of us was much more invested in our data and our ideas since it was our work – not a product of a research conglomerate. It was at the Liège meeting that we had several wild parties – including a famous one given by Paul Janssen and his company, with pink tents!

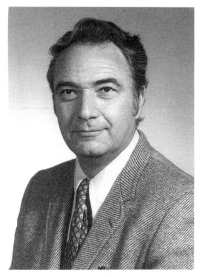

Leonard Cook

One of my main points in these early years was that drugs could be used to differentiate behaviours that seemed similar. The best example was that anxiety (as measured by Len Cook's conditioned avoidance paradigm) was not anxiety (as measured by Joe Brady's conditioned suppression paradigm); was not anxiety (as measured by Irv Gellers' conflict paradigm). Conditioned avoidance could be blocked by most drugs, but conditioned suppression could be blocked only by reserpine, and conflict behaviour could be blocked by meprobamate and other "minor tranquilizers." I was one of the few individuals using all three paradigms in the same laboratory and I summarized my work in the following table in the Liège report (4):

DRUGS	EXPERIMENTAL PROCEDURES		
	AVOIDANCE	SUPPRESSION	CONFLICT
Chlorpromazine	Decreases	No effect	No effect
Reserpine	Decreases	Increases approach responses during shock-paired stimulus	No effect
Meprobamate	Decreases	No effect	Increases shock-paired approach responses

In the late 1960s I expanded my research into learning and memory and also into genetic effects on several classes of behaviour. A change in academic position also moved me into clinical administration. These two changes took me away from the CINP for over a decade and it was the mid-1980s before I returned to active involvement with the organization. That story is told elsewhere.

REFERENCES
1. Stein, L. and Ray, O.S. (1959). Self-regulation of brain-stimulating current intensity in the rat. *Science,* 130: 570-572.
2. Ray, O.S. (1967) Preclinical approaches to clinical psychopharmacology. In H. Brill, J.O. Cole, P. Deniker, H. Hippius, P.B. Bradley.(eds.) *Neuro-psycho-pharmacolgy. Proceedings of the Fifth International Congress of the Collegium Internationale Neuro-Psychopharmacologicum.* (vol. 5. pp. 480-488). Amsterdam: Excerpta Medica Foundation.
3. Ray, O.S. (1966) Behaviour analysis of drug actions. P. Monteganna and F. Piccinini (eds.) *Methods in Drug Evaluation,* Amsterdam: North-Holland Publishing Company.
4 Ray, O.S. (1970) Animal behaviour. (Discussion). *The Neuroleptics.* In D.P. Bobon, PAJ Janssen and J. Bobon (eds.). *The Neuroleptics.* (pp 85-108). Basel: Karger.

Neurophysiological Profile

ELECTROGRAPHY MARKS THE SIXTIES

Richard P. White

In the 1960s electrography rose to prominence as a means of identifying functions of the brain and as an index of drug action. The electroencephalograph (EEG) was used extensively in clinical work and as a research tool. Many researchers were quantifying the stages of sleep with the EEG. I remember visiting the private laboratory of R. Hernandez-Peon in Mexico City in 1965 and being surprised to see chronic sleep experiments performed on iguanas. Hernandez-Peon was an independently wealthy neurologist who did not tolerate the petty politics of academia, but who contributed much to our understanding of cholinergic pathways involved in sleep and emotions.

Philip B. Bradley, a founding member of the CINP, exemplifies the interest in electrography in the 1960s. At that time he and his colleagues, used the EEG records of evoked potentials, involving those from single neurons, to define the effects of putative neurotransmitters and drugs. Many articles appeared that featured titles such as "EEG patterns of cyclazocine," and reports dealing with neuronal responses elicited by microelectrophoresis were common. A shift away from electrography after the sixties is evident when we compare the indices of psychopharmacological compendia of 1968 and 1978 (1, 2). The earlier edition has eight times more entries for the EEG and, overall, six times more entries concerning electrographic data than the 1978 edition.

In 1964 the Nobel laureate John C. Eccles published an excellent text that dealt with changes in the electrical activity of neurons. Today, it would generate little interest among neuroscientists (3). The newer patch-clamp method for studying ion channels has done much to keep electrography alive, but the electrophysiological methods so dominant in the sixties have taken a backseat to newer approaches.

I was introduced to electroencephalography as a student at Kansas by G.N. Loofbourrow, who had studied under Ernest Gellhorn. Gellhorn knew German better than English, and Loofbourrow helped him to write a clinically oriented neurophysiological text on emotions in English (4). Loofbourrow enjoyed teaching medical students about the old methods that C.S. Sherrington had used to study synaptic activity. He emphasized that Sherrington was eighty-five, when he became the oldest recipient of the Nobel Prize (1932). He was enthralled with the 1949 report of Moruzzi and Magoun (5), who followed potentials from peripheral nerves to the cortex and showed that EEG arousal (and consciousness) did not occur unless the

---

Richard P. White was born in Gary, Indiana, in 1925. He received his PhD from the University of Kansas. In 1959 he obtained a Career Development Award from the National Institutes of Health, which fostered his interest in electrographic and behavioural studies. He later also devoted time to cerebrovascular research and served as an editorial board member for *Circulation Research* from 1977 to 1983.

White was elected a fellow of the CINP in 1968. He presented a paper on "Neuropharmacologic comparison of subcortical actions of anticholinergic compounds" (White and Rudolph) at the 5th Congress.

impulses excited neurons scattered throughout the brainstem. It was world-class work that few know of today. Many neurophysiological studies followed to ascertain whether anesthetics and other drugs affected consciousness by inhibiting neurons of the brainstem. When I moved from Kansas to Galesburg, Illinois, to work in the laboratory of Harold E. Himwich, I found that such studies were performed to examine the role that cholinergic neurons played in the EEG mesodiencephalic activating mechanism (6).

I began to work in Himwich's laboratory in 1954. He was among the best-known neuro-scientists of that era and a pioneer investigator. In 1929, with L.H. Nahum, he had reported that the respiratory quotient of the brain was 1.0 (7). While teaching at Cornell in 1928, he introduced the unheard-of subject of neurochemistry to medical students, one of whom, Irvine H. Page, later revealed the presence of serotonin in the brain. Himwich was relatively short in stature but without the proverbial Napoleonic complex. He had the ability to summarize his thoughts with one-liners such as, "Leo Hollister diagnosed mental illness with the precision of an anatomist," "Percival Bailey is my patron saint," "The brain is an acetylcholine factory," "New methods make new science," and "Drugs, not psychiatrists, send patients home." Nathan Kline agreed with this last statement, although other psychiatrists at the time argued that neuroleptics only enabled physicians to gain access to troubled minds. Himwich went to bed promptly at 10:00 p.m. and to work in the morning long before others. His wife, Williamina Armstrong, was an innovative biochemist, and at their home the conversation revolved about neuroscience and scientists. He published a book on brain metabolism and cerebral disorders in 1951, which was updated with the help of others and republished in 1976, the year of his death at age eighty-two. Williamina died in 1993.

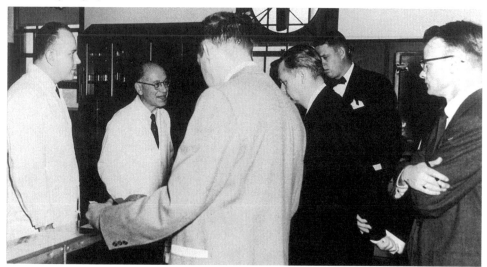

In Himwich's laboratory at Galesburg State Hospital (Illinois, USA): Richard P. White (left) and Harold E. Himwich (right), facing group

The laboratory of the Galesburg State Research Hospital was named Thudichum after the father of neurochemistry, J.L.W. Thudichum, who died in 1903. The hospital was unique for the time in that basic animal and human research was conducted at the same locale. It was truly amazing to see the beneficial effects of chlorpromazine in so many patients. Seminars in clinical and basic research by invited speakers were presented each week, and the hospital soon became a centre of learning in the corn fields of Illinois.

Himwich immediately put me to work to determine which part of the brain seemed responsible for the circling (turning) of animals produced by the injection of the cholinesterase inhibitor and nerve poison di-isopropyl-fluoro-phosphate (DFP) into one carotid artery. We found that microinjections of DFP into one caudate nucleus produced turning in rabbits and localized the site of action by determining cholinesterase activity of different brain regions. Our report was the first to show that stimulation of cholinergic neurons in the caudate nucleus produced movement (8).

It was Morrie Aprison who showed me how to measure cholinesterase activity. He later helped to identify glycine as an inhibitory neurotransmitter (9). In the 1950s acetylcholine was the neurotransmitter considered to be the workhorse of the brain.

Himwich had received funds from the U.S. army to evaluate the EEG and behavioural effects of anticholinergics, e.g., toxic delirium induced by atropine (10). He encouraged independent studies, and I performed one for a former mentor, Fred Samson, which showed that butyric acid was far more potent in producing EEG and behavioural signs of deep sleep than acetone, indicating that diabetic or hepatic coma is likely due to an increase in free fatty acids (11).

Erminio Costa arrived from Italy shortly before I left Galesburg in 1956. He hit the laboratory like a cyclone. One of his fertile experiments, using isolated rat uteri, challenged work of the renowned bioassayer J.H. Gaddum and taught me the value of in vitro experimentation (12). Costa, also a member of the CINP, soon became internationally known. In 1980 he invited me to present a seminar in Washington, DC, where we enjoyed recalling events of twenty-four years earlier. The interest in cholinergic drugs that I gained at Galesburg ultimately brought me into contact with other members of the CINP during the 1960s. These especially included Edward Domino, Albert Hertz, Vincenzo Longo, Louis Sokoloff, Zdenek Votava, and Philip Bradley.

While in Himwich's laboratory I also learned from Franco Rinaldi procedures for using rabbits for EEG studies. The relationship between cholinergic drugs, EEG activation, and evoked potentials occupied my research after I left Galesburg for Memphis. It soon became evident that cholinergic drugs such as physostigmine produced motor and EEG signs of arousal, but did not stimulate behaviour nearly as well as adrenergic drugs such as amphetamine. We found that drugs such as atropine, which do not primarily produce sleep but antagonized physostigmine, were used to treat Parkinsonism or motion sickness. Also, that drugs in the atropine category did not prevent the behavioural effect of amphetamine, but did have an effect on the EEG. On the other hand, drugs such as chlorpromazine would block all EEG and behaviour effects of amphetamine, but not the EEG effects of physostigmine (13, 14).

The best explanation of these findings was advanced by V.G. Longo, who electrostimulated parts of the brainstem and concluded that atropine mainly affected corticopetal activity (EEG arousal), but not centrifugal activity associated with muscle movements (15). Longo came to Memphis in 1965, and everyone enjoyed his visit. He wrote a comprehensive review of cholinergic pharmacology (16) and published an excellent stereotaxic atlas of the rabbit, which we used in our studies. Prior to these studies it was commonly taught that atropine was mainly a stimulant and scopolamine a CNS depressant, and that rabbit blood contained an atropinase.

I had questioned these assumptions while working with Himwich, and our study showed that these anticholinergics had effects that were qualitatively similar and that serum atropinase was unimportant (17).

Interest in cholinergic mechanisms and the brain waned rapidly after the fifth meeting of the CINP, held in Washington in 1966, which focused on anticholinergic drugs (18). In attendance were Himwich, Bradley, Fink, Longo, Votava, and many others. That year Bradley stayed at our house and we made tentative plans for my working in his laboratory in Birmingham, England.

Throughout the sixties I visited many investigators to learn first-hand about new procedures. These contacts also facilitated my comprehension of their reports. Klaus Unna, who discovered opioid antagonists, told me that administrators felt naked unless they were clothed in reports. He trained medical students in neuropharmacology during their summer break, and later I became well acquainted with two of them, Ed Domino and Bill Martin. I have followed Domino's reports so closely that I believe I could identify him by the "paw of the lion" as a reviewer of my manuscripts. I think that he arranged for my participation in a workshop on antidepressant drugs held in Washington on a snowy day in January 1966, which was hosted by Seymour Kety and Daniel Efron at the National Institutes of Health (19).

At that time some researchers thought that cholinergic neurons played a role in depression because imipramine antagonized acetylcholine in the brain (but enhanced actions of norepinephrine). It was also known that the administration of physostigmine made depressed patients worse, but antagonized mania; and that cholinergic activity might also contribute to the negative symptoms of schizophrenia.

In any case, the discussions were lively, especially between Julius Axelrod and his former mentor, Bernard Brodie. Axelrod told us that imipramine, but not chlorpromazine, inhibited the uptake of radioactive norepinephrine given into the lateral ventricle, and he discussed diurnal changes in the pineal gland. In 1970 he was awarded the Nobel Prize, and his work on the pineal gland ultimately led to the current use of melatonin as an aid to sleep.

About that time Max Fink was using cyclazocine to treat opioid addiction. Because he believed the drug had antidepressant effects, he asked me to compare the effects of cyclazocine and imipramine in animals. While I was in New York City, he nonchalantly gave me morphine and heroin in envelopes to take back to Memphis. I could only think of my future if I happened to be arrested, so I insisted that he write a covering letter for me to take on the journey. To my surprise, cyclazocine did produce some of the cardinal effects of imipramine in animals (20).

I visited Albert Herz in Munich in 1961. He expressed his concern that attitudes at the university had not changed since the war. I also spoke with R.J. Ilyutchenok in Stockholm that year through a morose Soviet interpreter. He was amiable and later sent me a signed copy of his text in Russian, published in 1965. He was invited by Zdenek Votava to a symposium in Prague, where his basic work was published in English (21). Votava toured the United States in a used taxi purchased in New York, and in 1967 spent time with us on his way to California. He seemed more American than most of us, having been a boy scout and played cowboys and Indians as a youngster. We had planned to meet in Prague, but the Russian army intervened in 1968.

With a Burroughs Wellcome Travel Scholarship and amino acids in my pocket, I went to England to learn more about neuropharmacology in the laboratory of Philip Bradley. The absence of one of these amino acids, cystathionine, was associated with seizures. I wanted to see if it might cause sedation in intact animals and whether its metabolites also had effects.

Bradley gave Brian Key the task of making the protocols needed for the study. Key used the *encéphale isolé* to establish the doses and basic effects of the amino acids when injected into the lateral ventricle. Later we studied the effects in free-moving animals. Key took care of the needs of visiting investigators and often introduced me as "our foreign visitor of the year" or as "the visitor from the colonies." He seemed to appreciate my efforts and the fact that I wrote the report on our work. Authorship was by alphabetical order, but Key was first-rate in any study. Our results showed that cystathionine induced EEG and behavioural sleep, while its immediate metabolite, cysteine, surprisingly produced marked excitatory effects (22). This was apparently the first report which showed that a simple amino acid could produce effects that resembled those of amphetamine. Recently, cysteine has been implicated in neurodegenerative disease as a neuroexcitant (23).

One study that Key was conducting measured prostaglandins released from the cortex during EEG and behavioural arousal. Prostaglandins were a new subject then, not mentioned in the textbooks, but thanks to this introduction, a fresh avenue of research opened to me. When I returned to the United States in 1969, two neurosurgeons, Francis Murphey and James T. Robertson, asked me to study a clinical phenomenon called cerebral vasospasm, an offer I could not refuse. The effects of prostaglandins on cerebral arteries were unknown then. We therefore began laboratory studies to determine if prostaglandins known to dilate peripheral arteries could be of value as vasodilators in cerebral vasospasm and whether those that constricted might be a cause of the spasm (24). The procedures used initially were new to me, and before publication I invited Louis Sokoloff to speak in Memphis and to evaluate the results (25, 26, 27). Fortunately, he accepted my invitation, even though he had just returned from a year in Moscow. At that time very few academicians were interested in vasospasm.

When I visited England in 1981, Bradley and Key said that they had seriously considered studying the phenomenon and were surprised to learn from the literature that I had been working in the area for a decade. Bradley had become chair of Pharmacology at the medical school by that time, and the cold quarters of the Neuropharmacologic Institute, which Joel Elkes had originally opened, were now closed. But I shall always remember Bradley as the quintessential proponent of electrography in the sixties.

REFEENCES
1. Efron, D.H., Cole, J.O., Levine, J., and Wittenborn, J.R. (eds.) (1968). *Psychopharmacology: A Review of Progress 1957-1967.* Public Health Service no.1836. Washington: U.S. Government Printing Office.
2. Lipton, M.A., Di Mascio, A., and Killam, K.F. (eds.) (1978). *Psychopharmacology: A Generation of Progress.* New York: Raven Press.
3. Eccles, J.C. (1964). *The Physiology of Synapses.* New York: Academic Press.
4. Gellhorn, E., and Loofbourrow, G.M. (1963). *Emotions and Emotional Disorders: A Neurophysiological Study.* New York: Harper and Row.
5. Moruzzi, G., and Magoun, H.W. (1949). Brainstem reticular formation and activation of the EEG. *Electroenceph. Clin. Neurophysiol.,* 1: 455-473.
6. Rinaldi, F., and Himwich, H.E. (1955). Cholinergic mechanism involved in functions of mesodiencephalic activating system. *Arch. Neurol. Psychiat.,* 73: 396-402.
7. Himwich, H.E., and Nahum, L.H. (1929). Respiratory quotient of the brain. *Proc. Soc. Exper. Biol. Med.,* 26: 496-497.
8. Werman, R., Davidoff, R.A., and Aprison, M.H. (1967). Inhibition of motoneurons by iontophoresis of glycine. *Nature,* 214: 681-683.
9. White, R.P., and Himwich, H.E. (1957). Circus movements and excitation of striatal and mesodiencephalic centers in rabbits. *J. Neurophysiol.,* 20: 81-90.
10. White, R.P., Rinaldi, F., and Himwich, H.E. (1956). Central and peripheral nervous effects of atropine sulfate and mepiperphenidol (Darstine) on human subjects. *J. Appl. Physiol.,* 8: 635-642.
11. White, R.P., and Samson Jr, F.E. (1956). Effects of fatty acids on the electroencephalogram of unanesthetized rabbits. *Am. J. Physiol.,* 186: 271-274.
12. Costa, E. (1956). Effects of hallucinogenic and tranquilizing drugs on serotonin-evoked uterine contractions. *Proc. Soc. Exper. Biol. Med.,* 91: 39-41.
13. White, R.P., and Westerbeke, E.J. (1962). Relationship between central anticholinergic actions and antiparkinson efficacy of phenothiazine derivatives. *Int. J. Neuropharmacol.,* 1: 213-216.

14. White, R.P. (1966). Electrographic and behavioral signs of anticholinergic activity. *Recent Adv. Biol. Psychiat.,* 8: 127-139.
15. Longo, V.G. (1956). Effects of scopolamine and atropine on electroencephalographic and behavioral reactions to hypothalamic stimulation. *J. Pharmacol. Exper. Ther.,* 116: 198-208.
16. Longo, V.G. (1966). Behavioral and electroencephalographic effects of atropine and related compounds. *Pharmacol. Rev.,* 18: 965-996.
17. Bradley, P.B., and Fink, M. (eds.) (1968). Anticholinergic drugs. *Progr. Brain Res.,* 28: 1-184.
18. White, R.P., Nash, C.B., Westerbeke, E.J., and Possanza, G.J. (1961). Phylogenetic comparison of central actions produced by different doses of atropine and hyoscine. *Arch. Int. Pharmacodyn.,* 132: 349-363.
19. Efron, D.H., and Kety, S.S. (eds.) (1966). *Antidepressant Drugs of Non-MAO Type.* U.S. Public Health Service, Workshop Series Pharmacol. no.1. Washington, DC.
20. White, R.P., Drew, W.G., and Fink, M. (1969). Neuropharmacological analysis of agonistic actions of cyclazocine in rabbits. *Biol. Psychiat.,* 1: 317-330.
21. Votava, Z., Horvath, M., and Vinar, O. (eds.) (1963). *Psychopharmacological Methods.* Oxford: Pergamon Press.
22. Key, B.J., and White, R.P. (1970). Neuropharmacological comparison of cystathionine, cysteine, homoserine and alpha-ketobutyric acid in cats. *Neuropharmacology,* 9: 349-357.
23. Heafield, M.T., Fearn, S., Steventon, G.B., Wing, R.H., Williams, A.D., and Sturman, S.G. (1990). Plasma cysteine and sulphate levels in patients with motor neurone, Parkinson's and Alzheimer's disease. *Neuroscience Letter,* 110: 216-220.
24. White, R.P. (1990). Responses of isolated cerebral arteries to vasoactive agents. In M. Mayberg (ed.), Cerebral vasospasm, *Neurosurg. Clin. North Am.,* 1: 401-416.
25. White, R.P., Heaton, J.A., and Denton, I.C. (1971). Pharmacological comparison of prostaglandin F_2", serotonin and norepinephrine on cerebrovascular tone of monkey. *European J. Pharmacol.,* 15: 300-309.
26. Denton, I.C., White, R.P., and Robertson, J.T. (1972). The effects of prostaglandins E_1, A_1, and F_2^α on the cerebral circulation of dogs and monkeys. *J. Neurosurg.,* 36: 34-42.
27. Pennink, M., White, R.P., Crockarell, J.R., and Robertson, J.T. (1972). Role of prostaglandin F_2^α in the genesis of experimental cerebral vasospasm: angiographic study in dogs. *J. Neurosurg.,* 37: 398-406.

PHARMACO-ELECTROENCEPHALOGRAPHY
A Debate in Psychopharmacology

Max Fink

A salutary interaction between psychopharmacology and electroencephalography began in 1929 soon after the discovery by Hans Berger of the rhythmic electrical activity of the human brain. His first studies included the effects of psychoactive drugs. The discipline of pharmaco-electroencephalography (pharmaco-EEG) – the study of the effects of drugs on brain functions as recorded in the electroencephalogram – was already established at the time of the first meetings of the CINP in 1958, and was well represented in the initial presentations at that meeting. Scientists focused their interest either on a favoured animal species, on patients with psychiatric illnesses, or on normal volunteers. Each population had its advantages and its limitations for study. Broad

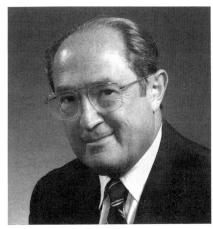

Max Fink

principles were sought as the effects of drugs differed in animal species and in man. Soon a debate developed, whether the findings in animals could explain the clinical and research

Max Fink has been in academic research since 1954 when he developed an interest in quantitative electrophysiology and in electroshock at Hillside Hospital in New York. He developed a theory of the association of EEG and behaviour which is the basis for a classification of psychotropic drugs. He has actively sustained public interest in electroconvulsive therapy by publishing a textbook, developing educational videotapes, editing the journal *Convulsive Therapy,* and organizing educational CME programs. He is professor of psychiatry and neurology at SUNY at Stony Brook and attending psychiatrist at the Long Island Jewish-Hillside Medical Center.

Fink was elected a fellow of the CINP in 1958. He presented on "EEG and behavioural effects of psychopharmacologic agents," on "Comparative studies of chlorpromazine and imipramine. II. Drug discriminating patterns" (Fink, Pollack, Klein, Blumberg, Belmont, Karp, Kramer and Willner), on "Clinical neurophysiology," on "Anticholinergic drugs and brain function in animals and man" (Fink and Bradley), on "Anticholinergic hallucinogens and their interaction with centrally acting drugs" (Fink and Itil), and on "Narcotic antagonists and substitutes of opiate dependence" at the 1st, 3rd, 4th, 5th, and 6th Congresses respectively; and coauthored papers on "Neuropsychological response patterns of some psychotropic drugs" (Pollack, Karp, Krauthamer, Klein and Fink), on "Comparative studies of chlorpromazine and imipramine. III. Psychological performance profiles," on "Treatment of chronic psychotic patients with combined medications" (Itil, Holden, Fink, Shapiro, and Keskinar), and on "High and very high dose of fluphenazine in the treatment of chronic psychoses" at the 2nd, 3rd 5th and 6th Congresses respectively. Fink was also a formal discussant of the 1st symposium (The problem of antagonists to psychotropic drugs) at the 2nd Congress, and presented the moderator's report of the 2nd Working Group (Experimental and Clinical Neurophysiology) at the 4th Congress.

experiences in man. By 1966, students of anticholinergic drugs concluded that electrophysio-logic observations in animals could not predict the action of drugs in man (1). Such a conclusion limited the interest in pharmaco-EEG to those scientists who could study patients or human volunteers. As the cadre of students shrank, interest in pharmaco-EEG shifted from the CINP to other societies, notably the International Pharmaco-EEG Group (IPEG)

PHARMACO-EEG

Hans Berger recorded rhythmic electric oscillations from the scalp of normal subjects and psychiatric patients. The rhythms changed with fluctuations in attention, eye closure and eye opening, mental calculations, and after the administration of drugs. In his third paper, Berger (2) described how the amplitude of alpha rhythms increased several times after the subcuta-neous administration of 30 mg cocaine, at a time when the pupils were dilated, pulse rate increased, and psychic processes enhanced. After 20 mg morphine and 1.0 mg scopolamine in an agitated psychiatric patient, EEG alpha activity decreased and the record desynchronized. With chloroform anesthesia, amplitudes progressively decreased as narcosis deepened, and increased again as narcosis waned. Berger concluded that:

> ... there was mutual correspondence between the changes in the alpha-waves of the EEG and the effects on mental processes; whenever a significant action of the drug upon the latter failed to occur, visible alterations of the alpha-waves of the EEG were also lacking.

He described also other associations between changes in EEG and behaviour. In the behaviour-al excitement which followed injections of scopolamine in patients, EEG beta-wave frequen-cies increased; and when behavioural sedation occurred, as after large doses, the mean frequency of the alpha-waves slowed. After oral coffee and intravenous caffeine, the EEG was desynchronized. In schizophrenic patients, the EEG records were normal before insulin coma, only to show a marked increase in very slow waves during coma. Upon awakening, the subject's records were again normal (3).

Berger's reports of re-cording electrical brain ac-tivity from the intact skull of man were confirmed by Adrian and Matthews (4). Soon an enthusiastic scien-tific community looked to the EEG as a window to the brain (in the same way that researchers today look at PET, SPECT, and MRI imaging). Descriptions of EEG changes with aging, psychological state, and mental performance chan-ges, as well as after psychotropic drug admin-istration and other psychi-

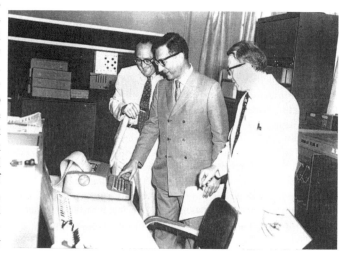

First computer center for EEG analysis at the Missouri Institute of Psychiatry. From left: Max Fink, Charles Shagass, and Turan Itil

atric treatments became commonplace. Some authors, notably Shagass (5), showed that there was a relationship between the mental state and the EEG response to a set dose of intravenous amobarbital.

The discoveries of the antipsychotic activity of reserpine and chlorpromazine encouraged an unparalleled enthusiasm in clinical psychiatry. Discovery of effective anxiolytic and antidepressant substances soon followed. Since EEG facilities were already active in psychiatric research hospitals, the effects of these new drugs on brain functions were explored. The EEG patterns became a basis for classifying psychopharmacologic drugs and predicting their clinical applications, a discipline that is still active today. The theoretical basis for this research, as well as for the major technical developments necessary to use the EEG for classifying psychotropics, i.e., quantitative EEG with statistical analytic methods, were done by Itil, Herrmann, Saletu, Shapiro, Irwin, Sannita, and Bente. The quantitative methodology helped screen for clinically active compounds during their initial studies in humans. Compounds that changed the human EEG were later found to have effective clinical activity. Compounds that failed to elicit changes in the human EEG were clinically inactive.

CINP MEETINGS

The first pharmaco-EEG reports were presented at the CINP meeting in Rome in 1958. Leo Abood, Brian Ackner, Dieter Bente, Turan Itil, Herman Denber, and Max Fink described the EEG changes of hallucinogens (LSD, piperidyl benzilates, psilocybin, megimide) and neuroleptics (chlorpromazine, reserpine). The observations from different laboratories were so similar that the scientists could have exchanged their slides and given the same presentation.

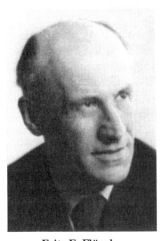
Fritz E. Flügel

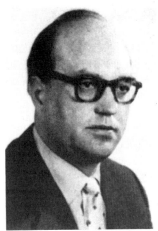
Dieter Bente

The replications showed that the findings had a physiologic basis and were not happenstance.

At the CINP meeting in 1960, antagonists to psychotropic drugs were described. The blocking effects of neuroleptics on mescaline-induced states, and the effects of anticholinergic drugs on electroshock-elicited EEG slowing were described by Denber and by Fink. These reports showed the merits of EEG measures in studying drug interactions.

By the late 1950s, electronic quantification provided detailed numeric measures that became the basis for quantitative pharmaco-EEG. Subsequently, high correlations between the EEG and psychologic test score changes were reported at the 1962 meetings. Reports on the EEG effects of the tricyclic and MAOI antidepressant drugs by Fink, Flugel, Itil, Helmchen, Kunkel, and Nakajima extended the catalog of drug classes identified by EEG. A new emphasis on defining therapy-resistance using EEG criteria also made its appearance. The effects of drugs on averaged evoked potentials, another new methodology to assess the brain's electrical activity, were described by Feldman.

A working group on experimental and clinical neurophysiology was organized by Longo and Fink with participation by Balestrieri, Herz, Hoffmeister, Itil, Kobayashi, Koknel, Monnier, and Shagass at the 1964 CINP meeting. It was at this time that the contrasts in EEG between animals and man in the area of behaviour surfaced. The changes in the animal EEG differed materially from those recorded in the human EEG, so much so that the investigators disagreed on the usefulness of EEG methods in clinical psychopharmacology. Human studies showed a predictable association between the changes induced by drugs and clinical observations, while animal studies failed to find such relationships. These differences became an active conflict in the pharmacologic studies of anticholinergic drugs.

The effects of centrally active anticholinergic drugs are dose-related. At pharmacologic doses of atropine and scopolamine, the animal EEG shows increased amplitudes and slowing of frequencies. At such times, animals are restless and those examined in restraining halters exhibit running movements. Superficially the EEG patterns are similar to those seen in deep sleep (6). The seemingly purposeful movements associated with "sleep-like" EEG records in dogs led Wikler (6, 7) to see an "EEG-behavioural dissociation," and to extend his view to a general theory of the relationship of EEG and behaviour. His strongly-held views were confirmed in other animal species, encouraging a widespread acceptance of the dissociation hypothesis among pharmacologists (8, 9, 10, 11, 12).

On the other hand, studies in man allow greater precision in describing the relations between EEG and behaviour. Low doses, such as 1 to 2 mg atropine, induce tension, irritability, and anxiety. Subjects are aware of changes in perception and mood, and they make repeated errors on cognitive tests. The EEG exhibits an increase in fast frequencies, accompanied by decreases in the mean alpha frequency and in the amplitude of the dominant (alpha) frequencies. These effects are accompanied by an increase in heart rate, salivation, and skin conductance (13, 14).

With higher dosages, such as 10 to 30 mg, or repeated administrations of atropine, human subjects become delirious and restless, exhibit impaired motor, sensory, and cognitive functions, and report illusory sensations, hallucinations, and delusions. Heart rate is increased, with dry mouth and dry skin, decreased urination, and difficulty in near vision. In the EEG, the percent-time slow waves increase, the mean frequency decreases, as do the percent-time and amplitudes of alpha activity. There is an accompanying increase in the EEG fast frequencies, which are seen to be "riding" on the slow waves. Both the EEG and the behavioural effects may be modified by the concurrent administration of other drugs. Thus, atropine (or Ditran) and chlorpromazine elicit a deep stupor (allowing surgery without pain responses), which is accompanied by persistent EEG high voltage slow waves and decreases in fast waves. When Ditran and yohimbine, or Ditran and imipramine, are given together, restlessness increases, with an accompanying increase in the relative amounts of fast waves to slow waves in the EEG. When patients who exhibit a toxic delirium to Ditran or atropine are given tetrahydro-aminoacridin (or THA), the stupor is relieved and both the slow and the fast EEG frequencies decrease.

In animal studies, anticholinergic drug doses are consistently much larger than in human studies. The animals develop a delirium, in which the EEG shows not only the high voltage slowing observed in stages of deep sleep, but also excessive amounts of very fast frequencies. Under these conditions, the animals are restless, exhibit increased motor movements, and their sensorium is clouded. They are able neither to carry out normal commands nor to make their usual responses to sensory cues. Learning behaviour is altered. The EEG is easily distinguished from that of normal sleep. In fact the "dissociation" reported by pharmacologists resulted from the error of limited observations – limiting behaviour to motor functions, and limiting the EEG analyses to visual measures emphasizing the gross character of heightened slow wave activity. The conclusion that the EEG of delirium is equivalent to that of normal sleep is erroneous.

The contrast in observations in animals and man fostered a debate. In man, the researchers saw a direct association between the amount of EEG fast waves and the degree of behavioural restlessness; the amount of EEG slow waves correlated with the severity of stupor and cognitive defects. Human studies of anticholinergic drugs are consistent with an "association" hypothesis formulated in the study of clinically important psychoactive drugs.

The debate was the central issue in the 1966 CINP symposium organized by Bradley and Fink with the proceedings published in the relevant journal (1).

The debate reduced the interest of psychiatrists in electroencephalography. Pharmaceutical companies had set up large laboratories dedicated to animal EEG studies. These studies proved unfruitful and within a decade most of the laboratories were closed. Despite our understanding of the origins of the discrepant observations and the source of the erroneous conclusions, the "dissociation" hypothesis dominated the thinking of electrophysiologists and pharmacologists for decades; indeed, it remains a feature of discussions today and is the basis for the rationalization among neuroscientists that EEG studies have little to offer and should be ignored.

At the 1968 CINP meetings, the effects of drugs on evoked potentials were described by Itil and by Shagass, and the effects on sleep by Itil. EEG methods were extended in reports by Vinar, Matousek, Roubicek, Volavka, Itil, and Ulett.

Reports on electrophysiology became fewer, and interest in subsequent CINP meetings waned. Yet, the technical methodology for pharmaco-EEG progressed rapidly with the introduction of digital computer methods of analysis of the EEG. While the initial methods depended on large computers and were expensive, the introduction of personal computers with the rapid increase in computer processing speed, increase in memory storage, and astonishing decrease in cost made it possible for on-line, real-time quantitative processing of EEG records.

The first quantification of human EEG used a passive frequency-analyzer originally developed by Grey Walter in 1943 and made available in the U.S. by George Ulett. After the development of a digital computer method at M.I.T. in 1960, the method was applied to pharmaco-EEG studies by Fink, Ulett, and Itil at the Missouri Institute of Psychiatry in St. Louis in 1963 and later extended at the New York Medical College in 1967. The computer methodology became increasingly sophisticated and soon real-time analyses were feasible for one and later multiple EEG leads. Present technology is based on two principal algorithms, period analysis and power spectral density analysis. Sophisticated technical equipment for such studies is now widely used. But these observations are now of little interest to psycho-pharmacologists (and the CINP). That is unfortunate because the EEG is a safe, effective, repeatable, and sensitive measure of the brain's activity. It is easily recorded in man, without discomfort or risk. Quantification methods are reliable.

CONCLUSIONS

The scalp-recorded EEG bears a message that is important for understanding the mental behaviour of our patients. Berger's observations of drug effects became the basis for the science of pharmaco-EEG which, with modern techniques of EEG quantification, using multi-lead recording and brain mapping, is a quantitative science with much to contribute to psychopharmacology. The associations between EEG measures and specific aspects of human behaviour warrant further study. Many of the findings and the principal debates were features of early meetings of the CINP.

REFERENCES
1. Bradley, P. and Fink, M. (eds.) (1968). Anticholinergic Drugs and Brain Functions in Animals and Man. *Prog. Brain Res.* 28: 184
2. Berger H. (1931). Über das Elektroenkephalogramm des Menschen. *Arch. Psychiat. Nervenkr.* 94: 16-60.
3. Berger H. (1938). Über das Elektroenkephalogramm des Menschen. *Arch. Psychiat. Nervenkr.* 106: 577-584.
4. Adrian, E.D. and Matthews, B.H.C. (1934). The Berger rhythm. Potential changes from the occipital lobes in man. *Brain* 57: 355-385.
5. Shagass C. (1956). Sedation threshold. A neurophysiological tool for psychosomatic research. *Psychosom. Med.* 18:410-419.
6. Wikler A. (1952) Pharmacologic dissociation of behavior and EEG "sleep patterns" in dogs: Morphine, n-allylnor-morphine and atropine. *Proc Soc exp Biol.* 79:261-264.
7 Wikler A. (1952). Clinical and electroencephalographic studies on the effects of mescaline, n-allylnormorphine and morphine in man. *J Nerv Ment Dis.* 120:157-175.
8. Bradley P and Elkes J. (1957). The effects of some drugs on the electrical activity of the brain. *Brain* 80:77-117.
9. Funderburk, W.H. and Case T.J. (1951). The effect of atropine on cortical potentials. *Electroenceph. Clin Neurophysiol.* 3:213-233.
10. Longo VG. (1966) Mechanisms of the behavioural and electroencephalographic effects of atropinic and related compounds. *Pharmacol Rev.* 17: 965-996.
11. Rinaldi F. and Himwich H.E. (1955) Alerting responses and actions of atropine and cholinergic drugs. *AMA Arch Neurol Psychiat.* 73:387-395.
12. Wescoe W.C., Green R.E., McNamara B.P. and Krop S. (1948). The influence of atropine and scopolamine on the central effects of DFP. *J. Pharmacol exp. Therap.* 92:63-72.
13. Andrews P.A., Miller R.D. and Gordon A.S. (1955) Evaluation of atropinization by various routes in humans. *Chemical Corps Laboratories Contract Report* No. 59, July, 1955.
14. Wechsler, R. and Koskoff, Y.D. Effect on humans of moderate doses of atropine. *Chemical Corps Laboratories Contract Report* No. 54, 1955.
15. Fink, M. (1985) Pharmaco-electroencephalography: A note on its history. *Neuropsychobiology* 12:173-178.

FIRST USE OF PLACEBO

Turan M. Itil

"Placebo control? Why do we need it? If there is a therapeutic effect, I would know it. I don't need sugar pills to justify my conclusions." That was the response of Professor Fritz Flügel to Professor Wirtz. The year was 1955. Their exchange took place at one of the regular meetings between the scientists of Bayer Pharmaceuticals of Leverkusen and clinicians of the Department of Neurology and Psychiatry at the University of Erlangen in Nuremberg, Germany. Professor Flügel was the only Ordinarius (Chairman) Professor in the conservative German academic world involved in drug research, considered a second-class endeavour by German academicians. Professor Wirtz was the chief of worldwide clinical research and development of Bayer.

I had just completed residency training in neurology and psychiatry, and was a Bayer research fellow. After working for four years as an extern, without pay, I was happy to be supported by Bayer for monitoring and coordinating their drug research at the Erlangen clinic.

Bayer had a licensing agreement with Rhône-Poulenc, the company which developed chlorpromazine, to study a series of their new phenothiazines. The objective of our clinical research was to identify those drugs

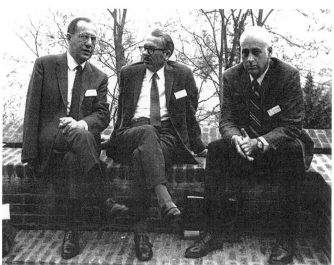

First meeting of the German Psychopharmacology Working Group in Erlangen (1961). From left: P. Borenstein (France), T. Itil (Germany), and R. Wittenborn (USA)

from the series which were therapeutically more effective than chlorpromazine or have fewer side effects such as sedation. The Bayer scientists had grown desperate in trying to convince Professor Flügel that the "real" thererapeutic effects could only be considered established if drug effects were statistically significantly greater than that of the placebo. However, Professor

Turan M. Itil is currently chairman of the New York Institute for Medical Research and Clinical Professor at New York Medical Center. He is a member of the World Health Organization's International Scientific Advisory Board on Alzheimer's Disease research. He has been a professor at the universities of Erlangen, Nuremberg and Missouri as well as at New York Medical College. He is the author of seven books and more than 500 publications.
Itil was elected a fellow of CINP in 1962. He presented papers on "EEG sleep state after anticholinergic drugs," on "Treatment of chronic psychiatric patients with combined medications" (Itil, Holden, [contd.]

Flügel, my boss, who was one of the most astute clinicians I had ever met, was absolutely against the use of placebos. He could not understand how placebos could help to determine the therapeutic effects of a drug. He used to say that every good clinician should be able to recognize whether a drug is effective or not, and he accused the Bayer scientists of Americanizing clinical research.

As a foreigner and a junior clinician-researcher I was a silent observer of the discussions between Professor Flügel and Professor Wirtz. By then, brainwashed in the conservative, clinical tradition of Germany, I had learned to agree with the opinion of my "big boss." If the drug is effective, a good clinician would know it! A placebo is needed only for the scientist who does not know his or her patients and who does not trust anyone!

Although I kept my opinion to myself, in reality I was coming in those days closer and closer to agreeing with the Bayer researchers. By reading the English and American research literature as much as I could with my limited knowledge of English, I recognized the possible need for a placebo. I also had a supporter in Dieter Bente in the department who was explicitly a "friend" of the placebo. He was my senior by only one year and both of us had come to join Professor Flügel from the famous Kretschmer clinic in Tübingen. But since he was German by birth, he had considerably more influence at the clinic than I did. Regardless, it took years before we could convince our colleagues to conduct our first placebo-controlled clinical trial in normal, healthy volunteer subjects (not in psychiatric patients) at the clinic.

I had been involved in clinical research prior to the discovery of chlorpromazine. It was pain research, testing promethazine's therapeutic effectiveness in phantom ("brain") pain, mainly in soldiers who had lost their arms or legs (1). The promethazine study had a profound effect on my career, because it was in this study that I had to learn how to use the EEG to test the hypothesis that in treatment-refractory patients the drug did not reach the target organ (thalamus), evidently by failing to pass the blood-brain barrier. The hypothesis was formulated by Dr. Betz, my boss at the time, and was based on the findings of Berger – who was the first to record the electrical activity of the brain by EEG – that drugs which affect human behaviour also produce effects on the EEG.

While I was learning how to use the EEG, chlorpromazine's behavioural effects were published. As soon we heard of this publication, Bente and I procured chlorpromazine to study its effect on the EEG. We published (2) our findings in 1954. (It helped me to get the Bayer fellowship.) In the absence of automated quantification of the EEG, it was extremely time-consuming and tedious to evaluate drug effects with the device. Originally, we used chlorpromazine as a standard reference (control) drug in our EEG studies with psychotropics. But

---

Fink, Shapiro, and Keskinar), on "Effects of psychotropic drugs on computer sleep-prints in man," and on "Quantitative pharmaco-electroencephalography in assaying new antianxiety drugs" at the 5th (twice), 6th, and 7th Congresses, respectively. He also coauthored papers on "A comparison of the action of various phenothiazine compounds on the human EEG" (Bente and Itil), on "Klinische und elektroencephalographische Untersuchungen in der Reihe der acylierten piperazine-phenothiazin Derivate" (Flügel, Bente, Itil und Molitoris), on "Klinische und elektroencephalographische Untersuchungen bei Therapieresistenten schizophrenen Psychosen" (Flugel, Itil und Stoerger), on "Anticholinergic hallucinogens and their interaction with centrally active drugs" (Fink and Itil), on "A clinical and EEG study of the withdrawal syndromes in schizophrenic patients" (Ulett, Holden, Itil and Keskiner), on "High and very high dose fluphenazine in the treatment of chronic psychoses" (Polvan, Yagcioglu, Itil, and Fink), and on "Psychotropic drug-induced alterations in somatosensory evoked responses in schizophrenic patients" (Jones, Itil, Keskinar, Holden, and Ulett), at the 1st, 2nd, 3rd , 5th, and 6th (three times) Congresses respectively.

as soon as we established the different CNS effects of reserpine, we recognized the need for a placebo to discover "real" drug effects.

By the late 1950s, when the organization of meetings dedicated specifically to psychotropic drugs began, I was already involved in studying the effects of psychotropic drugs on the EEG. At the first such meeting, the Milan Symposium on Psychotropic Drugs, organized by Dr. Garattini in 1957, Bente and I presented our findings on the effect of reserpine (3), methamphetamine and LSD-25 (4) on the EEG. The second international symposium on psychopharmacology was organized by Nathan Kline in 1957, in Zurich, during the Second World Congress of Psychiatry. In his preface to the proceedings of that symposium, published under the title *Psychopharmacology Frontiers,* Kline characterized the Zurich symposium on psychopharmacology as follows:

> This was the first scientific meeting many had attended which consisted almost entirely of unprepared, unrehearsed discussion, the intention of which was to bring together individuals with different points of view and to have them argue much as one would in private conversation. After the initial shock had worn off, some of them entered so enthusiastically into the spirit that a very junior man ended up berating the Herr Professor from his own clinic.

The Zurich symposium and the first congress of the Collegium Internationale Neuro-psycho-pharmacologicum, held in Rome in 1958, helped some European clinicians to appreciate the methodology of drug research, the need for the use of placebos in research, and last but not least, the fact that psychopharmacology is not a second-class field of research. To free up dialogue between senior professors and junior doctors, decades of many national and international meetings were required.

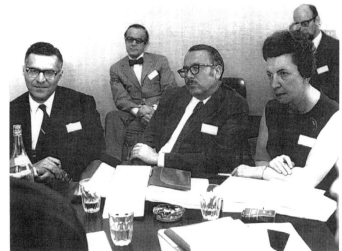

Annual meeting of the Early Clinical Evaluation Units (1972). From left: Ozcan Köknel (Turkey), Fritz Freyhan (USA), Turan Itil (USA), and Alice Leeds (USA)

Our research with Bayer resulted in the development of butaperazine, one of the most potent neuroleptics (5). In 1963, during the search for better monitoring of drug effects in the brain, I joined Max Fink in St. Louis (USA) while on my sabbatical year from the University of Erlangen (where I was associate professor by that time). Max, whom I had first met at a meeting in Rome, was at the time the director of a newly-established research clinic there, the Missouri Institute of Psychiatry (MIP). The MIP was created by George Ulett, a creative researcher and great administrator. It had everything: a lot of space, patients, money, and a creative group of researchers whom Fink had recruited. Included among them were Sam Gershon, Amedeo Marrazzi and Sol Garfield. Max Fink and Ulett could even manage to get one of the first computers for our EEG research. With funding from the Early Clinical Drug Evaluation Unit (ECDEU) of the National Institute of Mental Health created by Jonathan Cole, we had an opportunity to study almost every psychotropic drug before it was marketed.

While I learned of the scientific necessity of placebo, a new limitation was placed on their use in the 1960s. As a result of public pressure, Institutional Review Boards (IRBs) considered the use of placebos as unethical, particularly in psychiatric patients. Suddenly, we returned to the era in Germany in the 1950s when I was conducting clinical trials without a placebo. At our ECDEU meetings in Florida, which were closed for at least one day to the pharmaceutical industry, Nate Kline used to go to the blackboard and ask the audience, "Who would put his or her money on this drug?" With a majority of votes, it was decided whether or not a drug would survive.

While we helped to develop many new drugs, we also missed opportunities with others. In 1966, for example, Max Fink, Sam Gershon and I demonstrated that tetrahydroaminacridine (THA) was very effective in reversing anticholinergic drug-induced delirium (6). But we were not perceptive enough to try THA in dementia. The substance was renamed as Tacrine and marketed well over thirty years later.

Similarly, in 1972, we discovered the antidepressant properties of mianserin (7), but lost the patent rights due to an overeager publication two weeks before the deadline. The use of lisuride in organic brain syndromes (8) and alcoholism (9), mesterolone (10) and estradiol valerate (11) in depression, d-nogestrel in anxiety (12), were all discovered by the quantitative-EEG (QEEG), with patents assigned to companies that supported our research.

QEEG is now used to determine the pharmacodynamics of psychotropic drugs and to monitor their effects in a safe and economic fashion. The brain is the most vulnerable organ in our body because it has no pain receptors. The psychiatric patient is the most vulnerable of all in the absence of adequate judgment and insight. With the help of psychotropics, knowledgeable doctors can achieve marvellous results. On the other hand, inexperienced psychopharmacologists can also cause a lot of harm. It is part of the mission of organizations such as CINP to help psychiatrists to become better doctors.

REFERENCES
1. Bente, D. und Itil, T.M. (1934). Periphere Anästhesie und Schmerzgeschehen. *Acta Neuroveg.* 7 : 258-262.
2. Bente , D. und Itil, T.M., (1954). Zur Wirkung des Phenothiazin Körpers Megaphen auf das menschliche Hirnströmbild. *Arzneimittel Forschung* 4:418-423.
3. Bente, D. und Itil, T.M., Elecktroencephalographische Veränderungen unter extrem hohen Reserpindosen. In S. Garattin, and V. Ghetti, (eds.) *Psychotropic Drugs* (pp. 294-206), Amsterdam: Elsevier.
4. Bente, D. und Itil, T. M. (1957). Vergleichende klinisch elektroencephalographische Untersuchungen mit Pervitin und LSD-25. In S. Garattin, and V. Ghetti (eds.) *Psychotropic Drugs* (pp. 284-285), Amsterdam: Elsevier.
5. Flügel, F., Bente, D., Itil, T.M., and Molitoris, B. (1961) Klinische und elektroencephalographische Untersuchungen in der Reihe der acylierten Piperazino-Phenothiazin Derivate. In E. Rothlin (ed.). *Neuro-Psychopharmacology* (Vol. 2., pp. 236-243). Amsterdam: Elsevier.
6. Itil, T.M. (1966). Quantitative EEG changes induced by anticholinergic drugs and their behavioral correlates in man. In J. Wortis (ed.)., *Recent Advances in Biological Psychiatry.* (Vol. 8, pp. 151-173). New York: Plenum Press.
7. Itil, T.M., Polvan, N. and Hsu, W. (1972). Clinical and EEG effects of GB 94, a tetracyclic antidepressant (EEG Model in Discovery of a New Psychotropic Drug). *Current Therapeutic Research* 14:395-413, 1972.
8. Itil, T.M. (1976): Use of Lisuride and Physiologically Acceptable Salts Thereof to Achieve Psychic Energizer Effects I. United States Patent No. 3954 988, May 4, 1976. German Patent No. 2359128 Appl. published. Assignee: Schering AG, West Berlin (p. 1551)
9. Itil, T.M. (1978): Lisuride in Alcoholism. United States Patent No. 4096266, June 20, 1978.
10. Itil, T.M., Michael, S.T., Shapiro, D.M., and Itil, K.Z. (1984): The Effects of Mesterolone, A Male Sex Hormone in Depressed Patients. *Methods and Findings*, Vol. 6, No. 6.
11. Itil, T.M., and Herrmann, W.M. (1978): Use of Estradiol Valerate as an Antidepressant. United States Patent No. 972626, December 1978.
12 Itil, T.M., and Herrmann, W.M. (1987): Neuropsychiatric Agents and Their Use (l Nogestrel), United States Patent No. 4089952, May 16, 1987.

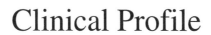
Clinical Profile

THE AMDP SYSTEM

Hanfried Helmchen and Bernd Ahrens

The introduction of chlorpromazine, a neuroleptic, in psychiatric therapy was the starting point for the development of the new science, psychopharmacology. With supporting research from other disciplines such as biochemistry and neurophysiology, psychopharmacology as neuropsychopharmacology has become one of the most active areas of basic research in pharmacology.

Shortly after the introduction of chlorpromazine in 1952 in France, a steadily growing number of potentially effective psychotropic drugs were developed. As this process continued, it became increasingly apparent that there was a need for a comprehensive evaluation of these new drugs, as well as for studies which compare the newly developed drugs with the older ones having proven value in treatment.

It also soon became apparent that studies were needed that were specifically designed to evaluate the efficacy of new psychotropic drugs. The studies required methods (assessments, tests) that could generate reliable and standardized data on benefits and drawbacks.

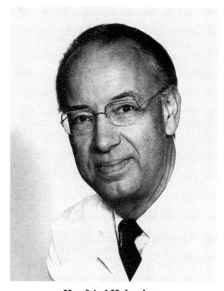

Hanfried Helmchen

Psychotropic drugs not only quantitatively affect a psychopathological condition but may also induce important qualitative changes. Therefore, the development of a comprehensive inventory covering a wide spectrum of clinical symptoms was of utmost importance. Much

Hanfried Helmchen has been head of the Department of Psychiatry at the Free University of Berlin since 1971. His research interests are clinical pharmacology and methodology, depression, dementia, and medical ethics.

Helmchen was elected a fellow of the CINP in 1964. He presented papers on "EEG-Langschnittuntersuchungen bei der Pharmakotherapie von Psychosen" (Helmchen und Kunkel), on "Zur Analyse elektroencephalographische Veränderungen unter psychiatrischer Pharmacotherapie" (Helmchen und Kunkel) and on "Syndromegenese psychischer Nebenwirkungen der psychiatrischen Pharmakotherapie" (Helmchen) at the 3rd, 4th, and 5th Congress respectively; he also coauthored a paper on "Documentation clinique en psychopharmacologie le systeme A.M.P." (Angst, Battegay, Bente, Berner, Broeren, Cornu, Dick, Engelmeier, Heimann, Heinrich, Helmchen, Hippius, Lukacs, Pöldinger, Schmidlin, Schmidt and Weis) at the 6th Congress. Helmchen was a formal discussant of Working Group 4 (Pharmacological and Clinical Action of Psychotropic Drugs) at the 4th Congress.

valuable information may be lost on unexpected changes and side effects if only a specific
syndrome is being considered.

At the end of the 1950s, five university departments of psychiatry in Germany decided to
collaborate on the development of a method for
the collection and documentation of data suitable for psychopharmacological research. The
participating departments were in Erlangen (D.
Bente), Mainz (K. Heinrich), Berlin (H. Helmchen and H. Hippius), Münster (M.P. Engelmeier), and Homburg/Saar (W. Schmitt). After
constructing an instrument for documentation
to be used by all five participating departments,
several multicentre trials were carried out to
test it in practice with a view to describing the
therapeutic effects of various new psychotropic
drugs. The results of these studies were first
published by Bente and his associates in 1961
(1).

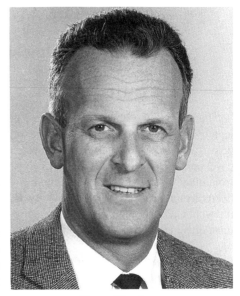

Hanns Hippius

A similar development took place in Switzerland at about the same time. The five
participating university departments in Switzerland were in Zürich (J. Angst), Bern (F. Cornu),
Geneva (P. Dick), Lausanne (H. Heimann), and Basel (W. Pöldinger) (2). Somewhat later, the
department of psychiatry in Vienna (Berner) joined the group.

The aim of the Swiss and German investigators was to understand the course of psychiatric
illness during treatment with psychotropic drugs. It was also to assess the entire field of
psychiatric findings, including demographic and anamnestic data for each patient, rather than
concentrating on specific psychopathological syndromes, such as the depressive syndrome.
The concept of "documenting" the data was also important.

The system was made public at the 5th Congress of the CINP in Washington in 1966 (3).
The first German edition of the *AMP Manual* appeared in 1971 and the first English edition
in 1982 (4). Since the initial workshop on translations of the system, which was held during
the 10th CINP Congress in Quebec City in July 1976, the *Manual* has been translated into
French, Italian, Japanese, Croatian, Portuguese, Spanish, Danish, Russian, and Estonian.

The group first called itself AMP and later AMDP (Arbeitsgemeinschaft für Methodik und
Dokumentation in der Psychiatrie, or Association for Methodology and Documentation in
Psychiatry). The original acronym did not refer to the concept of documentation, and this was
an unfortunate omission, because even at the beginning, the importance of accurate documentation was emphasized. Since then, the main goal of the AMDP has been to identify the kind
of data relevant to psychiatry, to develop methods for recording these data, and to render the
recorded data available for statistical processing.

The AMDP documentation system originally consisted of four data collection forms,
designed for optical evaluation in order to be used in digital processing by computer. The
number of the data collection forms was later increased to five. The system was different from
other psychiatric documentation systems in terms of the comprehensiveness of the recorded
information.

The AMDP system contains the following documentation structure:

1. Anamnesis – demographic data (e.g., education, level of employment)
2. Anamnesis – life events (e.g., death of spouse/partner)
3. Anamnesis – psychiatric history (e.g., birth and childhood, previous psychiatric episodes)
4. Psychopathological symptoms (100 items; e.g., incoherence, delusional ideas, depressed mood)
5. Somatic signs (40 items; e.g., interrupted sleep, nausea, dizziness).

Documentation of the anamnesis contains such details as the patient's working career and information about the patient's family, including the number and gender of siblings. The disease anamnesis covers the family history with regard to psychiatric disorders in the biological family of the patient, life events in patient's familial situation during childhood (e.g., divorce or separation of the parents), and the patient's psychosocial development, including such factors as drug abuse, aggressive behaviour, or suicide attempts. Furthermore, past psychiatric treatments and their efficacy, as well as diagnosis according to the International Classification of Diseases (ICD), are recorded.

The core of the AMDP system is the data collection forms that cover psychopathological symptoms and somatic signs. The symptoms described on these two forms were derived from classic descriptive psychopathology, familiar to the psychiatric community in German-speaking countries.

What is usually referred to as the "Homburg experiment" (5) took place prior to the publishing of the data collection forms. It consisted in part of a meeting of the representatives of all participating departments for a first interrater reliability session to determine to what extent their assessments correspond with each other. The Homburg experiment also tested the scientific validity of the clinical description of the selected symptoms. At the meeting of interrater reliability testing, agreement was reached on the decision-tree to be used for assessing the psychopathological state of patients. The actual decision-making process was represented by a logical model consisting of four judgmental steps: accessibility, certainty, presence or absence of a symptom, and severity.

Accessibility of an item exists when the necessary information required for judgment is available (e.g., a stuporous or mute patient cannot provide the necessary information for assessing disturbances of orientation, attention, memory, thinking, etc.). Certainty refers to the confidence that the assessor has in the information provided (e.g., negativistic behaviour on the part of a patient may cause uncertainty as to whether the patient is or is not hallucinating). The presence or absence of a symptom is coded if the question of certainty has been resolved (e.g., by interviewing a patient suffering from senile dementia, an assessor can usually ascertain the presence or absence of disorientation). Severity refers to the degree to which a symptom is present and is estimated as mild, moderate, or severe. Assessment of severity is based on a combination of intensity, significance, and frequency.

It was also necessary to produce a manual with operationalized descriptions of the symptoms covered. Objective sources of information included the following: observations made during the interview, observations of behaviour made by the doctor and nursing personnel, and remarks made by the patient's relatives, as well as subjective information obtained from the patient. The symptoms had to be presented descriptively, as far as possible without taking the anticipated or previous diagnosis into account. Similarly, the presence or absence of a symptom had to be decided upon without consideration of a suspected diagnosis.

The AMDP system falls into the category of observer-based assessments in which judgments regarding the presence and severity of symptoms are based mostly on assessors' observations of patients' behaviour, and patients' descriptions given to the assessors about their pathological experiences. Nevertheless, to ascertain clarity about the source of the recorded information it was originally marked in the AMDP whether a symptom was a purely observable one (O=observer/others), or a self-experienced and reported symptom (S=self/patient), or a combination of the two. After discussions with experienced users of the AMDP system, it was decided that each symptom would be classified as follows:

S = self-judgment alone is used;
O = the judgment of the observer or others alone is used;
SO= self-judgment and that of the observer are of equal value;
sO = self-judgment is of less importance than that of the observer;
So = self-judgment is of more importance than that of the observer.

One of the difficulties in developing the AMDP system was in defining the degree of precision necessary for the documentation. A related difficulty concerned repeated testings to ensure reliability. The difficulties were resolved by stipulating a certain training for the users of the AMDP system. The training program was to include at least ten interviews, with subsequent documentation of the findings (particularly for data collection forms 4 and 5), and with the interviews covering the whole range of symptoms contained in the *Manual*, particularly symptoms 1-100.

The AMDP system is based on the "classic" psychopathology of the nineteenth and early-twentieth centuries, when psychiatrists and neurologists tried to describe the "abnormal" behaviour of mental patients and focus on "pathognomonic" signs for the categorization of syndromes or even disease entities. However, the AMDP system went a step beyond by standardizing psychopathological symptoms for comparative use.

The development of the AMDP system reflects a change in scientific methodology and documentation: the transition from information gained for individual use to its universal application. When assessing the psychopathology of patients, psychiatrists record discrete patterns of behaviour that diverge from the normal and are formally characterized as symptoms. However, when a strategy for treatment is decided upon, it is usual for the treating psychiatrist to categorize the patient's condition according to one or another psychiatric syndrome or disorder. Although this procedure is suitable for clinical practice, it has many drawbacks when used as a method for gathering psychopathological data in psychiatric research. By using the AMDP system, the assessor must concentrate on phenomena less complex than the complete "Gestalt," that is, on the specific symptoms presented by the patient, and record these in a standardized manner so that this information can be readily transformed into data and used in scientific investigations.

To date, the important steps in the development of the AMDP system are the following:

• The publication of a statistical manual with a summary of the findings in the reliability and validity studies (6). The evaluations show that the AMDP system is a practical documentation system, the application of which is not limited to the field of psychiatry (e.g., it might be used in the examination of cardiac patients).

• The generation of syndromes by means of mathematical-statistical approaches. Factor analyses based on data from 2,313 patients resulted in stable, reliable, and sample-independent syndrome scales. Eight syndromes could be extracted by the different factor analyses:

paranoid-hallucinatory, depressive, psycho-organic, manic, hostility, autonomic, apathy, and obsessive-compulsive. The syndrome scales satisfy statistical test criteria (7).

- The publication of a comprehensive textbook for the English user of the system (8).
- The publication of a semi-structured interview for the system (9).
- The publication of a revised manual with instructions relevant to the completion of the anamnestic sheets and definitions of the psychopathological symptoms and somatic signs (10).

The AMDP system provides the necessary uniformity in the international assessment of psychopathological symptoms for diagnostic and research purposes. It is a uniquely rich system in phenomenological descriptions.

REFERENCES

1. Bente, D., Engelmeier, M.P., Heinrich, K., Hippius, H. and Schmitt, W. (1961). Zur Dokumentation medikamentöser Wirkungen bei der psychischen Pharmakotherapie. *Arzneimittel-Forsch.* 11: 886-890.
2. Angst, J., Battegay, R., and Pöldinger, W. (1964). Zur Methodik der statistischen Bearbeitung des Therapieverlaufes depressiver Krankheitsbilder. *Methodik Inform. Med.* 3: 54-65.
3. Angst, J., Battegay, R., Bente, D., Cornu, F., Dick, P., Engelmeier, M.P., Heimann, H., Heinrich, K., Hippius, H., Pöldinger, W., Schmidlin, P., Schmitt, W., and Weis, P. (1967). Über das gemeinsame Vorgehen einer deutschen und schweizerischen Arbeitsgruppe auf dem Gebiet der psychiatrischen Dokumentation. *Schweizer Arch. Neurol. Neurochir. Psychiat.* 100: 207-211.
4. Guy, W., and Ban, T.A. (transl. & ed.) (1982). *The AMDP System.* Berlin: Springer.
5. Poeldinger, W. (1969). Über Notwendigkeit und Möglichkeiten standardisierter Befunderhebungen in der Psychiatrie. In H. Kranz (ed.). *Psychiatrie im Übergang,* Stuttgart: Thieme.
6. Baumann, U., and Stieglitz, R.D. (1983). *Testmanual zum AMDP-system: Empirische Befunde zur Psychopathologie.* Berlin: Springer.
7. Pietzker, A., Gebhardt, R. Strauss, A., Stockel, M., Langer, C. and Freudenthal, K. (1983). The syndrome scales in the AMDP-System. In D. Bobon, U. Baumann, J. Angst, H. Helmchen, and H. Hippius (eds.). *The AMDP-System in Phamacopsychiatry* (pp. 88-99). Basel: Karger.
8. Bobon, D., Baumann, U., Angst, J., Helmchen, K. Hippius, H. and Schmitt, W. (1961). Zur Dokumentation medikamentöser Wirkungen bei der psychiatrischen Pharmakotherapie. *Arzneimittel-Forsch.* 11: 880-890.
9. Fahndrich, E. and Stieglitz, R.D. (1989) *Leitfaden zur Erfassung des psychopathologischen Befundes Halbstrukturiertes Interview anhand des AMDP-Systems.* Berlin: Springer.
10. Arbeitsgemeinschaft fur Methodik und Dokumentationen in der Psychiatrie (AMDP) (1997). *Das AMDP-System: Manual zur Dokumentation psychiatrischer Befunde.* 6. Auflage, Göttingen: Hogrefe.

MEMORIES OF DRUG DEVELOPMENT

Eugene S. Paykel

My research has been mainly into depression, and I am a product, psychiatrically speaking, of the antidepressant era. I started my psychiatric training at the Maudsley Hospital, London, in 1962. By that time several tricyclics were available, and they were in widespread use. There were also some MAO-inhibitors: the discovery of the cheese reaction and the consequent marked reduction in the clinical prescribing of this class of drugs all over the world was yet to come. The treatment of depression had by 1962 become effective and routine. To a young psychiatrist sharing the therapeutic optimism which these comparatively new treatments had generated, it was only a fact of distant history that, not many years before, none of these medications had been available. I did talk later to an elderly psychiatric nurse who remembered the 1930s, before even ECT had been introduced. Then there had been much

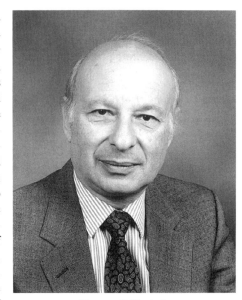

Eugene S. Paykel

suffering among severely depressed, hospitalized patients, although many did in the long run recover.

There was also much that we did not know. For instance, it had not yet been demonstrated that treatment usually needed to be continued beyond the acute episode, that higher doses were required in some patients, and that, from the point of view of research, controlled trials of antidepressants needed to be at least six weeks long, rather than two to four weeks, to be sure of showing superiority over placebo. Controlled trials were being carried out aplenty: in the United Kingdom the influential Medical Research Council study confirmed the efficacy of imipramine and of ECT, but not, to some consternation, of phenelzine (probably, in retrospect,

Eugene S. Paykel was born in New Zealand in 1934. He qualified in medicine there and trained in psychiatry in Britain. From 1966 to 1971, he worked at Yale University, serving as co-director and later director of the Depression Research Unit. He then returned to Britain to work at St Georges Hospital Medical School, London, where he subsequently became professor of psychiatry. Since 1985 he has been professor of psychiatry and head of department at Cambridge University. Dr. Paykel has been president of the British Association of Psychopharmacology, and chairman of the pharmacopsychiatry section of the World Psychiatric Association.

Eugene S. Paykel was elected a fellow of the CINP in 1970.

because of suboptimal treatment length and dose). I started my first controlled trial while still in training, together with equally young colleagues.

In September 1966 I moved across the Atlantic to Yale University, to undertake full-time research. Initially, I planned to stay for two years, but I remained almost five. I went to work with Gerald Klerman, who had not long been at Yale, and together we set up the Depression Research Unit. Over the next two years we were joined by Brigitte Prusoff and Myrna Weissman. This was an exciting and productive period, and it marked the heyday of American clinical psychopharmacology. Under the aegis of Jonathan Cole, the first large NIMH (National Institute of Mental Health) collaborative trial of neuroleptics in schizophrenia had already been undertaken, and from his Psychopharmacology Research Branch at NIMH, there flowed encouragement for good ideas, and usually the funds to support them. At the CINP and the American College of Neuropsychopharmacology (ACNP) meetings, reports of controlled trials and other clinically-based studies predominated.

At Yale we set up a broad-based program of studies in depression. Our interest was not so much in new drug development as in establishing what was important for the good clinical use of the drugs. At that time, questions about the pharmacotherapy of depression were as inextricably intertwined with questions regarding its classification and causes as they are today with its neuroendocrinology, brain functional neuroimaging, and molecular genetics. We aimed to resolve some of these issues at the same time as addressing its treatment. Particularly salient were debates about the endogenous-reactive and psychotic-neurotic classifications, their component features, and the place of life-event stress.

To address these questions, we set out to collect a large and fairly representative sample of depressives in various treatment facilities in New Haven. The considerable number of papers resulting from this study dealt with several main themes, including the classification of depression. We undertook statistical studies of classification by factor analysis, replicating the endogenous dimension, but without clear separation into a categorical diagnosis (1). We showed that inpatient and outpatient facilities tended to have individuals with different features. One of the first studies applying cluster analysis found a psychotic group, but three, rather than one, non-psychotic groups (2), indicating the heterogeneity of so-called neurotic depression. We examined some specific clinical features, including the depressives characterized by increased appetite, who are now known as atypical depressives.

In order to study the etiologic role of life events, we undertook the first large-scale comparison with control subjects from the general population. In what subsequently became a citation classic, we showed clearly increased rates of life events prior to onset of depression, particularly for events characterized as undesirable, and exit events (3).

All this work was intended as preliminary to our main aim: to undertake the first controlled trial of continuation of antidepressants versus early withdrawal after acute treatment. By 1966 it was becoming apparent that the usual pattern of three months' antidepressant treatment was sometimes followed by relapse on withdrawal. It was not clear whether the relapse represented a pharmacological effect of the termination of drug treatment or a psychological consequence of the approaching termination of treatment. We first designed a trial in which initial treatment with amitriptyline was followed by continuation to nine months, or by double-blind withdrawal to placebo after a total of three months, or by open withdrawal to no drug. We then decided that the study would be much enriched by addition of a comparison between psychotherapy and low contact in each of these three drug groups in a factorial design. A model of individual therapy by social workers was devised which was, in effect, the first use of interpersonal therapy (IPT). In a collaborative study with Alberto DiMascio in Boston, we found potent effects of continuing antidepressants, but not of psychotherapy, on relapse reduction and less strong, but significant effects of psychotherapy on improving social function and interpersonal relationships. Another citation classic ensued (4).

The design of this study led the way to controlled trials by other workers with different psychotherapy modalities (e.g., marital or group). By employing the factorial designs we used with antidepressants in these studies it was shown that the methods of clinical psychopharmacology could be successfully adapted to the evaluation of efficacy of psychotherapy. It also led in due course to much subsequent work on IPT.

Another productive offshoot of the study concerned social adjustment. Originally derived from the need to develop and validate an outcome measure for psychotherapy, this work extended into a series of papers and a book (5) detailing the social and interpersonal maladjustments of depressed women compared to normals in the general population and the impact of depression in different areas, its dimensions, and its course over time. Another offshoot was the recognition of carbohydrate craving and weight gain as a side effect of long-term tricyclic antidepressant treatment, with the first conclusive demonstration and attempt to study mechanisms (6).

In 1970 Gerald Klerman moved to the Massachusetts General Hospital, and I inherited the role of director of the Depression Research Unit. We had meanwhile extended the work on life events into similar controlled comparisons of events prior to episodes of schizophrenia and suicide attempts (7, 8) and of events and depressive relapse (9). We also undertook a scaling study of events in collaboration with E.H. Uhlenhuth in Chicago (10) and carried out a study of suicidal feelings in the general population (11, 12). In addition we began with the collection of new samples, including a sample of suicide attempters to study epidemiology and treatment (13) and a sample of medically ill subjects with depression (14). The material from the earlier studies was used for the analysis of predictors of antidepressant response, detailed work on rating scales, and rating procedures.

In 1971 I returned to London and established a new program of work on depression and antidepressants. The Depression Research Unit continued and developed strong work in interpersonal therapy, epidemiology, and genetics.

When I look back on the 1960s and the earlier 1970s, I see them as the best of times for clinical psychopharmacology. A first generation of effective drugs had already revolutionized treatment in psychiatry. They generated many fundamental questions best answered by well-designed controlled trials. There was a mood of excitement and a sense of new important findings waiting to be uncovered. The most salient reports at psychopharmacology conferences were of clinical trials and other clinical studies. Many of the findings which ultimately produced today's clinical guidelines were established. Later the climate changed. The clinical studies became more routine, and basic science studies more exciting, as they opened up new areas. With some notable exceptions, new drug development comprised minor modifications of existing drug classes, rather than new departures. The clinical methods of biological psychiatry did continue to improve, receiving new impetus in the later 1970s with the advent of neuroendocrine-challenge techniques and receptor binding. But for new drug development, it would be another twenty years before fresh generations of pharmacologically different antidepressants and neuroleptics restored the balance.

REFERENCES

1. Paykel, E.S., Prusoff, B.A., and Klerman, G.L. (1971). The endogenous-neurotic continuum in depression: Rater independence and factor distributions. *Journal of Psychiatric Research* 8: 73-90.

2. Paykel, E.S. ((1971). Classification of depressed patients: A cluster analysis derived grouping. *British Journal of Psychiatry* 118: 275-288.

3. Paykel, E. S., Myers, J.K., Dienelt, M., Klerman, G.L.. Lindenthal, J., and Pepper, M. (1969). Life events and depression: A controlled study. *Archives of General Psychiatry* 21: 753-76.

4. Klerman, G.L., Di Mascio, A., Weissman, M.M., Prusoff, B. A., and Paykel, E.S. (1974). Treatment of depression by drugs and psychotherapy. *American Journal of Psychiatry* 131: 186-191.

5. Weissman, M.M., and Paykel, E.S. (1974). *The Depressed Woman: A Study of Social Relationships.* Chicago: University of Chicago Press.

6. Paykel, E.S., Mueller, P.S., and de la Vergne, P.M. (1973). Amitriptyline, weight gain and carbohydrate craving: a side effect. *British Journal of Psychiatry* 123: 501-507.

7. Jacobs, S.C., Prusoff, B.A., and Paykel, E.S. (1974). Recent life events in schizophrenia and depression. *Psychological Medicine* 4: 444-453.

8. Paykel, E.S., Prusoff, B.A., and Myers, J.K. (1975). Suicide attempts and recent life events: A controlled comparison. *Archives of General Psychiatry* 32: 327-337.

9. Paykel, E.S., and Tanner, J. (1976). Life events, depressive relapse and maintenance treatment. *Psychological Medicine* 6: 481-485.

10. Paykel, E.S., Prusoff, B.A., and Uhlenhuth, E.H. (1971) Scaling of life events. *Archives of General Psychiatry* 25: 340-347.

11. Paykel, E.S., Myers, J.K., Lindenthal, J.J., and Tanner, J. (1974). Suicidal feelings in the general population: A prevalence study. *British Journal of Psychiatry* 30: 771-778.

12. Paykel, E.S., Hallowell, C., Dressler, D.M., Shapiro, D.L., and Weissman, M.M. (1974). Treatment of suicide attempters: A descriptive study. *Archives of General Psychiatry* 31: 487-491.

13. Prusoff, B.A., and Myers, J.K. (1975). Suicide attempts and recent life events: A controlled comparison. *Archives of General Psychiatry* 32: 327-337.

14. Moffic, S.H., and Paykel, E. S. (1975). Depression in medical inpatients. *British Journal of Psychiatry* 126: 126:346-353.

MONITORING CENTRAL ACTIVITIES BY PERIPHERAL MEANS

Walter Knopp

When I resumed my medical education in Heidelberg in 1947, after the Second World War, I did so to become "physician of the soul" (*Seelenarzt*). It was only for a short period of time, while still a medical student, that I would have liked to combine cardiology with psychosomatics. It happened when a senior cardiology professor was asked by one of my fellow students "What IS the average optimum dose of digitalis?" The professor replied that "There is no average dose, each heart has its own optimum dose." The impact of the reply was further enforced by the publication of a junior professor. He published a graphically documented study showing that by monitoring peripheral symptom change, such as heart rate, urinary output, body weight, size of liver, etc, the cardiologist could establish an optimum "heart level" of digitoxin.

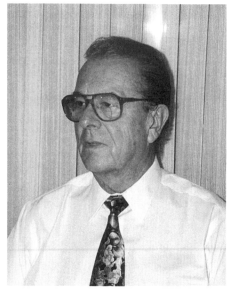

Walter Knopp

My intention of combining psychiatry and cardiology was short-lived. Instead, just about the same time that chlorpromazine was introduced, I began my psychiatric residency in a state hospital affiliated with several academic institutions. When chlorpromazine appeared on the scene I can still recall my supervisors pointing out that it was distinct from the old sedatives in that it could produce "sedation without impairment of intellectual functioning." Very soon, by the time trifluoperazine was released for clinical use, it was also recognized that the new drugs can decrease the intensity, frequency, distinctness, and "reality impact" of hallucinations and delusions.

In 1959 I decided to study trifluoperazine (TFP) by monitoring the changes in 12 TFP-treated schizophrenic patients. The improvement was impressive, but in the absence of a generally accepted method of quantifying the changes, I had to describe the changes encoun-

Walter Knopp, who was born in Czechoslovakia and received his medical training in Germany, is now professor emeritus of Ohio State University. His "heart" is "made in Czechoslovakia," his "brain" is "made in Germany," and his "homeostat" is made in America.

Knopp was elected a fellow of the CINP in 1968. He presented a paper on "Electronic pupillography in medical students and in patients before and during neuroleptic treatment" at the 6th Congress.

tered in patients day by day. It was in the course of this process that I realized that, in the same way as the cardiologist in cardiac decompensation could establish the "heart level" of digitoxin by monitoring peripheral cardiac symptom changes, I could establish in psychotic decompensation the "brain level" of TFP by monitoring peripheral psychopathological symptom changes. I felt that there should be a more sophisticated way to figure out the dose requirement of TFP, or in general of an antipsychotic in case of psychotic decompensation, and asked my colleagues to collaborate with me on some research to find it. Since neither at the hospital I was working at, nor at the university I was affiliated with, were any of the psychiatrists interested in collaborating, I decided to accept an instructorship at the Ohio State University Hospitals, with the hope that at least in one of the local hospitals I would find someone with a similar interest to mine. It was not to be the case.

The only colleague who was ready for a "joint venture" was a chemist, whose name was Fischer. He had a senior academic position at Ohio State University and was interested in testing the hypothesis that there is a linear relationship between the sensitivity of the local receptors for taste and "systemic sensitivity" for developing hypokinetic extrapyramidal side effects (HEPSE). In simple terms we assumed that patients with higher taste sensitivity, because of their higher systemic sensitivity, would develop HEPSE with lower cumulative doses of trifluoperazine than patients with lower taste sensitivity and vice versa.

We tested our hypothesis by treating forty-eight patients on the basis of an almost identical treatment (dose) regimen of TFP for twelve days, followed by optimizing the dose in each patient. Our findings were supportive of our hypothesis with a statistically significant level of probability.

Encouraged by these findings, I decided to pursue matters further and try to find a more sophisticated way for the detection of the optimal dose for individual patients than describing changes in their psychopathology, and a more comprehensive way of defining "systemic sensitivity" than in terms of the HEPSE. To achieve these ends I administered, after a one to six day observation period, TFP in almost identical doses for twenty days or until the detection of HEPSE, whichever came first, to thirty-two newly admitted acutely ill schizophrenic patients, while monitoring their "brain stem triad" (as defined by Reichardt and cited by Cornu), psychomotor system, autonomic nervous system (ANS) and "psychic system." The psychomotor system was monitored by the planimetric determination of handwriting area (PDHA), originated by Haase and modified by Fischer; the ANS by electronic pupillography (EPG), originated by Lowenstein and Loewenfeld and modified by Hakerem; the "psychic system" by the brief psychiatric rating scale (BPRS), target symptom rating (TSR), and global assessment. The findings of this study indicated high intra-individual consistency with inter-individual variability. The latter was so great that it prevented finding at the time a more sophisticated way of detecting dose requirements for individual patients, or finding a more comprehensive way to define systemic sensitivity. There was also a promising lead for further research: in those patients who were able to cooperate with all the testing, there was a

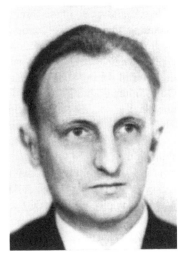

H.-J. Haase

trend for correlations between the PDHA and the extent of contraction of the pupil (EC) with the HEPSE.

In 1965 Bielecki, a child psychiatrist at the local state hospital, referred a sixteen-year-old male patient with Tourette's syndrome (TS) to me for treatment. The patient had been treated for fourteen years with dynamic psychotherapy, sedatives and anticonvulsants without success and Bielecki and I were aware of the successes with haloperidol in Europe in such cases. Haloperidol (H) at the time was still an experimental drug in the United States. I accepted the challenge with the clear understanding by all those concerned that the patient would be a subject in a double-blind, crossover, longitudinal study that would place great demands on patient, parents, staff, and myself; that at the end of the study, the patient and his parents would be told the details of the study and the reason for undertaking it; and that the family would not be charged any fees by either the hospital or myself. Since the parents had incurred $20,000 in expenses between 1951 and 1965, they were willing to accept my conditions. The patient (to be referred to as patient number 1) remained in the study from October 25, 1965, to May 28, 1966.

One month after Bielecki's referral of patient number 1, another TS patient, a nineteen-year-old female (to be referred to as patient number 2) was included in the "study." For two months these two patients were studied concomittantly on different H dosages, but according to the same experimental design. The results appeared to be a dream come true. Their PDHA ("psychomotor system") showed a one to one relationship with TSR ("psychic system") trends, i.e., improvement on H and reversal of the improvement on placebo. Their EPG (autonomic nervous system), however, was a great disappointment at first. Thus my expectation that the pupil would "behave" the same way as the PDHA did was very much thwarted. However, this particular finding turned out to be of great theoretical importance later on, when we evaluated our findings further.

A third TS patient (patient number 3) was admitted to the study before we had completed the evaluation of the first two. He was a forty-four-year old male with small PDHA prior to haloperidol and no PDHA response to the drug. He failed to respond to H, but eventually showed moderate improvement on 75 mg of imipramine daily.

In summary, two of our three TS patients responded whereas one remained refractory to H treatment. One of the responders was studied on two occasions almost exactly a year apart. Both responders showed dramatic clinical improvement, with decrease of PDHA without HEPSE. In neither of the two patients was there a response to haloperidol in the dark-adapted diameter of the pupil (ID). Their extent of contraction was 0.3 mm and 1.8 mm respectively. On optimum dose of haloperidol (9 mg and 5 mg respectively), by an increase of EC in patient number 1 and a decrease in patient number 2, their EC was the same, i.e., met in the middle. The EC of the non-responder moved away from the middle.

At this point it might be helpful to spell out what was being measured by EPG and to clarify some of the findings. EPG is a method for continuous infrared scanning and recording of the largest diameter of the pupil without touching the eye. In our procedure 1 second of light was followed by 4.9 seconds of darkness with the readings of five trials averaged. The extent to which the pupil contracts (EC) depends on stimulus intensity, frequency, and duration, as well as on the state of the retinal adaptation and the state of supranuclear inhibition (SNI) at stimulus impact. By keeping the first four conditions constant, the SNI is measured. After dark adaptation, there is no parasympathetic influence upon the Edinger-Westphal nucleus (EWN). In this state the dark-adapted pupil (ID = initial diameter) reflects the state of ANS balance in the hypothalamic modulatory area of the brain, i.e., in the hypothalamic central ANS balance where norepinephrine (NE) and serotonin (5-HT) are the main neurotransmitters. The light reflex, on the other hand, is modulated in the EWN of the mesencephalon. The effect of SNI upon the EWN is overwhelmed by the parasympathetic light stimulus falling on the retina. The EC reflects the state of ANS balance in the mesencephalic modulatory area of the brain, i.e., the mesencephalic central ANS balance between dopamine (DA) and 5-HT.

In patient number 1, the pre-H EC was very small. Within a day and a half of treatment, however, it increased to that of normal subjects. Since H is an antidopaminergic drug, it was reasonable to assume that the SNI of patient number 1 was very strong because of the excessive amount of "functional" DA in TS. I was excited about this possibility. But patient number 2 dampened my enthusiasm. Her pre-H EC was very large (thus her SNI was very weak), and it decreased slowly within twenty-five days to that of normal subjects. My assumption regarding the linear relationship between "functional" DA concentrations and of SNI strength did not make sense anymore. I rationalized that the technician must have made some mistakes. However, one year later, after six months without H, patient number 2 returned for treatment with H again. The technician was right and I was wrong! The second graph was almost identical with the first. In consideration of these findings I hypothesized, that the propensity towards TS becomes clinically manifest when the SNI is out of balance in either direction from the middle. H's therapeutic impact lies in the modulation of the mesencephalic central ANS balance (0.3 vs 1.8) towards the middle, which corresponds with the EC of normal subjects (0.8). In patient number 3, the patient who remained refractory to H, the pretreatment corresponded with the pretreatment EC of patient number 2, who responded to the drug. In variance with patient number 2 whose EC moved towards the middle with H treatment, in patient number 3, EC moved further away from the middle in the course of unsuccessful treatment with the drug. It has been suggested that the pupillary light reflex arc functions like nature's implanted electrode in the EWN. My findings are in line with this contention.

While the evaluation of PDHA, EPG, and the clinical response to H in TS were nearing completion in 1968, the twenty-four-hour urine collections from our three patients had to remain in the deep freeze, with the faint hope that one day a pharmacologist would become interested in carrying out a collaborative project with me, a clinician. While about two years passed and nothing happened, in 1970 Dr. Crane invited Hakerem, one of my collaborators and myself to present our work at the National Institute of Mental Health. There he introduced me to a pharmacologist named Messiha, who was looking for a clinician to collaborate with. The collaboration with Dr. Messiha further enriched our TS findings. The urinary DA excretion of patient number 1 (responder) had previously been elevated, but returned to normal within eleven weeks of H treatment. On the other hand the also elevated urinary DA excretion of patient number 3 (refractory) remained high in the course of H treatment. From patient number 2, no urine was collected.

Another finding I would like to comment on is the discrepancy between the TSR completed by the nurses and the BPRS which was completed by me on a single blind basis. Apparently the TSR rating of the nursing staff showed a 1 to 1 relationship with the dosages of H and (with minor exceptions) with PDHA. On the other hand, my own BPRS total morbidity scores turned out to be an embarrassing disaster: they showed no relationship either with the doses of H, or with PDHA. To save face, I began to look for some reasonable explanation for my failure to perform at the level of the nursing staff. I noticed that, in the first one and a half weeks, my ratings were consistent with PDHA and the nursing ratings, and only thereafter did the dissociation begin. Furthermore the dissociation between the ratings of the nurses and mine seemed to be somehow related to the unexpected increases in PDHA in weeks 3 and 4 and again in weeks 5 and 6. These were the weeks that were marked by severe emotional upheavals (Christmas, etc).

Was it possible that my "incompetence" could be due to the nature of the BPRS total morbidity score? Thus, I divided the total morbidity score empirically and used the BPRS factors 3, 5, and 9 separately. What I found was that Factor 9 (mannerisms and posturing) remained in keeping with the nurses' ratings whereas Factors 5 (tension and anxiety) and 3 (guilt and dread) went their own way. I was relieved.

With my BPRS findings I started to speak of cognitive-sensory-motor and intrapsychic-int-rapersonal-social-environmental factors and decided to subject the behavioural ratings done on the LORR scale we used with Fischer in our "taste study" to a similar analysis. To make a long story short, again I found a dissociation in improvement between the "cognitive-sensory-motor" items and the "interpersonal-social-environmental" items: that only the first set responded within the first twelve days of treatment with TFP. Obviously, hospitalization beyond twelwe days was needed to help the patients with their emotional and social readjust-ment (from two to one hundred days).

At about this time I became aware of Yakovlev's work in neuropathology and MacLean's in neurophysiology and began to think in terms of the "tripartite brain." I had not yet heard MacLean's much more appropriate term, "triune brain."

When I discussed my findings with my very senior colleague, Samuel Corson, he said, "This looks like more evidence of what Horsley Gantt [the prominent Virginian who by that time was one of the last living direct disciples of Pavlov] called 'schizokinesis' – a split between the psychomotor and visceral functions."

In view of all these experiences, I have resolved always to pay attention to the issue: does the improvement (or the lack of it) appear to be at the level of the visceral (hypothalamic – NE and 5 HT) integration or the psychomotor (mesencephalic – DA and 5 HT) integration? Each level calls for different therapeutic modalities to be applied.

In the past twenty-five years I have practised with this dichotomy in mind as a consultant and later on as a primary therapist (locum tenens), without precise documentation but with considerable success in different settings, including a general hospital with outpatients and acute in-patients, and four state hospitals with chronic and semi-chronic in-patients. In my opinion, optimum results in individual patients would be enhanced if permanent, detailed, quantitative, graphically-represented records of these and other variables relevant to patients' illnesses were available to study successes and failures. Isolating and comparing these two groups would be an important step in improving what is commonly called "titrating the individual patient's optimum dose."

PSYCHOPHARMACOLOGY AND BIOLOGICAL PSYCHIATRY
Pacemakers Towards a Scientific Psychopathology

Herman M. van Praag

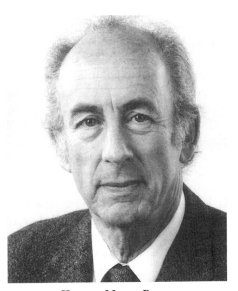

Herman M. van Praag

Between the early 1950s and the 1960s, psychiatry was the scene of two miracles. The first was the purely fortuitous discovery of four novel pharmacotherapeutic principles: the antipsychotic, the antidepressant, the mood-stabilizing, and the anxiolytic. The second miracle was the birth of a generation of psychiatrists willing, even eager, to measure and study empirically and systematically the phenomena they observed in psychiatric patients caused by psychotropic drugs – changes in both psychopathology and biology. Until then, psychiatrists had been primarily theoreticians, basing their views on a few observations and largely trusting the validity of those observations at face value. They had little motivation to verify empirically their ideas about diagnosis and treatment. Psychiatry was predominantly an essayistic discipline: psychologizing, with psychoanalytic ideas as the culminating point; philosophizing, an approach exemplified by anthropological psychiatry; and aestheticizing, particularly within the context of phenomenological psychiatry, where the handsomely formulated

Herman van Praag was the first professor of biological psychiatry and the first head of the Department of Biological Psychiatry at the University of Groningen in the Netherlands from 1966 to 1976. He subsequently became chairman of the Department of Psychiatry at the University of Utrecht, the Netherlands, and at the Albert Einstein College of Medicine in New York. Over the years, his research has mainly focused on biological psychiatry, psychopharmacology, and the psychopathology of affective disorders.

Van Praag was elected a fellow of the CINP in 1968. He served as Councillor of the 9th and 10th executive and as Vice-President of the 11th and 12th. Van Praag presented papers on "Some aspects of the metabolism of glucose and non-esterified fatty acids (NEFA) in depressed patients," and on "Influencing human indoleamine metabolism by means of a chlorinated amphetamine derivative with antidepressive action (p-chloro-N-methylamphetamine)" (Van Praag, Korf, Van Wondenberg and Korf) at the 5th and 6th Congresses respectively; and participated in Working Group 1 (Experimental and Clinical Biochemistry) as a formal discussant at the 4th Congress.

phrase to describe an experiential state often seemed more important than its clinical relevance. Psychiatry was a fascinating discipline, a discipline of ideas – sometimes brilliant ideas – but a discipline where one hypothesis was heaped with great ease on the next, and with little desire to test them.

It was psychopharmacology and its twin, biological psychiatry, that bred a generation of psychiatrists determined to convert their discipline into an empirical science. Methodologically, however, the field was not ready for this change. Empirical research requires a precise definition of the object of study: its demarcation from adjacent diagnostic constructs and methods for its assessment and measurement. Such methods were not available: diagnosis was not operationalized or standardized. With some, but not too much, exaggeration, one could say that there were as many classification systems as there were textbooks. "Schools" largely determined diagnostic approaches and terminology, and these were numerous. In the United States, psychoanalysis reigned supreme. Psychiatric conditions were thought to be determined primarily by individual life history and circumstances. Diagnostic generalizations were therefore considered to be little more than artefacts. "No diagnosis at all" was the adage in those circles. To diagnose was above all to individualize; diagnoses had to be tailor-made.

Psychopharmacology, with biological psychiatry in its wake forced psychiatry to change direction. The evolution occurred slowly but irresistibly. Hamilton published his rating scale for depression in 1960. The first standardized, structured interview to be introduced in psychiatry, our vital syndrome interview, appeared five years later (1). Psychometrics soon became a discipline in its own right. The method of standardized interviewing was further elaborated in the present state examination in 1974 (2), and in the schedule of affective disorders and schizophrenia (SADS), in 1978 (3). Rating scales soon proliferated, to such an extent that now we are suffering from an excess. There is an urgent need to study them comparatively, sort out those that are most usable, and try to reach international agreement in promoting some as standard instruments.

In retrospect, psychopharmacology and biological psychiatry have, I believe, leaned too heavily on psychometrics. Other strategies to analyze and measure abnormal human behaviour have received insufficient attention. More specifically, we have not taken sufficient advantage of the methods developed by experimental psychologists and ethologists. Experimental psychology provides ways to measure psychological (dys)functions with great precision, and often quantitatively as well. It offers the prospect of challenging psychological functions, that is, ascertaining whether they function within, below, or above normal limits. Ethology, the study of animals in their normal conditions, has developed refined methods of analysing the structure of complex behaviours in a strictly quantitative way. Studies applying these methods to human behavioural pathology are promising but few, e.g. Bouhuys (4).

In the late fifties, in the context of a study of the therapeutic and biological effects of monoamine oxidase (MAO) inhibitors in depression, the first attempts were made to standardize and operationalize the diagnosis of several subtypes of depression (5). Further developments in making the process of diagnosis more reliable were slow to appear, and only in the seventies (1972) did the St. Louis Group publish the Research Diagnostic Criteria (6), a large-scale proposal for a criteria-based, and thus reproducible, psychiatric taxonomy. It constituted the foundation for the third edition of the DSM. Published in 1980, it was the first standardized and operationalized classification system of psychiatric disorders. From the start it was embraced by psychiatrists, clinicians, and researchers alike. The ICD-10 followed, but it still plays second fiddle, particularly in research circles.

The DSM system is firmly rooted in Kraepelinian soil. It conceives mental disorders as discrete entities, each with its own symptomatology, course, and prognosis and, in principle, its own causation – "in principle" because so far little is known about the causes of mental disorder. Consequently, biological psychiatry is geared towards the elucidation of "markers" and eventually causes of discrete disorders, such as major depression, schizophrenia, generalized anxiety disorder, and many others.

In psychiatry the nosological disease model has been accepted almost axiomatically, and too little attention has been given to its validity. Regrettably so, because, though the model seems self-evident, on closer inspection it reveals foibles (7). On the basis of the model, one would expect most patients to show the symptoms belonging to one disorder. The contrary, however, is true: most show several syndromes at the same time, or rather, a patchwork of parts of several syndromes. The DSM system got around this difficulty by accepting that x number out of a series of y symptoms would suffice to qualify for a particular diagnosis. The price to be paid for this solution is diagnostic inaccuracy, in that each diagnostic label covers a variety of syndromes. The predictability of course, the prognosis, and the causational factors for a particular psychiatric condition, moreover, are vague, to say the least. Take, for example, the diagnosis of major depression. It may appear once in a lifetime or recur; it may remit completely or leave residual symptoms; it may be precipitated or occur "out of the blue," and similar precipitants may lead to different psychiatric conditions; antidepressants may be effective or turn out to be therapeutic failures; psychological interventions may be efficacious or of no avail. Thus the question of whether the disorders that we distinguish are true entities is a cardinal one. If not, our biological studies are built on quicksand. The search for the biological determinants of invalid constructs will probably generate invalid and irreproducible results.

Mental disorders can be conceived of in a different way: not as discrete disorders separable from each other, but as reaction forms to noxious stimuli with considerable interindividual variability and little consistency. The noxious stimulus might be of a biological or a psychological nature, it might come from within or without, and it could be genetically transmitted or acquired in the course of a lifetime. Such factors have in common that an individual cannot cope with them, physically or psychologically.

Noxious stimuli will perturb a variety of neuronal circuits and hence different psychological systems. The extent to which the various neuronal circuits will be involved will vary according to the individual, and consequently psychiatric conditions will lack symptomatological consistency and predictability. For instance, mood lowering will be combined with fluctuating degrees of anxiety, anger, obsessional thoughts, addictive behaviour, cognitive impairment, and psychotic features. These characteristics will vary in intensity and prominence between subjects and, over time, within subjects. Hence, psychopathological conditions are as variable as the shapes of clouds in the sky. One recognizes a cloud; its shape, however, is changeable and unpredictable. According to the reaction form model, the co-occurrence of various discrete mental disorders is mainly in appearance. In fact, we deal with ever-changing composites of psychopathological features.

The kind and measure of neuronal disruption which a noxious stimulus will induce is variable, contingent as it is on a number of factors. Most important are the intrinsic qualities of the stimulus and the resilience of the brain. Pre-existent neuronal defects may cause certain brain circuits to function marginally. An equilibrium barely maintained under normal conditions could fail if the demands were increased. Greater vulnerability can also be conceptualized on a psychological level in that imperfections in personality make-up render some individuals more than others vulnerable to stimuli that cause psychological disruption.

The reaction form model, if valid, would have profound consequences for biological psychiatry. The search for markers and eventually causes of discrete mental disorders would be largely futile. The farthest that one could go would be to group the multitude of reaction patterns in a limited number of diagnostic "basins," such as the psychotic, the dementia, and the affective reaction forms, each of which, however, would show considerable heterogeneity. Just as it is futile to look for the antecedents and characteristics of the group of abdominal disorders, for instance, it would be equally unwise to hope for the discovery of the pathophysiology of the "basin" of affective reaction forms. Within the scope of this model, the focus of biological psychiatric research must shift from the alleged mental "disorders" to disordered psychological domains. Schizophrenia, panic disorder, or major depression as such would not be studied, but rather disturbances in perception, information processing, mood regulation, anxiety regulation, or impulse control, to mention only a few areas. A biology of psychological dysfunctions – as they occur in dysfunctional mental states – would thus be the ultimate goal of biological psychiatric research (8). The systematic study of alternative models to the nosological disease approach seems urgent. That model shows too many shortcomings to continue to be accepted unconditionally.

All in all, it is fair to say that the diagnostic process in psychiatry has evolved dramatically since, and thanks to, the introduction of modern psychotropic drugs. We here witnessed the birth – or rather, rebirth (in view of the neuroanatomical studies in psychiatry that took place in the last part of the previous century) of biological psychiatry. We have moved far along the road from clever personal interpretations towards scientific rigour. However, by no means have we approached the desired end point. Diagnosis lacks quantitative precision and is based on a model that is much in need of scrutiny.

REFERENCES

1. Van Praag, H.M., Uleman, A.M., and Spitz, J. C. (1965). The vital syndrome interview: a structured standard interview for the recognition and registration of the vital depression symptom complex. *Psychiat. Neurol. Neurochir.* 68: 329-346.
2. Wing, J.K., Cooper, J.E., and Sartorius, N. (1974). *Measurement and Classification of Psychiatric Symptoms.* Cambridge: Cambridge University Press.
3. Endicott, J., and Spitzer, R.L. (1978). A diagnostic interview: the schedule of affective disorders and schizophrenia. *Arch. Gen. Psychiat.* 35, 837-844.
4. Bouhuys, A. L., and Van den Hoofdakker, R.H. (1991). The interrelatedness of observed behaviour of depressed patients and of psychiatrist: an ethological study on mutual influence. *J. Affect. Disord.* 23: 63-74.
5. Van Praag, H.M., and Leijnse, B. (1964). Die Bedeutung der Psychopharmakologie für die klinische Psychiatrie. Systematik als notwendiger Ausgangspunkt. *Nervenarzt* 34: 530-537.
6. Feighner, J.P., Robbins, E., Guze, S.B., Woodruff, R.A., Winokur, G., and Munoz, R. (1972). Diagnostic criteria for the use in psychiatric research. *Arch. Gen. Psychiat.* 26, 56-62.
7. Van Praag, H.M., and Leijnse, B. (1964). Die Bedeutung der Psychopharmakologie für die klinische Psychiatrie. Systematik als notwendiger Ausgangspunkt. *Nervenarzt* 34, 530-537.
8. Van Praag, H.M., Uleman, A.M., and Spitz, J.C. (1997). Over the mainstream: diagnostic requirements for biological psychiatric research. *Psychiat. Res.* (in press).

COUNTRY
MEMOIRES

In this section thirty-three clinicians and researchers involved with psychopharmacology present a personal memoir of the 1960s. The authors responded to the editors' invitation to write a first-person account of their participation in psychotropic drug development during this period.

The contributors are from a variety of countries and backgrounds. About two-thirds of the memoirs are from psychiatrists and one-third from other disciplines, including organic chemistry, neuropharmacology, psychophysiology and experimental psychology. The contributors have in common only that all were eye witnesses, and most were active participants, in the rise of psychopharmacology.

The vast majority of these memoirs are from psychopharmacologists elected to membership in the CINP during the first seven Congresses. To round off the story, the others were invited from countries which had no representation in CINP during the 1960s.

Scientific publication stresses impersonality. Yet these accounts, records of individual trajectories in the world of science, are anything but impersonal. The authors retain their distinctive voices. The editors have intervened minimally, and we hear in these memoirs the echo of national scientific traditions, of cultural context (one author describes his adventures in a "disco"), and of individual personality. Although the individual stories may differ, they are all tied together in their response to international psychotropic drug development in the 1960s. With this brief introduction, let the memoirs speak for themselves.

Memoirs from Around the World

PSYCHOPHARMACOLOGY IN ARGENTINA

Ronaldo Ucha Udabe

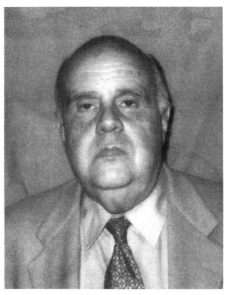

Ronaldo Ucha Udabe

I graduated from the Faculty of Medicine at the National University of Buenos Aires in 1958. My initial interest was in clinical neurology and I began my professional activities in this field at Ramos Mejía Hospital in Buenos Aires with two outstanding professors, José Pereyra Kafer and Gustavo Poch. Since at the time we did not have a psychiatric service in general hospitals, a high proportion of my patients were psychiatric.

My research interest in neurology was in hepatolenticular degeneration (Wilson's disease), but I was also involved in studying Khaler's disease (multiple myeloma), the subject matter of my first publication. During my short stay in the field I was more involved in treating psychiatric than neurological patients, and gained substantial experience in the use of chlorpromazine in the treatment of mania and schizophrenia. Another psychotropic drug we were using at the clinic was reserpine, a *Rauwolfia* alkaloid which was originally introduced in Argentina as an antihypertensive but promoted during the late 1950s by CIBA Laboratories for the treatment of depression. As we learned later on, it was a very dangerous practice, because electroconvulsive therapy may cause death in patients whose catecholamine and indoleamine stores are depleted by reserpine. Another psychotropic drug I recall using was prochlorperazine, a piperazine side chain containing phenothiazine we prescribed for psychotic patiens. Some years later I noted that prochlorperazine in the United States was marketed as an antiemetic drug.

In 1959 I received a scholarship from the Spanish government which allowed me to work for a year with Professor Juan José Lopez Ibor at the hospital which was to become the Reina Sofía Centre. Prior to my departure for Madrid I attended the International Congress of Physiology which was held in Buenos Aires that year. From the numerous excellent presentations, I found Erspamer's on serotonin one of the most stimulating.

I arrived in Madrid in October 1959 and shortly after my arrival I learned that Professor Lopez-Ibor was participating in a multicenter clinical trial with a new investigational drug that had similar therapeutic effects to chlorpromazine. It was one of the first clinical trials with the

Ronaldo Ucha Udabe is Past President of the Argentine Psychopharmacological Society. He coauthored the first handbook on psychopharmacology in Argentina.

butyrophenone, haloperidol, synthesized less than two years before in the laboratories of Janssen Pharmaceuticals in Beerse, Belgium. We had a distiguished guest lecturer every Wednesday in Professor Lopez-Ibor's department and one of these distinguished speakers during my stay was Roland Kuhn, who just about two years previously had reported on the antidepressant effects of the iminodibenzyl, imipramine.

The Madrid experience had a major impact on my future career development. On my return to Argentina in 1961, instead of continuing with neurology I obtained a position in the psychopharmacology laboratory of Borda Hospital in Buenos Aires. The director of the laboratory was Edmondo Fischer, a Hungarian exile, who was also for some time the head of the Department of Pharmacology at the University of Buenos Aires and at another time a consultant to Szabo Laboratories, an Argentine pharmaceutical company with an interest in psychotropics. Fischer became internationally known for his research with bufotenine in schizophrenia and phenylethylamine in depression. A large number of clinical and basic researchers and psychiatrists worked with Fischer. They included Spatz, Smolovich, Heller, Melgar, Fernandez Labriola, and others. My assignment in the laboratory was to do some basic research on alcoholic polyneuritis in animal models, in collaboration with Muchnik.

By the end of 1962 psychiatric services were established in all of the general hospitals in Buenos Aires, and I was appointed chief of the service at Rawson Hospital, a gigantic institution with sixteen hundred beds and a distinguished surgical tradition. I was still only thirty-years-old. It was while at Rawson that I became actively involved in clinical investi-gations with psychotropic drugs including multicenter clinical trials with diazepam (the second study in Latin America) and tranylcypromine, a monoamine oxidase inhibitor. We were among the first in Latin America to study desipramine (oral and intravenous), fluphenazine (in low and high doses), perphenazine, perphenazine enanthate, thioridazine and trimipramine in intravenous perfusion. We also were the first to use metronidazole in the treatment of alcoholism, as well as magnesium pemoline and diethylaminoethanol in minimal cerebral dysfunction.

The Argentine Society of Psychopharmacology was founded in 1963 and I became its first general secretary. The first president of the Society was Albert Bonheur and the first Vice President, Edmondo Fischer. I was to serve as president of the Society eight years later in 1971.

In 1964 and '65 my wife, Nora Portes, a professor of psychology, and I spent two years in France on a scholarship from the French government. We were based at Saint-Maurice with Henri Baruk, but once a week we attended the lectures given by Professors Delay, Deniker, Pichot, and Thuillier at Sainte-Anne Hospital. It was in 1964, during our stay in Paris, that the *Handbook in Psychopharmacology* I coauthored with Edmondo Fischer and Gustavo Poch was published. It was one of the first texts in psychopharmacology in the Spanish-speaking countries and the first text in psychopharmacology in Argentina.

I returned to Buenos Aires at the end of 1965 and resumed my activities at the hospital. In 1967 however, looking for a different kind of experience, I decided to retire temporarily from the hospital and accept first the position of consultant with a local pharmaceutical company and later on, the position of medical director with a multinational. During my years in industry, I participated in the launching of L-dopa and pimozide. I also served in 1968 as president of the Argentine Society of Psychosomatic Medicine. The founding of the International College of Psychosomatic Medicine was my proposal.

The International College became a reality and it was at the first meeting of the College, held in Guadalajara (Mexico), that I first met Thomas Ban. In those years, he was director of the World Health Organization-sponsored training program for teachers in psychopharmacology at McGill University in Montreal (Canada). I participated from July 1972 to April 1973 in the program and we have continued our collaboration in different research projects ever since. While in Montreal I was also in contact with Heinz Lehmann, who at the time was chairman of McGill's department of psychiatry. After Juan Peron's return from Spain and re-election as president of Argentina in April 1973, I was appointed director of the Argentine Food and Drug Administration and served in this position until Peron's death about a year later. I had known Peron since my childhood, through my father, who had a long and cordial relationship with him. My father was an engineer, who became rector of the National Technological University.

The rest of the story is outside the scope of this memoir. During the past twenty-five years I have been actively involved in clinical psychopharmacological research, and recently, the director of a program of the Barcelo Foundation which is dedicated to training professionals for doing clinical research in psychopharmacology.

THE 1960s: A REMINISCENCE
(Austria)

Otto H. Arnold

In the 1960s, European psychiatric research was practically identical with clinical research. It had been clinical studies that led to the discovery of neuroleptics and antidepressants. Compared to today, psychiatric research in the 1960s had distinct advantages and disadvantages. Among the disadvantages were the lack of standardized rating scales, and the absence of molecular-biological studies and electronic data processing; the minimal use of the double-blind design; and insufficient information on drug metabolism and on the effects of drugs on the electrical activity of the brain. (Pharmaco-EEG was still in an early stage of its development.) The advantages, on the other hand, included the availability of large sample sizes for clinical studies, the considerably better compliance of patients with treatment, the possibility for long-term follow-up with intensive clinical observations, and the close cooperation with internists to monitor side effects.

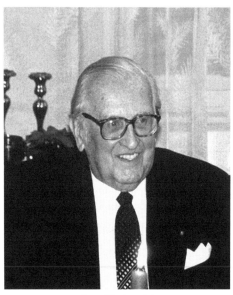

Otto H. Arnold

The exchange of experience was somewhat more difficult in the 1960s than it is today. The partition between the western countries and the eastern bloc impeded collegial contacts. I was very much aware of the need for such contacts and welcomed the opportunity to visit the Soviet Union as an "exchange professor" in 1964. Teaching at the psychiatric clinic of the Medical

Otto H. Arnold was born in Vienna, Austria, in 1917. He obtained his MD from the University of Vienna in 1942 and in 1962 became a professor of neuropsychiatry. Arnold has published books and 179 papers in the field of neuropsychopharmacology and schizophrenia. He is a founding member of the World Federation of Biological Psychiatry and a former consultant of the World Psychiatric Association.

Arnold was a founding member of the CINP and served as a secretary of the 4th Executive. He presented papers on "Der Einbau der Neuroleptica in die psychiatrische Therapie" (Arnold and Hoff) and "Psychopathologische und biochemische Untersuchungen zur Gruppe der Phenmetrazin-Psychosen (Ph. P)" (Arnold and Hofmann) at the 3rd and 6th Congresses respectively, and co-authored a paper on "Allgemeine Gesichtspunkte zur Pharmakopsychiatrie" (Hoff and Arnold) presented at the 1st Congress. He was a discussant in Working Group 6 (Dynamics and significance of psychopharmacological intervention in psychiatry) at the 4th Congress.

Academy of Sciences in Moscow made it possible for me to forge contacts between Russian colleagues and the World Psychiatric Association as well as with our Collegium. The close relationship with psychopharmacologists in Czechoslovakia that I established in those years contributed greatly to the organization of the CINP congress in Prague in 1970.

What I remember most about the 1960s was my fascination with the impact of the new antidepressants on patients whom I had known for many years. The feeling that we were engaged in pioneering work inspired us so much that we were ready to give up leisure time and holidays to pursue our research. I also enjoyed the personal nature of my early international contacts. It was due to my relationship with Professor Mezey of Merck, Sharp and Dohme, that I became in 1961 the first European psychiatrist to use amitriptyline; and it was due to my relationship with Professor von Euler that I was first to study the therapeutic effects of dibenzepine (Noveril) in depression. Furthermore, as a result of my contacts with Geigy, I was the first psychiatrist to study the therapeutic effects of clomipramine (Anafranil) in patients. In my mind, the fact that I was among the pioneers in testing those antidepressants which became the reference (standard) drugs was not due to chance, but the result of my personal relationships with people and my contacts with colleagues in the CINP and in the pharmaceutical industry.

For me the 1960s were characterized mainly by the rapid development of antidepressants. I was the head of a department at the University Clinic for Psychiatry and Neurology (directed by Professor H. Hoff) in those years. There were 100 hospitalized male patients in my department, which allowed me to observe and evaluate an average of thirty to forty patients suffering from various types of depression at any time. In collaboration with my associates I could study several new antidepressants concurrently. The following is an overview of my research in those years:

DRUGS	CASES	TOTAL SUCCESS	PARTIAL SUCCESS	NO EFFECT	ONSET	DELIRIUM
	N	%	%	%	DAY	%
Imipramine	185	38	50	25	10-14	0,55
Clomipramine	35	41	43	16	5-9	3
Desipramine	50	37	48	15	14-20	1
Opipramol	104	36	31	33	10-20	0
Amitriptyline	150	45	30	25	3-5	5
Protriptyline	100	48	36	16	1-3	9
Dibenzepine	85	38	39	23	8-14	0

The long-term follow-up periods in those days, which sometimes extended for years after the completion of the clinical trial or the acute phase of treatment, allowed for studying the effects of long-term therapy on the course of unipolar and bipolar depressive illnesss. We noted that the course of depressive illness treated with drugs in some patients displayed chronicity, i.e., continuous mild pathology, whereas in other patients it displayed lability, i.e., continuous variation of mood. A third alternative, seen in other patients, was "decoupling," i.e., separation of depressed mood from its seasonal or temporal dimension, a factor that influences the recurrence of depressive episodes.

For me the CINP congresses of the 1960s were intimately linked to stories which did not get into the records. One of these stories is from the Basel congress in 1960 where Hans Hoff was to become president elect. When he climbed the stairs to the rostrum to thank the Congress for voting for him, he lost his balance and, to avoid falling, took a big backwards step. While approaching the rostrum for the second time he made it clear that his step backwards should not be taken symbolically as refusing the honour bestowed on him.

In Munich two years later, Paul Hoch gave an impressive keynote speech during the gala dinner at the Bayerischer Hof. It lasted for well over an hour, and some

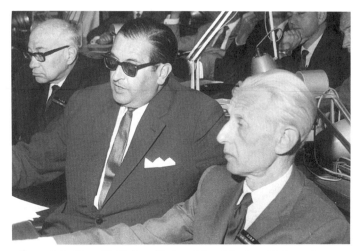

From left: Hans Hoff, Otto H. Arnold and Lothar Kalinowsky

of the audience simply fell asleep. The next day, Heinz Lehmann told us his story about sleepiness. Apparently after a day of intensive work, he had fallen asleep dead tired. Suddenly the phone rang, waking him. Still half-asleep, he answered it, "Lehmann sleeping" (instead of "speaking").

At the 1964 congress in Birmingham, Philip Bradley arranged lodging at the students' dormitory of the university. I spoke at the congress about the experimental induction of delirious states. The next morning while my wife and I were breakfasting with the Flügels, Professor Flügel said: "I slept very little last night because I've been wondering all the time why anyone would want to induce delirium artificially. It's bad enough watching it when it occurs spontaneously."

During the Washington Congress in 1966, Jean Delay delivered a speech at the gala evening in the Sheraton Hotel. He was followed by other speakers. There was then a short break before the dessert was served. I had finished my pipe and as usual was knocking it out on the ashtray. Suddenly the noisy hall fell silent; everyone was looking towards my table. All that remained to do for me was to stand up and say a few words of thanks to our American hosts.

In 1968, my wife and I participated in the CINP congress in Tarragona. On entering the hotel lobby, my wife said that she would like to call home from the post office to tell our family that we had arrived. I suggested asking for the post office at the reception desk. My wife had studied Spanish and had spoken the language quite well, but many years had gone by without using it. So when she asked the receptionist about the nearest post office, she used the word *corrida,* instead of *correos.* The receptionist was impressed by these Austrians, who immediately after their arrival in Spain, wanted to know about the next bullfight. They certainly provided us with detailed information.

In this manner, I experienced the 1960s as a kind of golden age of neuropsychopharmacology in which scientific rationality still seemed to be imbued with romanticism and worldly wisdom. We left it to the researchers of the future, starting from a much more developed scientific base than we did, to generate the findings which will eventually enable humanity to live a more stable, healthy, and happy life.

A BRAZILIAN EXPERIENCE IN PSYCHOPHARMACOLOGY

Elisaldo A. Carlini

My career in science started forty-five years ago when, in 1952 I enrolled in medicine at the Escola Paulista de Medicina in the city of São Paulo (Brazil), now the Federal University of São Paulo (UNIFESP). At that time I was pretty sure that my destiny would be to practise the "noble profession" in the Amazon area, nearly 4,000 kilometres from the city I was born in, treating poor people. But shortly after I began with my studies I attended a seminar of two professors, Jose Leal Prado and Jose Ribeiro do Valle, from the department of biochemistry and pharmacology, which had such a profound effect on me that I changed my plans. The two professors were rare examples in Brazil of medical doctors who did basic research instead of being successful (and wealthy) practitioners treating private patients. Their seminar dealt with the renin–hypertensinogen–hypertensin system (today the last two substances are called "angiotensinogen" and "angiotensin") and I was so fascinated by what I learned that I decided to dedicate myself to research that could save the lives of hypertensive people.

Led by this almost adolescent and naive dream, as a second-year medical student, I decided to begin with my research training in the department of biochemistry and pharmacology of the University; and several years later with two of my colleagues I published a paper on hypertensin I (1). It was one of the first reports on the "converting enzyme," the inhibition of which now represents an important therapeutic approach to the control of hypertension. In those years I also became interested in the research carried out by Professor Ribeiro do Valle, on *Cannabis sativa*. Maconha, the Brazilian folk name for the plant, was considered a "vice" of the poor and was very much used in north-east Brazil at the time.

About 1955 or 1956 I came across what was, I think, one of the first issues of a new journal, *Psychopharmacologia*, edited in Germany (now called *Psychopharmacology*). Looking at the journal I pledged to myself that I would publish a paper in it on my research on the behavioural effects of marijuana. It was not an easy promise to keep. At that time there was no research laboratory in experimental psychology in Brazil where I could find help in learning the methodology of behavioural research.

In 1960 I was given a golden opportunity in my scientific career: I was awarded a Rockefeller Foundation fellowship. After my arrival in the United States, I spent sixteen months in the biochemistry department of Tulane University in New Orleans, going later to the department of pharmacology of Yale University in New Haven, where I learned about a world that had been unknown to me. In Brazil I was used to the traditional gadgets of the pharmacologists, whereas at Yale every room had a Beckman DU spectrophotometer and the

Elisaldo A. Carlini was born in 1930. He obtained his medical degree in 1957 from the Escola Paulista de Medicina in São Paulo, Brazil, and his master of science degree in 1962 from Yale University. He was visiting research professor at the Mount Sinai School of Medicine of the City University of New York in 1970. He is currently full professor of psychopharmacology at the Federal University of São Paulo and director of the Brazilian Centre for Information on Psychotropic Drugs.

Carlini was elected a fellow of the CINP in 1978.

laboratory was equipped with the most advanced instrumentation modern technology could offer. Because of this, at a certain point I felt that I was running biochemical assays instead of doing "real" pharmacological experiments.

I was very fortunate to work under the guidance of Jack Peter Green, a competent scientist with keen intelligence and a great human being. I became part of an enthusiastic research team with three young American scientists for approximately two and a half years. During that time my assignment from Jack was to demonstrate the presence of histamine in synaptosomal fractions of rat brain. I succeeded with my task by using density gradient centrifugation together with a spectrofluorometric method and a biological assay on the guinea-pig ileum. The results were published in 1962 and 1963 (2, 3), and were to become frequently cited articles in the literature.

As time passed I became increasingly concerned about my return to Brazil. The laboratory in São Paulo lacked the equipment I had learned to use in United States, and there were no funds available in the foreseeable future to buy any. With consideration of my needs, Jack advised me to start attending meetings and conferences of other departments at Yale in order to see what I could adopt from there for Brazil. Encouraged by Jack, I began to attend the informal meetings of Neal Miller of the department of psychology, and the conferences of Daniel Freedman of the department of psychiatry. I also met Nicholas Giarman of the department of pharmacology with some regularity to exchange ideas. During a rather short period I became acquainted with many new ideas and came to realize that creative and interesting studies could be done using "home-made," simple equipment.

Upon my return to Brazil in 1964, I chose to study the effects of *Cannabis sativa* extracts on the behaviour of rodents. But I could not start with my research, because a few days after my arrival home the civilian government was overthrown by the military. Everything was turned upside down and it took me a few months to adapt to the new situation.

My first research project in Brazil was a study of the effects of cannabis on learning in rats. In this study I used a handmade Lashley III maze for testing. The results of this study, my first truly independent work, were published in *Psychopharmacologia* in 1965 (4). With this publication my pledge to publish in this journal was fulfilled. My first paper was followed by several others, including one with Karniol on the pharmacological interaction between cannabidiol and delta 9-tetrahydrocannabinol (5), another with Bueno on dissociation learning in marijuana tolerant rats (6), and others on the effects of psychotropic drugs on several parameters, using rather simple methodology adapted or developed in my own laboratory. Several of these publications have been frequently quoted in the literature, and one of them (5) was classified among the fifty most cited papers published in 1973 by scientists from the developing countries of the Third World.

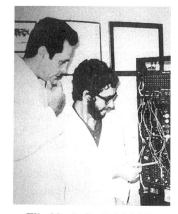

In the early 1970s I finally managed to obtain a grant from the Brazilian government to buy my first piece of "modern" equipment: an automatic Skinner box. It created an interesting situation because soon after the honeymoon phase with that fancy box, my scientific reasoning changed to "What kind of hypothesis shall I establish in order to run an experiment with this box?" instead of the reasoning I had

Elisaldo A. Carlini (right)

formerly used: "What kind of equipment do I need in order to test this hypothesis?" This sort of mental change brought about what I later called "equipment dependence" (like a drug dependence in which the patient's everyday life is determined by the substance). It is like a mental disease that takes over the scientist's mind.

Since I refused to be enslaved by any kind of equipment or methodology, I used to spend at least one hour every day at the library, reading bits and pieces of the scientific literature. I always found it great fun to leaf through an array of different sources, moving from clinical to biochemical journals. I strongly resist using the computer to retrieve only papers selected by keywords. I feel that such a mechanical search takes away pleasure and in the long run narrows knowledge.

During one of my daily visits to the library, I came across a picture of two aggressive rats that had previously been deprived of REM sleep and injected with amphetamine (7). The rats' behaviour displayed in that picture was quite similar to some aspects of aggressive display I had previously observed in rats chronically treated with cannabis extract and deprived of food. I decided to inject cannabis in REM-sleep-deprived rats and found that the rats became aggressive to the point that some deaths occurred. Since that time the relationship between REM-sleep deprivation, dopaminergic systems, *Cannabis sativa,* and aggressive behaviour has been an important line of research at UNIFESP, yielding several doctoral dissertations and published papers.

Parallel to my research activities, I have devoted part of my time to organizing the Brazilian Center for Information on Psychotropic Drugs (Centro Brasileiro de Informaçes sobre Drogas Psicotrópicas, or CEBRID), involved in the collection and dissemination of information on the non-medical use of psychotropic drugs in the country. CEBRID has already carried out four surveys on drug use among Brazilian students and street children, and has remained active to-date.

In 1994 I was chosen by the World Health Organization as a candidate for serving on the United Nations International Narcotic Control Board (INCB), and I was elected to this important post by the Economic and Social Council of the UN. Just after my election I was invited by our Minister of Health to become the national secretary of sanitary surveillance. I was nominated for this post by the president of Brazil and moved to Brasilia, the capital of the country. Unfortunately, by accepting this appointment I had to give up the INCB post.

After the completion of my assignment in Brasilia, I returned to the university and the directorship of CEBRID, resuming my research on Brazilian medicinal plants . As I am now sixty-seven years old, I have only a couple of years before I reach the age of compulsory retirement. But I will certainly be working enthusiastically for much longer than that, I hope that I am not too optimistic in saying, for the next fifteen or twenty years.

REFERENCES
1. Carlini, E.A., Picarelli, Z.P., and Prado, J.L. (1958). Pharmacological activity of hypertensin I and its conversion into hypertensin II. *Bull. Soc. Chim. Biol.* 40: 1825-1834.
2. Carlini, E.A., and Green, J.P. (1962). The subcellular distribution of histamine, slow-reacting substance and 5-hydroxytriptamine in the brain of the rat. *Brit. J. Pharmacol.* 20: 264-278.
3. Carlini, E.A., and Green, J.P. (1963). The measurement of histamine in brain and its distribution. *Biochem. Pharmacol.* 12: 1448-1449.
4. Carlini, E.A., and Kramer, C. (1965). Effects of Cannabis sativa (marijuana) on the maze performance of the rat. *Psychopharmacologia* (Berlin) 7: 175-181.
5. Karniol, I.G., and Carlini, E.A. (1973). Pharmacological interaction between cannabidiol and delta 9-tetrahydro-cannabinol. *Psychopharmacologia* (Berlin), 33: 53-70.
6. Bueno, O.F.A., and Carlini, E.A. (1972). Dissociation of learning in marijuana tolerant rats. *Psychopharmacologia* (Berlin), 25: 49-56.
7. Ferguson, J., and Dement, W. (1969). The behavioral effects of amphetamine on REM deprived rats. *J. Psychiat. Res.* 7: 111-118.

ANTIDEPRESSIVE MECHANISMS AND RESERPINE SEDATION – A MODEL FOR DEPRESSION?
(Germany)

Norbert Matussek

In 1961, with a fellowship from the National Institutes of Health (NIH) in Bethesda, I had the opportunity to spend a year with Dr. B.B. Brodie at the National Heart Institute. I had been rather discouraged about my work with Substance P at the Max Planck Institute in Munich and thought that this would be a good opportunity to shift the main thrust of my research to the study of schizophrenia.

I had first become interested in schizophrenia after Wooley and Shaw's formulation of their serotonin (5-HT) hypothesis of the disorder in 1954. Because in the early 1960s Brodie was

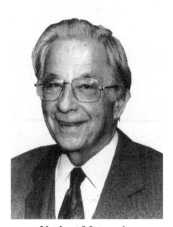

Norbert Matussek

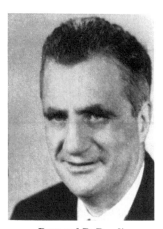

Bernard B. Brodie

one of the leading scientists in the neurochemistry of 5-HT, I was looking forward to working with him on the neurobiology of the disease.

Norbert Matussek was born in Berlin in 1927. After completing his studies in medicine and chemistry in Heidelberg, he worked with Professor Butenandt in Tübingen before joining the Max-Planck Institute of Psychiatry in Munich. From 1961-62 he was at the National Institutes of Health with B.B. Brodie, and from 1971-87, at the Psychiatric Hospital of the University of Munich. He is the recipent of several awards for his contributions to the understanding of the neurobiology of depression.

Matussek was elected a fellow of the CINP in 1964. He presented on "L-dopa in the treatment of depression" at the 7th Congress, and coauthored papers on "The effect of elctroconvulsive shock on norepinephrine metabolism in the brain and on behavior induced by certain pharmaca" (Steinhauff and Matussek), and on "Changes in tyrosine levels in affective disorders" (Benkert and Matussek) at the 6th and 7th Congresses respectively. Matussek was a formal discussant in Working Group 1 (Experimental and clinical biochemistry) at the 4th Congress.

Shortly after my arrival in Bethesda from Europe, still shaken from Hurricane Esther while crossing the Atlantic by boat, Brodie invited me to his house. He was sick that day, but still he outlined to me his concept of the neurochemistry of the ergotropic and trophotropic systems. It was a kind of brainstorming session and he seemed to be happy to talk to someone who would listen. And I did listen with reverence and respect even if, with my poor comprehension of English, I understood little. After he finished with his monologue, he asked me what I would like to do during the year. I was prepared for this question and expected that he would be excited about my interest in studying the circadian cycle of 5-HT in the brain and similar other ideas. He listened while I was talking, occasionally shaking his head. But when I stopped talking, he told me in a friendly manner to forget about whatever I proposed, and that I should first learn from Erminio (Mimo) Costa, his deputy chief (at the time), how to estimate 5-HT in the brain with the spectrophotofluorimetric method.

Later on, I learned that such nightly brainstorming sessions were customary for Brodie. Sometimes he would come to the laboratory in the late afternoon and ask me in a friendly way, "German boy," – I think my family name was too difficult for him to pronounce – "would you like to join me for dinner tonight?" Naturally I was flattered by his invitation, which actually meant that after work I had to drive him home in my old twenty-five-dollar Dodge. We had a brief dinner with Mrs. Brodie, who called her husband respectfully "Doctor," and after dinner brainstorming started, lasting until a couple of hours after midnight. For poor Mimo Costa it went on usually practically every night until the early morning hours.

In addition to the brainstorming sessions at his house at night, sometimes he might also invited people working on a specific project to his small office in the afternoon to discuss their findings and provide them with his interpretations of their data. I had the impression that he needed this kind of session to clarify his thinking and to develop new ideas. By participating in these discussions I got to know Brodie. He was a bright, intelligent, and creative scientist. His speculations were stimulating.

Brodie's circadian rhythm was practically reversed; he worked at night and came to the laboratory about noon. Sometimes when I was working at night I had to call and report to him my most recent findings, the results I just had obtained. On these occasions, he gave me instructions about how to continue the experiment. He was the most stimulating teacher I have ever had.

During the time I was in Brodie's laboratory, Fridolin Sulser and Marcel Bickel were carrying out some fascinating experiments. They found that desmethylimipramine (DMI) reversed sedation induced both by reserpine and by the benzoquinolizines. Prior to them in 1959, Domenjoz and Theobald from the Geigy Company found that imipramine antagonized the sedative effects of reserpine. Considering the findings in his own laboratory, Brodie suggested that imipramine's antagonism of reserpine-induced sedation was due to DMI, its active metabolite. At a certain point we all thought that the reversal of reserpine-induced sedation by imipramine or DMI was somehow connected to the mechanism of the therapeutic effect of antidepressant drugs.

Since DMI counteracted reserpine-induced sedation more rapidly than imipramine, I think Brodie also believed that DMI should have a faster therapeutic onset than imipramine in depressed patients. In keeping with Brodie's contention, psychiatrists at three Swiss psychiatric clinics – Pierre Dick in Geneva, Paul Kielholz in Basel, and Walter Pöldinger in St. Urbain – found that the onset of therapeutic effects of DMI (G35020) in many cases was more rapid than that of imipramine, i.e., within the first twenty four to forty-eight hours. This was reported together with some dramatic case reports in the proceedings of a colloquium held at Kielholz's clinic in Basel on August 29, 1961. Today, we still would be very happy if we had one such rapidly acting antidepressant drug.

I changed my plans and instead of continuing to speculate about schizophrenia I decided to pursue research in the field of depression. I asked Elwood O. Titus, a senior scientific assistant in Brodie's laboratory, to teach me the methodology of measuring H3-noradrenaline (NA) uptake in tissues. Titus was experienced in this methodology. It was one of those curious facts that Titus, in collaboration with H.J. Dengler, a visiting German scientist, discovered in Brodie's laboratory that imipramine inhibits H3-NA-uptake, at the same time and in the same building as Axelrod did in collaboration with G. Hertting, a scientist from Austria. Both groups published in 1961 practically the same results, one, Dengler's (1) in *Nature*, the other, Axelrod's (2) in *Science*. Later on usually the Axelrod paper was cited as reference for NA-uptake inhibition, which to me did not seem to be correct. Of course, Dengler and Hertting, as two German-speaking scientists, knew each other. Many years later I asked both whether they had talked about their experiments perhaps during lunch in the cafeteria of NIH or somewhere else. They said they had not.

Within this context, one of my conversations with Brodie might be relevant. I was to estimate a specific enzyme activity with a method which was used in Sidney Udenfriend's laboratory around the corner on the same floor. To get going more quickly, I asked Brodie whether I could ask Udenfriend to let me watch the particular method in question in his laboratory. Brodie looked at me shocked, and replied: "German boy, don't do that! Don't talk to anybody about what we are doing! You have enough time to learn the method by yourself." This kind of "paranoia" that somebody could steal your idea was not so rare in the NIH, as I learned later on. At the time I could not understand this mistrust. Nowadays we all know this is what happens in the scientific world.

It is regrettable that the relationship between these two great scientists, Brodie and Axelrod, was so strained. Axelrod was for a long time Brodie's technician, then left Brodie to study chemistry and to work alone. Many famous scientists in the field of neuropsychopharmacology are disciples of Brodie or Axelrod. Regrettably, only Axelrod got the Nobel Prize; many scientists feel that Brodie deserved it too. Kanigel, a scientific journalist, wrote extensively about the relationship between these two men (3). And in an interview with Axelrod by Healy (4), Axelrod himself talked about his relationship with Brodie.

After a stimulating year at NIH, during which I became somewhat familiar with psycho-pharmacology, I began to work in Munich on the mechanism of action of antidepressant drugs with several first-class junior associates, such as Manfred Ackenheil, Otto Benkert, Eckart Ruther, and others. Within our small group I instituted Brodie's tradition of brainstorming. Each day at around four p.m. we met for a coffee break and talked about the results of the experiments of the day. Some people did not like this, because they wanted to repeat each experiment five to ten times before discussing the result. But I was influenced by Brodie's methods of thinking and talking. We worked on the reversal of benzoquinolizine sedation with DMI and cocaine, which has in some way a similar effect to DMI on NA-uptake and reserpine sedation. I took some cocaine orally once, and it had no effect on me. I did not know that this drug had to be sniffed to be effective. Maybe this protected me from cocaine addiction during our work with this dangerous compound.

Paul Kielholz, at the time director of the University Clinic in Basel, proposed a special depressive syndrome. He called it "Erschöpfungsdepression" (exhaustion depression). My coworker Eckart Ruther thought that if the Sprague-Dawley-rats we worked with were to swim (which they usually don't do) until exhaustion, this might provide a good animal model for exhaustion depression. Although Kielholz and other psychiatrists were thinking of psychic rather than physical stress conditions, we began to study in our animal model the exhaustion syndrome by examining how they behaved, what happened with the amines in their brain, and how DMI, dopa and 5-hydroxytryptophan (5-HTP) affected them. After swimming, the poor rats were cataleptic. The NA was decreased in their brain, just as after reserpine administration, but in contrast to reserpine administration, their brain 5-HT increased. DMI and dopa counteracted the cataleptic state, whereas 5-HTP prolonged it. This so-called swimming test is also used today as a screening test for antidepressant properties like reserpine sedation. Sometimes the test is referred to as the Porsolt Test. But as the well-known and fair-minded pharmacologist Porsolt told Ruther, if it was to be called anything it should be called the Ruther Test.

In the early 1960s a lot of animal experiments with antidepressants focused on the importance of the NA-system in the brain in affective disorders. The findings of Everett and Toman (5) made us aware of the reversal of reserpine sedation in animal experiments; it seemed there might be a disturbance in catecholamine metabolism in depressed patients. Later on in the United States, two independent groups published their results about NA and depression at the same time (6, 7). I also published in a German journal at that time. Our experiments all converged on the same conclusion, that a NA-deficit in the nerve endings just as after reserpine administration or swimming is most probably responsible for the depressive syndrome in people (8). But none of us had any real evidence for this deficit in depressed patients. The methods for the estimation of NA and its metabolites in CSF were not yet available. In retrospect it is clear that 3-methoxy-4-phenylglycol (MHPG) determinations in the cerebrospinal fluid (CFS) of depressed patients did not yield to a breakthrough in terms of the NA-deficit hypothesis of depression. Yet we thought that at least we should examine whether dopa as the precursor of dopamine (DA) and NA could be an antidepressant, because it counteracts the reserpine and exhaustion induced cataleptic state after swimming. In Munich I had good relations with Walter Birkmayer of Vienna, who treated his Parkinsonian patients with L-dopa with great success. First we infused L-dopa, instead of administering it by mouth, to get more dopa in in the brain. Peripherally acting decarboxylase inhibitors were not yet available. Because we expected a stimulatory effect from L-dopa, we selected depressed patients with motor retardation and observed them for three to six hours. We expected a very fast antidepressive effect as in reserpinized animals or Parkinsonian patients. In eight out of ten patients we saw a clear activating effect – the patients talked more about their problems, and so on. It is perfectly understandable that the patients talked more than usual about their problems. In this big *Landesnervenkrankenhaus* (state hospital), where we sought our patients, the psychiatrists usually talked only very briefly with the patients during their rounds, whereas we in contrast spent hours and hours sitting with them in a kind of talking therapy. This was probably more important than the dopa-infusion. When a peripherally-acting decarboxylase inhibitor (Ro 44602), developed by the well-known pharmacologists A. Pletscher and M. Da Prada of Hoffmann La-Roche (Basel) was made available to us, we started a placebo-controlled study. Now we could administer dopa by mouth and treat our depressed patients who exhibited motor retardation with it for eleven to eighteen days. We felt this period should be enough to fill up the depleted NA-storage we postulated in the nerve terminals of the patients. In the sixties nobody was talking about down or up regulation at receptors and adaptation about the time we finished our study with thirty-one patients (eighteen treated with dopa and thirteen with placebo), Fred Goodwin and Biff Bunney from NIMH published the findings of their similar study on "Nine patients with predominantly retarded depression" in *The Lancet* (9). They found a clear improvement in three patients. In our study we found patients in each group with strong improvement but no significant difference between groups (10). Both groups presented their results at the CINP congress in Prague in August 1970.

This was about one year after the invasion by Russian troops of Czechoslovakia. I told Fred Goodwin about the events in my car on the way from Munich to Prague and back. The political situation was still quite tense, to the extent that one night in a disco the police arrived to make trouble. But Fred, as a member of NIH, had a diplomatic passport. When he showed his passport to the police, they immediately left the disco. It seemed they did not want political complications with the United States. On our journey back to Munich, the police at the border wanted to confiscate one of my books, written by an American communist about the Russian revolution, which I had brought with me from Germany. I protested vehemently and I believe they let me go with my book because an American "diplomat" was sitting in my car – namely Fred.

I was very disappointed that dopa had no antidepressant properties. Does this mean that catecholaminergic mechanisms are not disturbed in affective disorders? Arvid Carlsson, an outstanding neuropharmacologist, and his coworkers demonstrated that after using dopa, only dopamine increases in the brain, whereas NA does not. With Otto Benkert we enlarged this study and also found no NA increase in the brain. Menec Goldstein, a very bright and creative pharmacologist, told me later that he found an NA increase after dopa application only in some specific brain areas. Our conclusion, however, was that reserpine sedation, which could be counteracted by dopa, was not a good animal model for depression in humans, because otherwise dopa would have had antidepressant effects.

But the question regarding the antidepressant effect of 5-HTP, the precursor of 5-HT, still remained to be answered. Since Arvid Carlsson (11) found no reversal of reserpine-induced sedation with 5-HTP in 1957 (in contrast to dopa), I was sceptical about the usefulness of 5-HTP in depression. Arvid told me that Brodie had also been sceptical about it. But Alec Coppen, a well-known biologically-oriented psychiatrist from the UK, found that tryptophan contributed to the treatment of depression in patients who had received monoamine oxidase inhibitor (MAOI) (12). On the basis of his findings he postulated a disturbance in the 5-HT metabolism in the brain of depressed patients. After 5-HTP was made available in the seventies, Japanese psychiatrist, Professor Sano, published an enthusiastic paper about the strong therapeutic effect of 5-HTP. After three days of treatment the patients emerged from their depression.

Together with Otto Benkert, Eckart Ruther and Hanns Hippius (as principal investigator) we examined the antidepressant effect of 5-HTP in an open study. Independently of each other we observed our patients very carefully every day. We came to the conclusion that at the very best our patients must have been quite different from Sano's, because 5-HTP in Munich showed no antidepressant activity. At the same time Jules Angst in Zurich had similar results and so we published our findings together (13). I think today most psychiatrists would agree that 5-HTP is not an antidepressant. However, I learned from Herman van Praag's farewell lecture in Maastricht this year, that "5-HTP appeared to exert a therapeutic effect and, if chronically administered, a prophylactic effect on depression (14)." I met the main represen-tatives of the 5-HT-hypothesis, Alec Coppen and Herman van Praag, in a small group of about ten to twelve scientists, called the International Group for Study of the Affective Disorders (IGSAD). This group was founded by Jules Angst and Carlo Perris in about 1970. I became a member later on. We met every year at different locations around the world. Max Hamilton, Georges Winokur, Detlev von Zerssen, Paul Grof and others also belong to this circle. I was more convinced of catecholaminergic mechanisms, but Herman and Alec believed in the importance of 5-HT in affective disorders. Nonetheless, we have always been good friends. If we were psychoanalysts, each of us would belong to a different school and we would be antagonists who never talked to each other. After one of these IGSAD meetings in Canada, Herman and I had to give a lecture about our work in a small university in the early afternoon. Our host invited us to an excellent French lunch which, of course, included good, heavy, red wine. Herman, in the tradition of such abstainers as Manfred Bleuler or Emil Kraepelin, refused, but I enjoyed the Bordeaux. Directly after lunch we had to give our lecture. Herman spoke first and gave the transporter for the slides in the first row to me.

He started his lecture, which I knew very well. The lights were off. Two or three times I heard his voice: "The next slide, please." Then, however, I fell into a deep sleep and maybe I was dreaming of a joke because suddenly I heard all the people in the audience laughing and Herman's voice very loud next to me: "Next slide, please." Immediately, I woke up as if bitten by a snake and from then on I did not go to sleep any more during the rest of Herman's talk. Herman has forgiven me my lapse.

When I look back today on nearly forty years of research on the mechanism of action of antidepressive drugs, I think that we were on the wrong track in approaching the problem with the reserpine sedation reversal model. In affective disorders there is neither a 5-HT- nor a NA-deficit alone, as there is a dopamine deficit in Parkinson's disease. To understand mind and soul, or psychiatric disorders, is more complicated than we expected forty years ago, when I still thought it would be possible to find out the neurobiological disturbance of depression or the mechanism of antidepressant effects during my lifetime. Today it does not appear that the Decade of the Brain will solve these problems. Many years of neurobiological research will be necessary to clear up the pathophysiology of depression.

REFERENCES
1. Dengler, H.J.. Spiegel, H.E., and Titus, E. (1961). Effects of drugs on uptake of isotopic norepinephrine by cat tissues. *Nature* (London) 191: 816-817.
2. Axelrod, J., Whitby, L.G,.and Hertting, G. (1961). Effect of psychotropic drugs on the uptake of H3-norepinephrine by tissues. *Science* 133: 383.
3. Kanigel, R. (1980). *Apprentice to Genius*. New York: McMillan Publishing Company.
4. Healey, D. (1996). *The Psychopharmacologists, Interviews*. New York: Aftaman. An Imprint of Chapman Hall
5. Everett, G.M., and Toman, J.E.P. (1959). Mode of action of Rauwolfia alkaloids and motor activity. In: *Biological Psychiatry*, Vol 1 New York-London: Grune & Stratton.
6. Bunney, W.E. Jr., and Davis, J.M. (1964). Norepinephrine in depressive reactions. *Arch. Gen. Psychiatry* 14:83.
7. Schildkraut, J.J. (1965). The catecholamine hypothesis of affective disorders:a review of supporting evidence. *Am. J. Psychiatry* 122: 509.
8. Matussek, N. (1966). Neurobiologie und Depression. *Med. Wschr.* 20:109-112.
9. Goodwin, F.K., Brodie, H.K., Murphy, D.L. and Bunney, W.E. (1970) *The Lancet* 1: 908.
10. Matussek, N. Benkert, O., Schneider, K., Otten, H., Pohlmeier, H. (1970). L-dopa plus decarboxylase inhibitor in depression. *The Lancet* II: 660-661, 1970.
11. Carlsson, A., Lindquist, M., and Magnusson, T. (1957). 3,4-dihydroxy-phenylalanine and 5-hydroxy-tryptophan as reserpine antagonists. *Nature* 180: 1200.
12. Coppen, A., Shaw, D., and Farell, J.P. (1963). The potentiation of the antidepressive effets of a monoamineoxidase inhibitor by tryptophan. *The Lancet* II: 61-64.
13. Matussek, N., Angst, J., Benkert, O., Gmur, M., Papousek, M., Ruther, E., and Woggon, B. (1974). The effect of L-5-hydroxytryptophan alone and in combination with a decarboxylase inhibitor (Ro 44602) in depressive patients. *Adv. Biochem. Pharmacol.* 11: 399-404.
14. Schildkraut, J.J. (1965) The catecholamine hypothesis of affective disorders: a review of supporting evidence. *Am. J. Psychiatry* 122:509.

PSYCHOPHARMACOLOGY IN HUNGARY IN THE 1960s

Zoltán Böszörményi and Péter Gaszner

Chlorpromazine was introduced in the treatment of psychotic patients in Hungary in the mid-1950s. The great difficulties of obtaining it from abroad in those years restricted its use until Hibernal, the Hungarian brand of chlorpromazine, became available in 1960.

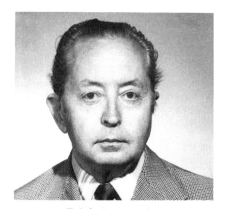

Zoltán Böszörményi

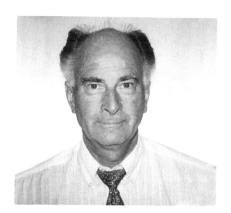

Péter Gaszner

Another event in the mid-1950s with a major impact on Hungarian psychopharmacological development was the isolation and synthesis of dimethyltryptamine (DMT), a psychomimetic substance, by Steven Szara, a Hungarian-born physician and biochemist. Szara began his

---

Zoltán Böszörményi was born in 1913 in Debrecen, Hungary. He graduated from medical school in 1938. Prior to his retirement he was director of one of the clinical services of the National Institute of Psychiatry and Neurology (Hungary).

Böszörményi was elected a fellow of the CINP in 1962 and served as councillor of the 7th and 9th Executives. He presented papers on "Psilocybin and diethyltryptamine: two tryptamine hallucinogens," on "Die Psychopatholgischen Reflexionen der extrapyramdalen Nebenwirkungen der Neuroleptica" (Böszörményi and Kardos), and on "Therapeutische Bedeutung spontaner Delirien und Vorbeugung pharmakogenen Delirien" (Böszörményi and Solti) at the 2nd, 3rd and 7th Congresses respectively. He coauthored a paper on "The favourable and unfavourable effects of psychopharmacology in the group-therapy of psychotics" (Solti and Böszörményi) presented at the 7th Congress. Böszörményi was a formal discussant of Working Group 4 (Pharmacological and clinical action of neuroleptic drugs) at the 4th Congress.

Péter Gaszner is director of psychopharmacology at the National Institute of Psychiatry and Neurology of Hungary. He served as Vice President of the European College of Neuropsychopharmacology. Gaszner was elected a fellow of the CINP in 1980.

research on DMT at the National Institute of Psychiatry and Neurology with a clinical and research team working in close collaboration with him.

In the mid-1950s, many still believed that an endogenous psychotoxic substance such as DMT was responsible for schizophrenic psychopathology. But by the time the research with DMT at the Institute concluded, we recognized that the DMT-induced psychosis is a nonspecific toxic psychosis.

In the late 1950s, an attempt was made to use DMT to facilitate psychotherapy. By the early 1960s, however, interest in DMT waned and was replaced by a steadily increasing excitement over the introduction of therapeutically-effective new psychotropic drugs. The sudden shift of interest was intimately linked to the fact that by 1960 the Hungarian national pharmaceutical industry was ready to embark on the manufacturing (for local use) of psychotropic drugs. Other possible contributing factors to the growing interest in psychopharmacology were the first Hungarian publications on lithium and imipramine respectively by Orthmayer and Szilagyi in 1959, and Angyal and Fenyvesi in 1960.

Prescription practices in Hungary during the 1960s were determined to a great extent by the drugs available from the national pharmaceutical industry. The most frequently used drugs in the treatment of schizophrenia in Hungary during the 1960s were Tisercin, Frenolon, and Luvatren, i.e., levomepromazine (an aminoalkyl-phenothiazine), metofenoxate (a piperazinyl-alkyl-phenothiazine) and moperone (a butyrophenone). Tisercin also had a low dose preparation, Tisercinetta, for the treatment of neuroses.

The first Hungarian antidepressant preparations were the tricyclic Melipramin (imipramine) and the monoamine oxidase inhibitor, Nuredal (niamide), introduced in 1963 and 1965 respectively. The first Hungarian preparations of "minor tranquilizers" were Andaxin (meprobamate), a propanediol, Trioxazine (trimetazine), and Grandaxin (tofisopam), a benzodiazepine. The shift from barbiturates to the propanediols, and from the propanediols to the benzodiazepnes, took place in Hungary considerably later than in the United States.

Probably the most important Hungarian contributions to psychopharmacology during the 1960s were the development of vincamine, the main alkaloid of Vinca minor, a cerebral vasodilator, and deprenyl, a Type B monoamine oxidase inhibitor. Vincamin, first isolated in 1953, was to become extensively used in Hungary during the 1980s with the view that it might prevent memory impairment in the aging process. Deprenyl, developed in the 1960s, was to become known as the monoamine oxidase inhibitor without the cheese effect. Its potential in the treatment of depression, however, still remains to be tested in properly designed clinical experiments.

MY MEMORIES OF DRUG THERAPY IN THE 1960s
(Japan)

Itaru Yamashita

In Japan, chlorpromazine and reserpine were first introduced and studied extensively by Professor Nauseam Suva, who was my predecessor as head of the Department of Psychiatry at Hokkaido University. He delivered a special report on psychotropic drugs at the Fifty-fourth convention of the Japanese Society of Psychiatry in 1957, which opened up the era of drug therapy in psychiatric practice.

The late 1950s and early 1960s were the period when the "prototype" psychotropic drugs were marketed in Japan. The first antipsychotic drugs, chlorpromazine and reserpine, became available in 1955. They were followed by perphenazine in 1957, levomepromazine in 1959, fluphenazine in 1960, thioridazine in 1962, and haloperidol in 1964. Among the antidepressants, imipramine was introduced in 1959, and both amitriptyline and isocarboxazid in 1961; and among the anti-anxiety drugs, chlordiazepoxide was introduced in

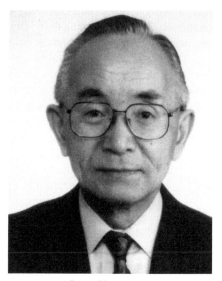

Itaru Yamashita

1961 and diazepam in 1964. We felt excitement and hope, but also bewilderment and caution in face of so many new drugs appearing in rapid succession.

The drugs brought hope because until then the only treatments that we could offer our patients were ECT, rehabilitation, and psychotherapy. I remember very vividly the joy and excitement I experienced when I saw my patients recovering from long-lasting delusions and hallucinations after taking small doses of chlorpromazine, or saw them gradually, but steadily relieved from depression by imipramine, or grateful for the prescription of chlordiazepoxide. (I graduated from medical school in 1953, and belong to the older generation of psychiatrists who know what mental hospitals were like before the introduction of psychotropic drugs, a subject that younger colleagues are often eager to hear about).

Itaru Yamashita was chairman and professor in the Department of Psychiatry at the Hokkaido University School of Medicine from 1976 to 1993. He is currently professor in the Department of Social Welfare at Kokusei Gakuen University.

Yamashita was elected a fellow of the CINP in 1978. He served as vice-president from 1990-92.

However, we also felt much bewilderment, particularly at the beginning of our clinical trials with these drugs. We had to be cautious because everything was new to us, and we did not know what would happen next. It was especially perplexing that the doses of psychotropic drugs recommended in reports from Europe and the United States often caused severe side effects in our patients. In the case of neuroleptics for instance, 300 mg or even 150 mg of chlorpromazine sometimes produced severe Parkinson's syndrome, which was just as much a surprise for the medical staff as for the patients. Moderate doses of perphenazine or fluphenazine frequently induced all kinds of acute dystonia. We soon learned that a gradual increase in the dosage and the simultaneous administration of antiparkinsonian drugs with neuroleptics were almost always necessary. In the case of antidepressants, imipramine helped patients, but it often also upset them by causing severe dry mouth, constipation, and sometimes acute gastritis. Only few could tolerate 150 mg of imipramine, in contrast with the 300 mg dose often recommended in the United States. Chlordiazepoxide caused sleepiness more readily than reported in other countries. The use of isocarboxazid and other monoamine oxidase inhibitor antidepressants was prohibited after a few years on the market because of the fatal liver damage they occasionally caused.

In 1963, as our clinical experience with psychotropic drugs increased, we (N. Suva, S. Morita, and myself) published a 285-page book entitled *Clinical Psychopharmacology: Theories and Practice* (Kanehara Publishing Company). The initial five hundred copies sold out quickly, and a second printing of five hundred copies was also soon exhausted, at a time when there were only about two thousand psychiatrists in Japan. (There are now about ten thousand.) Except for a few translations of foreign works, it was the first book available in Japan that dealt with the clinical use of such psychotropic drugs. I wrote the section entitled "Practice," in which I described my clinical experience in treating 34 patients. These patients exhibited various types of illnesses treated with a variety of drugs, some successfully and others not. Soon after our book was published, numerous other books dealing with psychotropic drugs in use in Japan were published. The revised edition of our work, prepared on the request of the publisher, was published in 1972. It was not as popular as the first edition and did not sell well. What I later regretted most about the book was that it conveyed the idea that psychotropic drugs were generally safe and their side effects transient. That idea was a reflection of my lack of clinical experience and the inadequate information available about the drugs in the early 1960s.

By 1965 Hollister had reported sudden death during treatment with phenothiazines, and Ban had observed ECG changes induced by the same group of drugs. In the late 1960s we too became aware of the question of safety problems with regard to psychotropic drugs, and we therefore conducted several studies to collect the necessary information. First, in 1967, I sent a questionnaire to all the psychiatrists in Hokkaido, nearly two hundred in number, asking about their experience of sudden death since phenothiazines had been introduced in their practices, and I learned that 29 cases of sudden death had occurred on the island. It would, of course, be presumptuous to consider the deaths to have been solely the result of the administration of phenothiazines. Two series of ECG studies were then carried out, the first with 252 cases and the second with 492 cases. The ECG data were analysed by a cardiologist who did not know the clinical condition of the patients. The results of the second study indicated that 54.4 percent of patients taking phenothiazines showed abnormal ECG findings. Nearly half of them had disturbances in cardiac rhythm, mostly sinus tachycardia of a benign nature; nearly 20 percent showed signs of myocardial damage; and more than 25 percent had a combination of various disturbances. The frequency in occurrence of abnormalities correlated closely with the doses and duration of drug treatment. Of 73 cases examined longitudinally, the ECG findings were aggravated in more than half the patients as the therapies were continued. Propranolol improved the sinus tachycardia markedly, but not the myocardial damage. These results attracted much attention among psychiatrists in Japan and have often been referred to in the studies of side effects that followed.

I was alerted to the abuse of benzodiazepines through Hollister's report on withdrawal reactions from chlordiazepoxide in 1961 and through my own experience with neurotic patients. In the first edition of our book, I described one patient who continued to take 180 mg of chlordiazepoxide in spite of my strong advice to reduce the dosage. These drugs could be freely purchased at drugstores in the 1960s. Cases of severe withdrawal symptoms from benzodiazepines were occasionally reported, and at the urging of many psychiatrists, legislation was enacted in 1971 to make them available only by prescription. Soon after, I conducted a survey in Hokkaido and found no cases of severe withdrawal reaction, but many colleagues commented that increasing numbers of patients were taking large amounts of benzodiazepines continuously.

It was after the 1960s that psychiatrists first became concerned about tardive dyskinesia, water intoxication, and other serious side effects. In 1968 our Department of Psychiatry at the Hokkaido University School of Medicine was appointed a collaborating centre for research and training in psychopharmacology under the World Health Organization, and Professor Suva became its head. Our task was to collect information and conduct investigations into psychoactive drugs, in close contact with other centres. The centre was not very active, however, until it became involved in the work of the WHO collaborating centres in biological psychiatry. At meetings of the heads of the WHO centres held every year, I had the opportunity to become acquainted with such figures as W.E. Bunney, A. Coppen, H. Hippius, P. Kielholz, J. Mendlewicz, G. Racagni, and O.J. Rafaelsen, each of whom served as president of the CINP. And as a result, I became involved in the organization and had the pleasure of knowing its distinguished members.

Looking back at the 1960s, I feel that the rise of psychopharmacology influenced my career as a psychiatrist to a considerable extent, and I believe that many psychiatrists of my generation had a similar experience. When I graduated from medical school, I had been planning to become a psychoanalyst after some years of clinical training. But in 1952 chlorpromazine was found to be effective in the treatment of schizophrenic symptoms, and that discovery stimulated psychiatrists, pharmacologists, and pharmaceutical companies to develop new drugs, design new treatments, and eventually establish a new philosophy of psychiatry. The 1960s were the years when the tide of psychiatry moved decisively from the psychodynamic to the biological. I was one of those swept along in this worldwide tide. But I could not isolate myself entirely from the psychodynamic way of thinking, and I was not young enough to begin biological studies in a laboratory. What I could do was remain a clinical psychiatrist with a keen interest in the progress of research in the social, psychological, and biological aspects of psychiatry and I could look at my patients from such a multifaceted viewpoint and try to help them accordingly. My younger colleagues have made a considerable contribution to clinical and basic psychopharmacology and the neurosciences, and I am proud of them.

PERSONAL RECOLLECTIONS OF PSYCHOTROPIC DRUG DEVELOPMENT IN NORWAY

Odd Lingjaerde

As the son of a psychiatrist, I grew up just outside a large psychiatric hospital or asylum, as it was called at that time. I still vividly remember the many strange and deeply disturbed people who lived inside its high fences. I later learned that many of them had been diagnosed as schizophrenic; some were manic-depressive, and a few were megalomaniacs suffering from general paresis. Most of them, notably the schizophrenics, were chronic inpatients with little hope of ever being discharged, although some had been given both insulin-coma treatment and later ECT. In the late 1930s a new treatment was introduced: leucotomy. Ten years later, leucotomy came to Norway. It has often been said that this treatment was a disaster which we would have been far better without. That was certainly the case for many patients, but there were some whose severe suffering diminished after the

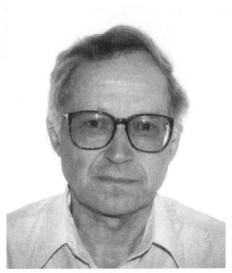

Odd Lingjaerde

surgery. In hindsight, psychiatrists were too slow to realize that, in practical terms, leucotomy had a beneficial effect only for those patients who were *subjectively* suffering from chronic depression, anxiety, delusions, or hallucinations.

In 1956, when I started my psychiatric career at the same hospital around which I had spent my schooldays, leucotomy was still in use and ECT was employed almost daily. But the neuroleptics had also arrived, and they soon became the preferred treatment for psychotic

Odd Lingjaerde was born in 1929 in Asker, Norway. He graduated in medicine from the University of Oslo in 1954 and became a specialist in psychiatry ten years later. He was professor of psychiatry at the University of Tromsö between 1972 and 1984. He was subsequently chief psychiatrist, and since 1990 head of the department of research and education at Gaustad Hospital in Oslo; he was also a professor at the University of Oslo until he retired from that position in 1994. His scientific interests include psychopharmacology at both the basic and clinical levels; biological psychiatry, particularly with blood platelets as a model system; and seasonal affective disorder and light therapy.

Odd Lingjaerde was elected a fellow of the CINP in 1974. He presented a paper on "Some clinical experiences with a new benzodiazepine" at the 6th Congress.

patients. They created a new optimism with regard to these patients' prognoses. In the beginning, chlorpromazine was the most widely used neuroleptic, but the *Rauwolfia* alkaloid reserpine was a serious competitor. Reserpine, however, gradually lost ground because it was generally less effective and because of its tendency to induce depression. New neuroleptics, mainly phenothiazine derivatives such as chlorpromazine, were introduced in rapid succession in those early days of the psychopharmacological era. My first contribution in the field, together with my colleague Arne Schjoth, was a double-blind, crossover comparison of perphenazine (Trilafon) and placebo in 77 female in-patients, which showed perphenazine to be significantly better than the placebo. This study, which was published in Norwegian in 1958, was, as far as I know, the first double-blind clinical trial in psychopharmacology performed in our country.

Perphenazine is still one of the most widely used neuroleptics, at least in Norway, whereas the next substance that I studied had a lesser fate, perhaps undeservedly so. It was tetrabenazine (Nitoman), which is a synthetic, simplified reserpine analogue with the ability to deplete neuronal storage granules of noradrenaline, serotonin, and dopamine. It was shown to be an effective antischizophrenic drug that worked sometimes in otherwise "drug-refractory" patients. But it was not considered interesting enough for the rather conservative drug company (Roche) to launch on a broad scale. Some years later tetrabenazine had a sort of renaissance in the treatment of choreatic disorders such as tardive dyskinesia (since it was believed not to provoke TD itself) and Huntington's chorea, but it never gained much popularity, even for these conditions. However, there have been anecdotal reports in recent years that tetrabenazine may sometimes be effective in schizophrenic patients who have not responded even to clozapine.

Speaking of clozapine (Leponex, Clozaril), this "atypical" neuroleptic was received with enthusiasm at the beginning of the 1970s and was fairly widely used until the report from Finland in 1975 of fatal agranulocytosis. However, some of us still used it for refractory patients together with regular checking of the white blood cells, often with excellent results. My colleague Christian Erlandsen published his favourable findings with the drug in a comparative double-blind clinical trial with haloperidol as early as 1981, long before clozapine was "rediscovered" in the United States.

As for the antidepressants, I remember when the late Professor Ornulv Odegaard from Gaustad Hospital in Oslo (where I now work) came back from the Second World Congress of Psychiatry in Zurich in 1957 and enthusiastically told us about Roland Kuhn's report on the unexpected antidepressant effect of imipramine. Although ECT was and still remains a very effective treatment in severe melancholic depressions, imipramine raised new hopes about what might be achieved with drug treatment in psychiatry. Somewhat disappointingly, however, some forty years later we still have no antidepressant drug with a better therapeutic effect than imipramine.

Shortly after imipramine was introduced, we got the first monoamine oxidase inhibitor, iproniazid (Marsilid), which was also very effective for some patients, but was later withdrawn because of serious complications. Before we learned that tricyclic antidepressants should not be combined with or given immediately after an MAO-inhibitor, I remember that we changed directly from iproniazid to imipramine in the treatment of two patients who had not responded to the former with excellent results after only two days and no complications! Sometimes, luck is on one's side.

Lithium and the anxiolytics also had an important impact on psychiatric practice in those early days, but they were generally not regarded as being of the same importance as the neuroleptics and the antidepressants.

Neuroleptics and antidepressants rapidly became the standard treatments for psychotic states and depressions throughout Scandinavia. Their use created the need for an international forum through which ideas and experiences in the field could be exchanged. When the CINP was formally inaugurated during the Second International Congress of Psychiatry in Zurich in 1957, Jan Odegard, then chairman of the Norwegian Psychiatric Association, was one of its founding members. Although there have never been many formal members of the CINP from Norway, the CINP congresses have become very popular among Norwegian psychiatrists and psychopharmacologists. Eighty-four specialists from Norway attended the nineteenth CINP congress in Washington in 1994. However, the scientific contributions from our country at these meetings have been rather few in number.

The Scandinavian Society of Psychopharmacology (SSP) was founded in 1960. It is linked to the CINP as one of its corresponding associations. In addition to organizing annual scientific meetings, always in Copenhagen, the SSP has done some important work through a standing committee called the *Utvalg for kliniske undersøkelser* (UKU), or Committee for Clinical Investigations. I was chairman of the UKU for twenty-five years, during which we, *inter alia*, developed the now well-known "UKU side effect rating scale" (published in 1987) and performed the first double-blind study showing lithium to enhance the therapeutic effect of antidepressants (published in 1974).

In the first few years after the introduction of the new drugs in Norway, comprehensive reviews of them were lacking. Since I had become interested in the potential of pharmaco-therapy in psychiatry with the new drugs early in my career, I took it upon myself to write some reviews for Norwegian doctors, the first one of which appeared in 1959. This endeavour led to the publication in 1966 of my book *Psykofarmaka: Den medikamentelle behandling av psykiske lidelser* (Psychotropics: Drug Treatment of Psychic Disorders). It was well received in Scandinavia and subsequently appeared in several revised editions.

Throughout the years I have been involved in numerous clinical drug trials, which I will not describe in detail here. But I would like to say, with reference to my many skilful clinical colleagues, that I am proud that Norwegian clinical studies in psychiatry have always been highly regarded.

Since this is intended to be a personal account from someone involved in the development of psychopharmacology in Norway, I will conclude by briefly describing my own work in a more basic field, notably, studies using blood platelets as a model system. In part drawing upon the work of my father, the late Ottar Lingjaerde, on carbohydrate metabolism and transport in schizophrenic patients, in the mid-1960s I decided to study the transport of serotonin in blood platelets, primarily with the aim of looking for abnormalities associated with schizophrenia and manic-depressive disorder. Before starting I had stimulating discussions with Alfred Pletscher and Mose da Prada in Basel, Arvid Carlsson and Bjorn Erik Roos in Gothenburg, and Matti Paasonen in Helsinki. Most important, however, was the fact that I had the opportunity to perform my studies in the research laboratory at the University Psychiatric Clinic, Vinderen, in Oslo, under the inspiring and highly competent supervision of Professor Elling Kvamme.

Soon after I started with my research however, I became aware that the basic mechanism of serotonin uptake in platelets was little known. It was here that I started. Serendipitously I stumbled on several new and interesting features of the "serotonin pump" (later shown to be identical in platelets and neurons). For example, I discovered that it is dependent on the presence of sodium and chloride ions, and stimulated in an allosteric manner by several monocarboxylic acids, such as lactate and pyruvate. In my later studies with the platelet model, carried out in Asgard Psychiatric Hospital at the University of Tromsö between 1972 and 1984, I studied serotonin transport in depression and schizophrenia and the effects of psychotropic drugs on serotonin transport. In the course of my research in depression and schizophrenia I was able to demonstrate that not only patients with endogenous depression, but also untreated schizophrenics, had a reduced capacity for serotonin transport into platelets. In my research with antidepressants, I found that different drugs had different effects on the kinetics of serotonin-uptake inhibition, with some, such as imipramine, exerting a pure competitive inhibitory effect, whereas others, including clomipramine, a non-competitive inhibitory effect. The therapeutic relevance of this differential effect has not yet been elucidated. I also found that clomipramine, in contrast with other tricyclics, had a retarding effect on the spontaneous efflux of serotonin from platelet granules. Again, it is not yet known whether this particular property of clomipramine has any therapeutic implication.

Since I returned to Oslo in 1984, I have been primarily involved with studying seasonal affective disorder. My research was inspired by Norman Rosenthal and his co-workers' now classic description of this disorder in 1984. However, from a psychopharmacological point of view, only two observations in this field are perhaps worth mentioning here: first, that the selective MAO-A inhibitor moclobemide (Aurorix) differs very little from a placebo in its effect on winter depression after treatment for three weeks; and second, that the effect of placebo tablets after three weeks shows a remarkable and highly significant negative correlation with the age of "winter-depressed" patients. (No such correlation was found for light treatment.)

During recent years, the University of Bergen has become the leader in basic psychopharmacological research in Norway. Young scientists such as Dr. Vidar Steen are conducting very interesting research projects there these days. I hope that this development will give a needed boost to this field of research in our country.

Memoirs from Canada

HARMALA ALKALOIDS, RABBIT SYNDROME AND LITHIUM BABIES

André Villeneuve

I arrived in Québec City (Québec, Canada) in July 1967 as a research psychiatrist with the responsibility of organizing a research unit at the Hôpital St-Michel-Archange (now the Centre Hospitalier Robert-Giffard), at that time a psychiatric hospital with slightly more than 5,000 beds located in Beauport, a suburban area. I had just finished many years of diversified training in psychiatry, which started with a psychoanalytically-oriented training program at the New York School of Psychiatry, headed by Sandor Rado, a dissident psychoanalyst who was a contemporary of Freud. I completed my training in New York in 1964, and between 1964 and 1966 I was at McGill University, where, as a postgraduate student, I did research under the supervision of Professor T.L. Sourkes. To obtain a Master of Science degree I studied the biochemical pharmacology of a harmala alkaloid, harmaline, in rats. (Harmaline is a naturally occurring ß-carboline found in the malpighiaceous vine *Banistereopsis caapi,* used by certain South American Indian tribes to prepare a hallucinogenic beverage.) From Montreal I went to France to pursue my training further, mainly in Paris. It consisted of clinical research with Professors J. Delay and P. Deniker at the Centre Hospitalier Sainte-Anne, working primarily with D. Ginestet and P. Péron-Magnan. In animal pharmacological research, I worked with Professor J.R. Boissier of the Department of Pharmacology and in the Faculty of Medicine, University of Paris, I worked primarily with P. Simon and J.P. Tillement. In Paris I participated in studies conducted in animals and humans on the action of flurothyl, a hexafluorinated ether that could be used clinically by inhalation for convulsive shock therapy. This "European experience" had a great impact on my life.

When I first arrived in Québec City, I must admit, I experienced feelings of isolation and loneliness. But fortunately I could rely on the friendship of my research colleagues both here and abroad, as well as on the clinical psychiatrists in my hospital. Professor C. Radouco-Thomas, a founding member of the Collegium Internationale Neuro-Psychopharmacologi-

André Villeneuve, born in 1932 in Chicoutimi, Québec (Canada), received his MD at Laval University (Quebec City) in 1958. In 1964 he completed studies in psychiatry at the New York School of Psychiatry under Professor Rado, a one-time associate of Freud. From 1967-85 he created and directed the research unit in neuropharmacology at Centre Hospitalier Robert-Giffard in Québec City. In 1977 he became a professor of psychiatry at Laval University and in 1983 was appointed Psychiatrist in Chief and Chief of the Neuropharmacological Section at Clinique Roy-Rousseau. His production of more than 150 publications, includes the editing of five books on neuropsychopharmacology. In 1991 he received an award for career achievement from the Québec Psychiatric Association. He left his hospital work in September 1997, and is currently involved with psychiatric research and forensic psychiatry.

Villeneuve was elected a fellow of the CINP in 1968. He presented a paper on "Lithium therapy in recurrent manic-depressive psychosis" (Villeneuve, Langlois, Chabot, Dogan, Lachance and Laurent) at the 7th Congress.

cum, who was from 1962 to 1975 the head of the Department of Pharmacology at the Université Laval, offered from the beginning unfailing support. At that time, in the province of Québec, there was also a very active group of researchers in neuropsychopharmacology. It included H.E. Lehmann, T.A. Ban, J.M. Bordeleau, and L. Tétreault, who met regularly under the auspices of the Québec Psychopharmacological Research Association (an organization that was dissolved after the Canadian College of Neuropsychopharmacology was founded in 1978).

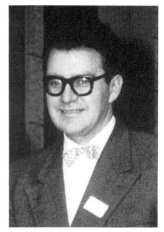

C. Radouco-Thomas

In those early years of psychopharmacology, one selected a particular area of central nervous system research on the basis of one's intellectual curiosity. Of course, some techniques were not yet available. The field of biogenic amines was still in its infancy and that of brain imaging was unthinkable. From the beginning, I had a particular interest in lithium therapy and in the extrapyramidal system, namely, in tardive dyskinesia, as well as in genetics.

With respect to lithium, in 1968 I succeeded in persuading a small Québec pharmaceutical laboratory to prepare the necessary supplies for me for a placebo-controlled study with lithium. With the supply in hand I began, in collaboration with two other clinicians, to study the effect of lithium therapy in manic-depressive psychosis. The selection of the initial patients was based on the indisputable diagnosis of mania. Other inclusion criteria were chronicity of illness, frequency of relapse, and unsatisfactory response to available treatments. The study protocol, for methodological considerations, included a placebo washout period. This created considerable worries and problems for the nursing staff and other attendants, because it was often accompanied by marked excitation. However, the spectacular results obtained in these refractory patients after about two weeks of lithium therapy created enthusiasm, confidence, and a great tolerance for the difficulties during the placebo washout period by the staff. The first trial with lithium was followed by studies with the substance on a larger scale and with the exploration of the effect of this treatment on various biological parameters, including antithyroid antibodies.

In the area of lithium teratogenicity, I was able to collaborate early in my career with Mogens Schou, who during his pioneering work with lithium established the Scandinavian Register of Lithium Babies for mothers exposed to the drug during their first trimester of pregnancy. This was followed in 1970 by the creation of an American Register of Lithium Babies by M.R. Weinstein and M. Goldfield and a Canadian Register of Lithium Babies by me. Our data were placed in a common pool called the International Register of Lithium Babies, and our first results were published in a paper in 1973. In this paper we cautiously reported on an abnormality that coincided largely with Ebstein's cardiovascular anomaly. Thereafter the Register was maintained primarily by Weinstein until his untimely death in 1979. To pursue my interest in lithium I had organized the First Canadian International Symposium on Lithium in Québec City in 1974, with contributors such as J. Angst, F.K. Goodwin, P. Grof, M. Schou, and others.

My research endeavour relevant to the extrapyramidal system began in 1967 with the development of a rating scale to study the incidence of tardive dyskinesia in my hospital. For many years, with my small research team, I studied the pathophysiology of this neuroleptic-induced complication, by means of a polygraphic technique, under various conditions, including vigilance, attention, concentration, sleep, and a number of different drugs. In 1970, at a scientific meeting in Montreal, I was first to report a new extrapyramidal side effect manifest in a perioral Parkinson-like tremor. I called it "rabbit syndrome" because it mimicked the movements of a rabbit mouth. When studied under the same polygraphic conditions as tardive

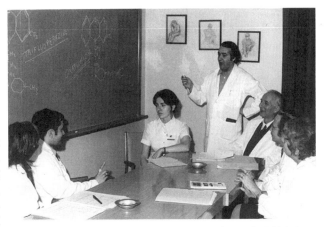

Staff meeting in the Research Unit at Hôpital St. Michel Archange (now Centre Hôpitalier Robert-Beauport), Québec, 1971. André Villeneuve (standing), Andrzej Jus (to his right), and Karolina Jus (far right)

dyskinesia, the "rabbit syndrome" proved to be distinct from it in many respects, especially by its favourable response to the administration of anticholinergic drugs. In the course of my research in tardive dyskinesia I found reserpine therapeutically effective. Finally, in the fall of 1975 on the referral of G. Crane from Baltimore, I was consulted by a then forty-nine-year-old woman who had developed a severe buccolinguo-masticatory dyskinesia, that moderately improved with the combined administration of reserpine and deanol. The patient's greatest improvement, however, coincided with a four month period of amenorrhea. Subsequently, a striking relationship was noted between the intensity of the dyskinetic movements and her menses, i.e., improvement during amenorrhea, worsening with menstruation. When her gynecologist prescribed her a progestogen agent (norethindrone), there was a marked aggravation of her dyskinesia. On the other hand, conjugated estrogens (Premarin), given for several weeks in increasing doses up to 2.50 mg, resulted in a striking improvement that persisted for almost a month after discontinuation of treatment. It was in this patient that I noted a mild tremor of her right hand while on the highest doses of estrogens. This serendipitous observation led in 1977, after some further investigations, to the first report I wrote in collaboration with P. Bédard and P. Langelier on the apparent antidopaminergic action of estrogens. To this day, this female patient, who was seventy-one years old in the summer of 1997, has remained markedly improved with respect to her tardive dyskinesia on a low dose of reserpine (0.50 mg daily) alone.

In addition to clinical trials with psychotropic drugs, my main research activities over the last decade have been in genetics. Here I have collaborated for the past fourteen years with a team headed by Professor N. Barden from the Neurosciences Unit at the Centre de Recherche, Pavillon Centre Hospitalier de l'Université Laval (Centre Hospitalier Universitaire de Québec). Our group is pursuing linkage studies of bipolar affective disorder in an attempt to detect a genetic marker in a very large sample of pedigrees from a homogeneous population in northern Québec.

I have been associated with the Collegium Internationale Neuro-Psychopharmacologicum since 1968, when I was elected a member at the sixth international congress, held in Tarragona. In 1976, as president of the local organizing committee, I contributed to the planning of the tenth CINP Congress (held in Québec City). Professor C. Radouco-Thomas served as president of the scientific program committee. I have been able to participate in and to witness the exciting development of the neurosciences and neuropsychopharmacology over three decades. Yet a challenging question still confronts us: how does the brain become the mind?

FROM CONDITIONING AND PSYCHIATRY TO PSYCHOPHARMACOLOGY

Thomas A. Ban

I arrived in Canada from Hungary, my native country, in early 1957. After a fellowship in neuroanatomy at the Montreal Neurological Institute, and a rotating internship, I enrolled in McGill University's training program in psychiatry. I already had two years of psychiatry in Hungary and – thanks to George Sandor, my service chief at the National Institute of Psychiatry and Neurology – some familiarity with the use of new psychotropics, such as chlorpromazine, reserpine, lithium and isocarboxazid.

During the 1950s, psychiatric residents at McGill were required to write a "thesis," and I was fortunate to have Dr. Heinz Lehmann of chlorpromazine's fame as my advisor.

My thesis dealt with Pavlov's original experiments and brain model in a modern (1950s) neurophysiological framework. It was based on the notion that conditional reflex variables are functional patterns of the brain; and focused on the need – created by the rise of psychopharmacology – to replace conventional psychopathologies with a functional psychopathology, in which mental illness is described in terms of conditional reflex variables instead of psychopathological symptoms.

As a follow-up to my thesis, we developed a diagnostic test procedure based on the conditional reflex method (1) and a conditioning test battery for the study of psychopathological mechanisms and psychopharmacological effects (2). Since the action of psychotropics could be characterized in terms of conditional reflex variables, with the battery in place, by the end of the 1960s the stage was set to develop a methodology for the matching of the pharmacological (conditional reflex) profile of drugs with the clinical (conditional reflex) profile of psychiatric patients.

In 1960 I received my diploma in psychiatry with distinction at McGill. *Conditioning and Psychiatry* was published in the mid-1960s (1964 in the US and 1966 in the UK) with a

Thomas A. Ban is emeritus professor of psychiatry at Vanderbilt University. A graduate of Semmelweis University (Budapest) in 1954, he was the founding director of the division of psychopharmacology at McGill University (Montreal) from 1970 to 1976, and subsequently, professor of psychiatry at Vanderbilt University (Nashville). Currently he is chairman of the First Multinational Corporation in Psychiatry.

Ban was elected fellow of CINP in 1962 and served as secretary of the 8th and 9th executives, as vice-president of the 10th, and as treasurer of the 12th, 13th, 14th and 15th. He presented papers on "Comments on the use of Sernyl", on "The effects of phenothiazines on the human electrocardiogram" (Ban, St. Jean and Desautels), on "Predictors of therapeutic responsivity to thiothixene in schizophrenia" (Ban, Lehmann, Sterlin and Saxena), and on "Methodological problems in the clinical evaluation of anxiolytic drugs" at the 4th (2x), 6th and 7th congresses respectively. Ban was formal discussant of G.V. Morozov's paper (Role of different structures of the brain stem in the genesis of catatonic stupor) at the 4th congress.

foreword by the late W.
Horsley Gantt, at the time
one of the last living pupils
of Pavlov. For the "battery,"
we received in 1969 the annual McNeil Award of the
Canadian Psychiatric Association.

In the early 1960s I joined
Heinz Lehmann as his co-
principal investigator in our
Early Clinical Drug Evaluation Unit (ECDEU) suppor-
ted by the US Public Health
Service. Ours was one of the
first units of the network,

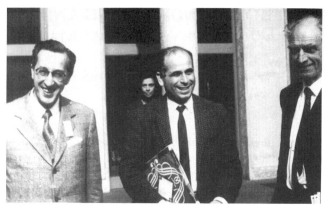

**From left: Carlo L. Cazzullo, Thomas A. Ban and
W. Horsley Gantt**

which met with some regularity to exchange observations and findings on new psychotropics.
The first meetings were chaired by Bertrum Schiele, the most senior member of the group, and
the key players of those meetings were Art Sugerman, George Simpson (at the time still an
associate of Nate Kline), and Don Gallant (at the time an associate of Bob Heath). Doug
Goldman, Max Fink, and Sid Merlis were present too, if my recollection is correct; so were
Dave Engelhardt, Leo Hollister, and Gerald Klerman. Others, like Turan Itil, Barbara Fish,
Don Klein and David Wheatley became ECDEU investigators later in the 1960s.

Although the nature of the research to be conducted in the units was not clearly defined,
the overall objective of the program was the development of an acceptable methodology –
acceptable to both the drug companies and the drug regulatory agencies – for establishing the
therapeutic efficacy of psychotropic drugs. To achieve this objective testimonials were
replaced by the idiosyncratic methodologies employed in the different units (e.g., we used the
Verdun Target Symptom and Depression Scales, the Psychopathological Symptom Profile,
and the Verdun Psychometric and Conditioning Test Batteries) during the leadership of Jon
Cole (the first half of the 1960s); and during Jerry Levine's administration (the second half of
the 1960s), these idiosyncratic methodologies were replaced by uniform, standardized data
collection, processing and analytic procedures. By the end of the 1960s the Early Clinical Drug
Evaluation Units, Biometric Laboratory Information Processing Sysytem (ECDEU-BLIPS)
was in place (5) to dominate the field during the 1970s.

From the beginning, our early clinical drug evaluation unit was very productive. Because
of the unique geographic position of Canada, we had been involved with most of the
psychotropic drugs marketed in North America during the 1960s and 1970s. I was in regular
contact with the late Tom da Silva, the conscientious officer of the Canadian Health Protection
Branch (the corresponding organization to the US Food and Drug Administration) responsible
for the CNS area, with Peg Milliken of the US Adverse Drug Reaction Reporting Program,
and with the pharmaceutical companies involved with the development of psychotropic drugs.

Each drug we worked with has its own story, which will need to be told elsewhere, and our
contributions – impressions, observations and findings – were mostly, but not always, further
substantiated by subsequent clinical investigations. In case of desipramine, the demethylated
metabolite of imipramine, for example, our impression that it had a faster onset of action than

its parent substance – reported in 1962 (6) – was not borne out. On the other hand, our observations that levomepromazine, an aminoalkyl phenothiazine, was somewhat distinct from the typical phenothiazine neuroleptics – reported in 1963 (7) – received further substantiation in recent years. The same as to levomepromazine applies to our finding with trimipramine, reported in 1964 (8).

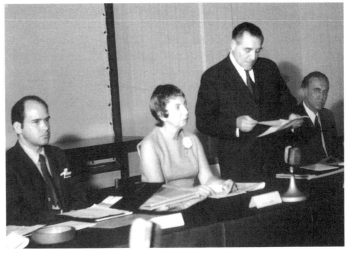

From left: Gaston Castellanos, Alice Leeds and Nenad Bohacek

We were among the first to conduct series of systematic studies, instead of just an isolated study, with a particular psychotropic, e.g., trimipramine (9), and with a group of psychotropics, e.g., the butyrophenones (10) or the thioxanthenes (11). Since we were just as much interested in exploring therapeutic effects as adverse effects, we were first to demonstrate cardiac conductance changes with thioridazine (12), the phenothiazine promoted for use in geriatrics. We were among the first to describe skin pigmentation and ocular changes with chlorpromazine (13).

With the steadily accumulating preclinical and clinical information in our unit, I became increasingly aware of the heterogeneity of the descriptions provided in the preclinical brochures; of the gap between the preclinical and clinical data; and of the lack of integration of clinical findings in clinical psychopharmacologic research. To overcome the difficulties and to create a common language, I decided to write *Psychopharmacology* (14). It became the first comprehensive text in the field. The writing was greatly facilitated by an invitation to conduct a workshop on "What preclinical information does the clinician expect to be given prior to conducting a clinical trial with a new drug" at the 1966 annual meeting of the American College of Neuropsychopharmacology (ACNP) (15). I also benefitted from the request to write a series of reviews on the different groups of psychotropic drugs for *Applied Therapeutics* (16, 17, 18, 19, 20, 21, 22). There was also my increasing involvement in teaching psychopharmacology to the residents at McGill. The material presented at the ACNP Workshop provided the basis of the first part of the book, General Psychopharmacology; the papers published in *Applied Therapeutics*, for the second part, Systematic Psychopharmacology; and the material used in teaching, for the third part, Applied Psychopharmacology. In my concluding remarks in *Psychopharmacology*, I pointed out that pharmacotherapy with psychotropics focused attention on the biological heterogeneity within the traditional nosologic categories in terms of therapeutic responsiveness; and postulated that progress in pharmacotherapy will depend on how fast this heterogeneity is resolved.

Psychopharmacology was published by Williams and Wilkins in 1969. It shared the 1970 Clarke Institute Annual Research Award with Harvey Stancer's contributions to the role of catecholamines in affective disorders.

Prior to the publication of *Psychopharmacology* I was very much involved in the activities of the Quebec Psychopharmacological Reserach Association (23,) that we founded with Lehmann in the early 1960s and with the coordination of the Canadian Mental Health Association's Collaborative Studies on Nicotinic Acid in the Treatment of Schizophrenia (24). In the late 1960s, after the publication of *Psychopharmacology*, I became increasingly involved with activities of the Mental Health Unit of the World Health Organization, under the direction of the late Boris Lebedev, and with activities of the International Reference Center Network on Psychotropic Drugs, a joint venture between the World Health Organization and the US National Institute of Mental Health, under the direction of the late Alice Leeds, but it's time to stop.

REFERENCES

1. Ban, T.A. and Levy,L. (1961). Physiological patterns: A diagnostic test procedure based on the conditional reflex method. *Journal of Neurophysiology* 2: 228-231.
2. Ban, T.A., Lehmann, H.E., and Saxena, B.M. (1970). A conditioning test battery for the study of psychopathological mechanisms and psychopharmacological effects. *Canad. Psychiat. Assoc. J.* 15: 301-308.
3. Ban, T.A. (1964). *Conditioning and Psychiatry.* Chicago: Aldine.
4. Ban, T.A. (1966). *Conditioning and Psychiatry.* London: George Allen and Unwin.
5. Guy, W. and Bonato, R. (1970). *Manual for the ECDEU Assessment Battery.* (2nd ed.). Washington: U.S. Department of Health, Education and Welfare.
6. Ban, T.A. and Lehmann, H.E. (1962). Clinical studies with desmethylimipramine. *Canadian Med. Assoc. J.* 86: 1030-1031.
7. Ban,T.A. and Schwarz, L. (1963). Systematic studies with levomepromazine. *J. Neuropsychiat.* 5: 112-117.
8. Ban, T.A. (1964). Trimipramine in Psychiatry. In H.E. Lehmann, M. Berthiaume, and T.A. Ban (eds.). *Trimipramine a New Antidepressant* (pp.95-98). Montreal: Quebec Psychopharmacological Research Association.
9. Lehmann, H.E., Berthiaume, M. and Ban T.A. (eds.). (1964). *Trimipramine a New Antidepressant.* Montreal: Quebec Psychopharmacological Research Association.
10. Ban, T.A. (1954). The butyrophenones in psychiatry. In H.E. Lehmann and T.A. Ban (eds.). *The Butyrophenones in Psychiatry.* (pp. 120-134). Montreal: Quebec Psychopharmacological Research Association.
11. Lehmann, H.E. and Ban, T.A. (eds.). (1969). *The Thioxanthenes.* Basel: S. Karger.
12. Ban, T.A. and St.Jean, A. (1964). The effectt of phenothiazines on the electrocardiogram. *Canad. Med. Assoc. J.* 91 : 537-540.
13. Ban, T.A. and Lehmann, H.E. (1965). Skin pigmentation, a rare side effect of chlorpromazine. *Canad. Psychiat. Assoc. J.* 10: 112-124.
14. Ban, T.A. (1969). *Psychopharmacology.* Baltimore: Williams and Wilkins.
15. Ban, T.A. What preclinical information does the clinician expect to be given prior to conducting a clinical trial with a new drug? (Abstract). *Bulletin of the American College of Neuropsychopharmacology.* Volume 4, 1966.
16. Ban, T.A. (1966). Clinical pharmacology of psychotropic drugs. *Appl. Therapeutics* 8: 145-175.
17. Ban, T.A. (1966). Clinical pharmacology of the phenothiazines. *Appl. Therapeutics* 8: 423-427.
18. Ban, T.A. (1966). Phenothiazines alone and in combination. *Appl. Therapeutics* 8: 530-535.
19. Ban, T.A. (1966). Clinical pharmacology of tricyclic antidepressants. Part I. *Appl. Therapeutics* 8: 779-785.
20. Ban, T.A. (1967). Clinical pharmacology of tricyclic antidepressants. Part II. *Appl. Therapeutics* 9: 66-75.
21. Ban, T.A. (1967). Clinical pharmacology of psychotropic drugs. The benzodiazepines. Part I. *Appl. Therapeutics.* 9: 366-371.
22. Ban, T.A. (1967). Clinical pharmacology of psychotropic drugs. The benzodiazepines. Part II. *Appl. Therapeutics.* 9: 677-680.
23. Lehmann, H.E. and Ban, T.A. (eds.). (1967). *Toxicity and Adverse Reaction Studies with Neuroleptics and Antidepressants.* Montreal: Quebec Psychopharmacological Research Association.
24. Ban, T.A. and Lehmann, T.A. (1970). Nicotinic Acid in the Treatment of Schizophrenias. *Canadian Mental Health Association Collaborative Study. Progress Report I.* Toronto: Canadian Mental Health Association.

Memoirs from Czechoslovakia

ORIGIN AND DEVELOPMENT OF THE CZECH PSYCHOTROPIC AGENTS IN THE 1960s

Miroslav Protiva

During the 1960s there was a concentrated effort in Czechoslovakia to develop new psychotropic drugs. I was in charge of the group responsible for designing new molecules with a potential for psychotropic effects at the Research Institute for Pharmacy and Biochemistry in Prague. It was my resposibility also to coordinate the activities of the pharmacologists, toxicologists and even clinicians involved with the early development of these drugs. I was supported in my activities by a team which included about 15 "synthetic" chemists.

I'm a 1946 graduate of the Institute of Chemical Technology of Prague. I began with my studies in 1939, but my education was interrupted for a few years, because the universities in Czechoslovakia were closed (during the German occupation). I was a postgraduate student in organic chemistry in Zu-

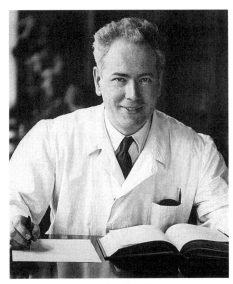

Miroslav Protiva

rich in the department of Prof. V. Prelog which provided me with the necessary background for leadership in the synthesis and development of new drugs.

My first task at the Institute was to develop new antihistamines, which would complement those developed at the end of the Second World War, such as promethazine and diphenhydramine, at the laboratories of Rhône-Poulenc in France and Parke-Davis in the United States, respectively. We used these two compounds as the prototypes and aimed at procuring through structural modifications more effective antihistamines with fewer central depressant effects. Our efforts produced two antihistamines, marketed with the brand names Alfadryl and Bromadryl in Czechoslovakia. Bromadryl was licensed to Smith, Kline and French and was marketed also in the UK. It was manufactured in great quantities in India.

Our objective of developing antihistamines without a central depressant effect was not fulfilled. In fact, some of our drugs, as for example moxastine teoclate – the molecular complex

Miroslav Protiva was born in Prague, Czechoslovakia, in 1921. He studied chemistry at the Institute of Chemical Technology in Prague and at the Laboratory of Organic Chemistry at the Institute of Technology in Zurich, Switzerland. Between 1948 and 1986 he was head of the Department of Organic Synthesis of the Research Institute for Pharmacy and Biochemistry in Prague, where he dealt mainly with neurotropic and psychotropic agents.

Protiva was elected a fellow of the CINP in 1972.

of Alfadryl with 8-chlorotheophylline, marketed as an antiemetic – was strongly sedating and had ataractic effects so pronounced that Vinar in 1958 tried it in the treatment of psychoses.

It was not our intention to enter the psychotropic field, but we slipped into it through further modifications of our antihistaminic prototypes. The drug which triggered the shift was propazepine, an isomer of imipramine, that was found independently by Votava in 1961 and Benesova in 1962, to share pharmacological properties with the tricyclic antidepressants. Although the drug was found to be therapeutically effective in depression by Vinar as early as 1961, it was not introduced into clinical use because its synthesis required the dangerous mixture of sodium azide with sulphuric acid.

Pursuing matters further in the field of psychotropics, Seidlova, a member of our team, synthesized a combination of imipramine and chlorprothixene, a substance which I named Proheptadien, but which became known as amitriptyline. Apparently, while our preclinical research with Proheptadien was still underway, amitriptyline was introduced by Roche.

The loss of amitriptyline was a big disappointment and prompted me to speed up the development of a completely new series of drugs, the 6,11-dihydrodibenzo(b,e)thiepins. The synthesis of the corresponding amitriptyline analogue of the series, which I named Prothiaden, was performed by Rajsner in 1961 in my team. After conducting the pharmacological and toxicological studies required at the time in Czechoslovakia, the substance was handed over for clinical studies to the psychiatric clinic in Plzen. By 1962, Vencovsky reported that dosulepin, which was to become the generic name of Prothiaden, was a "worthy" substitute for amitriptyline. My preliminary communication on dosulepin in 1962 was followed by reports from the teams of Boehringer-Mannheim and of Sandoz on the same compound, but in this case our compound was in a more advanced stage of development. We also succeeded in obtaining the US patent of dosulepin.

Getting approval for the introduction of Prothiaden into clinical use was not easy. It was the first time that we were required to do chronic (one year) toxicology in rats and dogs. Our first attempt ended as a disaster; the rats were fine, but the dogs showed excessively high mortality. At the time we only had "street dogs" available for testing, and they were often mongrels and full of infections. I was called to see the director of the institute in his office; he was with Z. Votava, the head of our departmant of pharmacology. They instructed me to discontinue any further research with Prothiaden because of the drug's toxicity. I disagreed, pleading that our findings were due to the sickness of the dogs and not to the toxicity of the drug. I won, and the toxicity study was repeated in English beagles. In the second study with healthy animals, Prothiaden was found to be clean! We were authorized to proceed and Prothiaden was released for clinical use in Czechoslovakia in 1967. Prothiaden is a therapeutically effective antidepressant with the distinct advantage over amitriptyline that it has no cardiovascular side effects.

Prothiaden was licensed first to Crookes Laboratories in the United Kingdom and then to the Boots Company (now Knoll AG) in Nottingham, with the provision that it be manufactured in Czechoslovakia. A similar arrangement was made with the Japanese firm, Kaken Pharmaceuticals. Cooperation with these companies greatly increased the information available about the drug. Special symposia on the drug were organized in Moscow (1972), Paris (1974), Prague (1977), and Vienna (1978). Boots introduced Prothiaden in all the countries of the British Commonwealth and, for many years, in some Commonwealth countries, the drug was the leading antidepressant in clinical use. It was the greatest success of the Czech pharmaceutical industry in the psychotropic field.

Some of the analogues of Prothiaden were found to have antihistaminic properties. Of them, the methyl derivative (Methiaden) and the thiophene isostere (Dithiaden) were introduced in Czechoslovakia for use as antihistamines. Both are still available for clinical use, Methiaden in the form of a parenteral preparation in combination with calcium glucoheptonate, and Dithiaden supplied as 2 mg tablets.

After we exhausted the dibenzo(b,e)thiepins, we turned our attention to the isomers of the series. Although the first substance, the Prothiaden isomer, was completely inactive, we had accessible intermediates which were sufficiently encouraging to proceed. It was in the course of this research that we got to 4-methyl-1-piperazinyl (Perathiepin), a substance with pharmacological properties shown by J. Metysova in 1964 to be similar to, but with a greater potency than, those of chlorpromazine. After its successful preclinical development in 1965, Perathiepin was ready to be used in clinical trials. The Czech psychiatrists O. Vinar and K. Nahunek found that the drug was a neuroleptic, but they did not consider it sufficiently effective in the treatment of schizophrenia to recommend further clinical development. Nevertheless, we thought that by structural changes of Perathiepin we could derive an effective drug for clinical use. Thus, it was Perathiepin which led us to octoclothepin, or clothiapine, the 8-chloro derivative of the substance, a safe and therapeutically effective antipsychotic which by now has been used for over 20 years in Czechoslovakia, primarily in the treatment of schizophrenia. Since octoclothepin represented the discovery of a new series of potent neuroleptics, I was invited to lecture on it at the 150th American Chemical Society Meeting in Atlantic City (USA) in 1965 and discuss it at a Symposium on CNS Drugs in Hyderabad (India) in 1966.

The dibenzo(a,d)cycloheptene analogue of octoclothiepine, chloroperaptene, was found to be as active in preclinical tests as the parent substance, but by the time we were to proceed with its development as a neuroleptic, I became aware of a growing number of patents by Rhône-Poulenc dealing with similar compounds. It seemed at a certain point that we will not be able to avoid a collision with a major competitor. But then in May 1967, I was invited to lecture about our work at the Centre de Recherches Nicolas Grillet of Rhône-Polenc, in Vitry-sur-Seine. I gave the lecture in French. It was very well received. While there, I was asked to join some of the leading researchers of the company in a private room with a large table; P. Viaud, R.M. Jacob, L. Julou, J.C.L. Fouché, R. Horclois were there, among others. We discussed the issue I was concerned about and worked out an agreement that I would stop working with the piperazino-dibenzo(a,d)cycloheptene and piperazinodibenzo(b,f)oxepin series, and they would stop working with our piperazinodibenzo(b,f)thiepin series. The agreement was sealed with a glass of delicious French champagne. I consider this episode the climax of my professional career. After returning to Prague, I could, of course, not report to the Communist bosses anything about this agreement because I was not entitled to negotiate with anyone. The "gentleman's agreement" worked and I felt that it was to our advantage to be able to continue quietly concentrating on one line of work rather than splitting our team into three.

After our first publications on octoclothepin, the Japanese company Fujisawa expressed interest and we sent them samples of the substance together with some documentation. Fujisawa's intent, as it turned out, was to develop a series of piperazine enamines, which differed from our series only by an additional double bond in the central ring. I was aware of the possibility of having a double bond in the central ring, but since I thought the stability of such compounds problematic in acidic media, such as the stomach, I kept on postponing their synthesis. We finally synthesized them in 1969, but at that point Fujisawa had the priority.

The enamines ("dehydroclothepin" was the name I gave for the enamine analogue of octoclothepin) were shown to share pharmacological properties with neuroleptics, especially potent on the catalepsy test. The concern that they might cause frequent and severe extrapyramidal signs was probably the reason that none of the enamines was ever released for clinical use.

To continue with octoclothepin, we found that the chlorine atom ("the neuroleptic substituent") in its structure may be replaced by different atoms or groups, e.g., bromo, iodo, methoxy, etc., without a decrease of activity. The 8-methylthio-derivative, methiothepin, attracted the interest of the Hoffmann-La Roche research group in Basel. Roche began with the furher development of the substance, but, because of the high frequency of extrapyramidal signs, at a certain point they abandoned it. In the meantime, however, W. Haefely revealed that methiothepin is a potent central serotonin antagonist. Because of this, it is still manufactured on a small scale for experimental purposes by BIOMOL Research Laboratories.

The replacement of N-methyl in the molecule of methiothepin with a 3-hydroxypropyl led to oxyprothepin, Since the late 1970s, oxyprothepin methanesulfonate (Meclopin) has been used in Czechoslovakia for the treatment of psychoses. It actually replaced octoclothepin on the market. Its ester, oxyprothepin decanoate, proved to be suitable for long-term maintenance treatment of schizophrenic psychoses. More recently, after a series of comparative studies with fluphenazine decanoate, fluspirilene, perphenazine enanthate, and clopenthixol decanoate –, oxyprothepin decanoate (Meclopin inj.) was rendered available for clinical use in Czechoslovakia. A single intramuscular injection was found to be active for three to four weeks.

Extensive metabolic studies with several of our compounds, but especially with octoclothepin, yielded findings that 3-hydroxy-octoclothepin (a strong neuroleptic) was an active metabolite of octoclothepin. In consideration of this finding I hypothesized that blocking hydroxylation with fluorine atoms could delay the breakdown and elimination of active compounds, and decided to synthesize fluorinated compounds in our series with the aim of developing orally administered long-acting neuroleptics. But the story of fluorinated compounds would take us into the 1970s and even the 1980s.

All I would like to add is that our choice for a long-acting preparation was the 3-fluoro-8-isopropyl-N-(2-hydroxyethyl) analogue of perathiepin (isofloxythepin). However, the drug has never reached the market. Already in the late 1960s the search for non-cataleptic, atypical neuroleptics began and isofloxythepin was not devoid of extrapyramidal side effects.

RELEVANT READINGS

The structural formulas of some of the drugs referred to in this paper are shown in the figure and the original references relevant to the preclinical and clinical research described in this paper are given in the following review articles:

1. M. Protiva (1970) *Pharm. Ind.* 32, 923-935.
2. M. Protiva (1973) *Activ. Nerv. Super.* (Prague), 15, 186-192.
3. M. Protiva (1976) *Farm. Obzor.* 45, 103-122.
4. M. Protiva (1978) *Lectures Heterocycl. Chem.* 4, 1-15.
5. M. Protiva (1979) *Pharmazie* 34, 41: 274-277.
6. M. Protiva (1986) *Pharmazie* 225-232.
7. M. Protiva (1991) *Collect. Czech. Chem. Commun.* 56: 2501-2771.
8. M. Protiva (1996) *J. Heterocycl. Chem.* 33, 497-521.

PSYCHOPHARMACOLOGY WAS MY DESTINY

Olga Benešová

I was elected a member of CINP in 1970 at the 7th Congress in Prague, but I was already an active participant at three previous CINP Congresses (1964 in Birmingham, 1960 in Washington, and 1968 in Tarragona). My interest in the physiology and pharmacology of the central nervous system dates back to my student years in the late 1940s at the Faculty of Medicine, Charles University in Prague, when I carried out in the Department of Physiology some experiments in rats concerning the action of glucose in the brain. Subsequently, with a UNESCO postdoctoral fellowship, I learned electrophysiological techniques (e.g., EEG and evoked potentials in cats with implanted electrodes) at the Laboratoire de Neurophysiologie Comparé of Prof. Busser, at the Faculté des Sciences, in Paris.

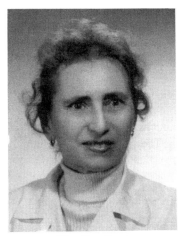

Olga Benešová

During my first appointment at the Pharmaceutical Research Institute (1948-1955), I used this experience for the evaluation of the central depressant effects in some new antihistaminic and narcotic agents. However, it was in 1955 that I started with pure psychopharmacologic research when I joined Prof. Z. Votava, who was head of the Department of Pharmacology at the Medical Faculty. We worked in close collaboration with the Research Institute for Pharmacy and Biochemistry on the testing of a new series of compounds with possible psychotropic effects, which were synthesized by the group of M. Protiva. The main problem was the differentiation of neuroleptic and antidepressant activity in animal experiments. Various experimental approaches were used: special

Olga Benešová received her MD from Charles University in Prague in 1948, followed by a doctorate in science in 1969. She became a professor of pharmacology in the Medical Faculty of Hygiene at the University, and since 1985 has been Head of the Laboratory of Brain Pathophysiology at the Prague Psychiatric Centre. She has conducted research in psychopharmacology, the neuropathology of aging, and drug-induced brain maldevelopment.

Benešová was elected a member of the CINP in 1970. She presented papers on "Pharmacological effects of proheptatrien, a new antidepressant drug of the dibenzocycloheptene group" (Benesova, Bohdanecky, Metysova, Metys and Votava) and on "The action of cocaine, atropine and tricyclic antidepressants on self-stimulation in rats" at the 4th and 6th Congresses respectively. She coauthored papers on "Experimental study on the mechanism of depressogenic action of apomorphine" (Benes and Benesova), on "The effect of octoclothepin and perphenazine on behaviours in rats with different exploration and defecation rates" (Kazdova, Dlabae, and Benesova), on "Influence of atropine, scopolamine and benactyzine on the physiostigmine arousal reaction in rabbits" (Votava, Benesova, Bohdaneczky and Grofova), and on "Comparison of pharmacological effects of some antidepressants of the imipramine type and their demethylated derivatives" (Votava, Metysova, Metys, Benešová and Bohdanecky), at the 7th (2x), 5th and 4th Congresses respectively. Benešová was also a formal discussant of the 5th Working Group (Pharmacological and clinical actions of antidepressive drugs) at the 4th Congress.

behavioural tests (e.g., self-stimulation in rats), electrophysiological techniques (e.g., EEG in rabbits with implanted cortical and subcortical electrodes), and biochemical analysis of the brain and its main parts (glucose metabolism, turnover of monoamine neurotransmitters).

Among the different psychotropics we identified and characterized, dosulepin (Prothiaden), synthesized by M. Protiva in 1961, was to become the most successful antidepressant of the Czechoslovak pharmaceutical industry. In 1962, I presented our results on self-stimulation in rats and on the EEG in rabbits, at the 27th "Tagung der Deutschen Pharmakologischen Gesellschaft" in Vienna. I remember well that someone from the audience was taking photographs of the structural formula of the drug and of other documentation. Some three weeks later, a letter from the Boots Co. in Nottingham arrived at my address, referring to my Vienna lecture and suggesting commercial collaboration on Prothiaden production and distribution. I passed the letter to M. Protiva, and this marked the very beginning of negotiations with Boots Co. on licensing Prothiaden.

The period from the late 1950s through the 1960s was a time of rapid growth for psychopharmacological research in Czechoslovakia. Since 1958, members of our Psychopharmacological Society (which includes chemists, pharmacologists, neurophysiologists, psychiatrists and neurologists) have met every year in early January at Jesenik Spa/Graefenberg in the Moravian mountains. The number of participants rose from around forty people in 1958 to five hundred in 1997. The popularity of these meetings is partly due to the favourable combination of scientific sessions in the morning and evening, with the opportunity for active recreation during the afternoon (skiing, scenic walks, curative water bath). Really, mental health care in practice!

In 1970 Professor Votava, who was the leading personality in our national psychopharmacological life and also an active member of CINP from 1962, was asked to organize the 7th CINP congress in Prague. The preparations started in the late 1960s. The leaflets with the advance information were printed, and it was my job to distribute them at the 6th CINP meeting, held in 1968 in Tarragona. The problems I encountered illustrate the difficulties in organizing international meetings in the divided Europe of those years.

First, even before I could confirm my registration as a participant at the Tarragona Congress, I had to apply to the Czechoslovak authorities for permission to travel abroad to a "capitalist country" and to buy a limited amount of foreign currency. Then I needed a visa for Spain since Spain had no diplomatic representation in Czechoslovakia. Then, my Spanish visa had to be mediated by the Swiss authorities. These transactions took several months. Further obstacles appeared when I arrived with my husband in our car at the French-Spanish border in Perpignan. For Spanish custom officers, we were, as all people from a Communist country, *a priori* enemies and spies whose car was subject to a special inspection. Their suspicion was confirmed when they found a parcel full of odd leaflets in English, which for them was a mysterious language. Our explanations in French, German and English were in vain because they understood only Spanish, and we knew only some Spanish phrases from the first page of the tourist's conversation guidebook. Consequently, the parcel and our passports were confiscated, we had to park our car on a layby and wait in the midday heat over three hours. At the end, the situation was resolved by the arrival of a higher official, who allowed us to continue on our way to Tarragona.

The CINP Congress in Tarragona was a success from both a scientific and a social point of view. With a sense of nostalgia, I look at the photo taken at the concert in the Roman Caves which we enjoyed together with Professor Z. Votava, who left us forever in 1990.

MY MEMORIES OF EARLY PSYCHOTROPIC DRUG DEVELOPMENT

Oldrich Vinar

PREHISTORY

In December 1949, I graduated in medicine from Charles University in Prague. I would have liked to specialize in neurology, but at the time in Czechoslovakia, it was the Ministry of Health that decided where a medical doctor had to work. So I was glad when I was sent to the State Hospital for Brain Diseases in Kosmonosy, about 60 kilometers north of Prague. When I arrived at the hospital, I was surprised to find that it was a psychiatric hospital with only one doctor for 1100 patients. The same doctor was the psychiatrist and the director of the hospital. He had to treat not only the mental disorders of his patients, but also their somatic conditions. He had to be their dentist, gynecologist and obstetrician. The situation that I found in the hospital was the consequence of the German occupation of Czechoslovakia, during which the universities had been closed for five years. The majority of psychiatrists perished in the Nazi concentration camps because they were Jews or in the resistance. Only about forty psychiatrists survived the occupation in a country of 12 million inhabitants. Many hospitalized psychotic patients had undergone a "special treatment" during the war in Czechoslovakia. They were castrated! It was referred to as "eugenics."

I was shocked while walking through the crowded wards, packed with aggressive and shouting patients approaching me with menacing gestures or crying, telling me that they were brought to this "prison" by mistake, and demanding from me their immediate discharge. I was advised never to enter a ward without being accompanied by one or two attendants, because

Oldrich Vinar, MD, DSc, has worked as a psychiatrist since his graduation in 1949. Clinical psycho-pharmacology has been his major field of interest, and he introduced the methods of controlled clinical trials in the former Czechoslovakia and elaborated several rating scales. He has also been involved in the development of several new psychotropic drugs. For forty years, he has organized Annual Psychophar-macological Meetings of the Czech and Slovak Society of Neuro-Psychopharmacology in Jesenik. Currently, he is head of the Joint Laboratory of the Institute of Organic Chemistry and Biochemistry of the Academy of Sciences and the State Institute for Drug Control. He works as a consultant in the Prague Psychiatric Hospital and lectures as assistant professor at Charles University.

Vinar was elected a fellow of the CINP in 1966. He presented a paper on "Conditioning in LSD-induced state and influence of neuroleptics," and on "Importance of some clinical and EEG criteria for drug selection" (Vinar, Matousek, Roubicek and Volavka) at the 5th and 6th Congresses respectively. He was a formal discussant of a paper by W.H. Bridger (Conditioning and psychomimetic drugs) at the 5th Congress, and a discussant from the floor of the second (The effects of psychotropic drugs on conditioned responses in animals and man) and third (The influence of specific and non-specific factors on the clinical effects of psychotropic drugs) symposia at the 2nd Congress. He was also a discussant from the floor of the paper by H. von Brauchitsch (The influence of thyroxine and insulin on the clinical effects of some neuroleptic drugs) at the 2nd Congress.

if I did, I was exposing myself to the risk of physical assault. All I was expected to do on my daily rounds was to approve the isolation of patients who had to be quieted down, and to identify the patients who required electroconvulsive treatment. This experience has always been a challenge for me and a source of my fascination with the psychotropic drugs that changed the scene so dramatically.

The years 1949-1960 were years of heavy Communist ideological oppression. The term *psychiatry* was not accepted because of the idealistic "psyche" in the word. The only research the state supported was based on the work of I.P. Pavlov and his Soviet disciples. The concept of "protective inhibition" had to dominate in all therapeutic activities. Conditioned reflexes were elaborated not only in experimental animals but also in patients. Various methods of sleep treatment were developed and even the effects of ECT and insulin coma therapy were interpreted in terms of protective inhibition.

PSYCHOTROPIC DRUGS

In 1952, I read about artificial hibernation and the effects of chlorpromazine. The concept of hibernation was criticized as pseudoscience. Fortunately, we succeeded in persuading Communist opinion leaders that the neuroleptics were compatible with the concept of protective inhibition, as the cortex is protected by such drugs from the influence of emotions which have their origin in the subcortex. Already in the mid-fifties, our chemists (Protiva, Jilek) had succeeded in the synthesis of new phenothiazines and synthetic *Rauwolfia* analogues. Czech pharmacologists (Votava, Metysova, Benesova) were well prepared to use their knowledge of the methods of conditioned reflexes and soon explored their effects in animals. Thus the clinicians (Nahunek, Vencovsky, Vinar, Vojtechovsky) could test the clinical properties of the new psychotropic drugs without delay. We began to organize annual psychopharmacological meetings in Jesenik as an interdisciplinary forum in order to exchange information about our experiences.

We had good results when treating patients with sleep therapy, combining small doses of hypnotics with antihistaminics. We knew that chlorpromazine (Largactil), the French miracle drug, was a potent antihistaminic. For political reasons it was very difficult to import a sufficient amount of Largactil. The amount of the drug sent to psychiatric institutions depended mainly on the political influence of the director. Not having enough Largactil, we treated our patients with a Czech compound, moxastin, an antihistaminic. Together with Vojtechovsky, we demonstrated quite good results with this drug in schizophrenia.

Our chemists synthesized prochlorperazine, perphenazine and thioridazine in the first half of the fifties. Because they used a different method of synthesis from the original producer, the production of these drugs by the Czechoslovak pharmaceutical industry began without any delay. The year 1956 was a turning point, when due to the widespread administration of phenothiazines, the number of psychiatric in-patients decreased dramatically.

Soon, our chemists began to synthesize original "me-too drugs." The first one was dichloropromazine. We reasoned that, since chlorpromazine was more efficacious than promazine (Sparine), adding another chlorine atom would increase the efficacy of chlor-promazine. We were disappointed. The drug had some tranquilizing properties but it had no antipsychotic effects. More interesting were the effects of another original compound, pheno-harmane. It was a synthetic analogue of reserpine and had a selective dysphoric effect in mania. Given to a manic patient, it induced dysphoria and even depression without decreasing psychomotor agitation. Its effects were spectacular if administered intravenously: a euphoric and happy patient became morose and depressed in 30-40 seconds. Since he remained agitated, we thought that the drug was interesting theoretically, but not suitable for practice.

Then, our chemists, Protiva, Jilek and their associates, became interested in the synthesis of new tricyclic antidepressants. Propazepine was the first of them. Pharmacologists found that it inhibited ptosis induced by reserpine and that it was not toxic. I performed the first double-blind trial with it in Czechoslovakia. After a placebo wash-out, we compared propazepine with imipramine and found that the average decrease in the scores of the rating scale was greater in patients on propazepine compared with those on imipramine, but the difference was not significant statistically. We used a newly developed Czechoslovakian rating scale for depression constructed according to the model of the Hamilton scale.

Since the validation of the scale was not ready before 1960, I was not allowed to publish my results by the "methodological board" of the Research Institute I was working in. I was so impatient to motivate psychiatrists to collaborate in controlled clinical research that I asked my wife, a psychiatrist who performed the trial with me, to publish the paper herself. I did not recommend the production of propazepine since I could not prove that it was better than the standard drug.

Another original antidepressant, dosulepine (dothiepine, Prothiaden) escaped the same fate thanks to E. Vencovsky, an influential university professor who recommended its production on the basis of his favourable experience with six patients and despite the fact that its superiority over imipramine was unproven.

In the fifties it was not difficult to develop a new drug. The chemists designed the molecule on the pattern of existing drugs, and pharmacologists performed some simple behavioural tests and predicted its therapeutic profile. Toxicology was restricted to finding the LD 50 in two animal species.

Human pharmacology consisted most often of a single experiment. It was usually Professor Votava, a pharmacologist, who ingested the drug and, based on his experience, the drug was given to the clinicians. The employees of the Institute for Pharmacy and Biochemistry in Prague knew that Protiva had synthesized a new drug whenever Votava was found in the corridor unconscious after an orthostatic collapse. I was usually the second subject to test the new drug, but I did it in a clinical setting and usually only at the dose which was given to patients as the initial one. Thanks to our enthusiasm, it sometimes took only three months before the newly-synthesized drug was given to the patients. Those who were considered capable of understanding were asked to give permission to be treated with a new drug. Usually, the response depended more on how much the patient trusted the doctor than on the information he or she got. It is my belief that this is still true today, when the patient reads pages of documentation and signs the informed consent.

Very early on, I began to organize multicenter-controlled trials. It was easy to find psychiatrists willing to cooperate since that was the way they got drugs which otherwise were difficult to obtain. The doctors were willing to be trained to use rating scales and they cooperated in their further education without expecting any payment.

CINP

I learned about the founding of the CINP from Professor Votava. We wanted to participate in the First Congress in Rome and to help other colleagues go there. Although it was very difficult to get permission to leave the country, a group of about twenty psychiatrists and pharmacologists succeeded in getting a passport and permission to go to Rome with a travel agency. It was a serious disappointment that we could not get an Italian visa in spite of the efforts of Votava, who contacted Professor Trabucchi several times.

We tried at least to get the program of the first congress. I got it from Professor Arnold (Vienna) who came to our meeting in Jesenik. We could see that many topics of the Rome congress were closely related to the work being done in Czechoslovakia. Therefore, it was an important event for me when, with the help of Professor Votava, I got permission to go to the second congress in Basel. This time, the Swiss visa was issued without difficulties. I could meet people whom I knew previously only from their publications. I was afraid to contact them with my poor English. Again, it was Professor Votava who helped me by reading a paper at the congress on the antiserotonin effects of LSD and of other synthetic ergot alkaloids. When I listened to his English, I realized that my English was not worse. Nevertheless, his paper was very well received by the audience and there was a vibrant discussion. This gave me more courage and I approached some speakers. I was surprised how interested people like Denber, Deniker, Fink, Shepherd, Pichot, Rickels, Carlsson and Itil were in our work. Particularly friendly to me were Heinz Lehmann, Nathan Kline, Max Hamilton and Donald Klein. I could discuss at length my experience relevant to the elaboration of conditioned reflexes in patients with W.H. Gantt, and Leo Alexander. Later, Horsley Gantt visited Prague and his lectures helped to persuade the Communist opinion leaders in Czechoslovak scientific institutions that cooperation with American and not only with the Soviet scientists could be useful.

My participation in the Basel Congress taught me how an international congress needs to be organized and so we held a symposium on psychopharmacological methods in Prague. The proceedings were published by Pergamon Press in 1963. Heinz Lehmann was the leading figure of this symposium. I suppose that the decision to organize the 7th CINP Congress in Prague was taken as a result of his influence.

I was not allowed to go to the congresses in Munich and Birmingham. My participation in the CINP congress in Washington was therefore very important to me. I had invitations to lecture at several United States psychiatric institutions and universities. Because they offered honorariums, I was able to persuade the Czechoslovak authorities that I would not need to exchange Czech crowns for dollars to be able to go to Washington. Thus, I got permission to leave Czechoslovakia for the United States. Unfortunately, my visa was issued only for six days, which was just sufficient to participate in the congress. The officials at the embassy in Prague assured me that it would be easy to prolong the visa in Washington. They were right – but I nearly missed three important sessions of the congress by going repeatedly to the immigration office.

That was my first trip to America. I was deeply impressed by the country, by the American people, and by the atmosphere of the research institutions. I was lucky to be able to buy the flight ticket for Czech crowns in Prague. I suppose that it was Professor Bente who advised me to buy also a "US ticket" when buying the flight ticket to Washington. The "US ticket" enabled me to fly to any destination in the United States for six weeks. It was relatively cheap. It saved me when I needed to travel from one institution where I had lectured to the next one. I had expected to get the honorarium immediately after my presentation, but to my surprise, instead of getting money, they asked about my bank account to which the honorarium would be sent. Of course, I had no bank account. It was a crime to have a bank account in a western country for a citizen of a "socialist" state. Being left without money in some places where I lectured, I used my American air ticket. I went to the airport and flew to a very distant place overnight. I was well fed on the plane and was able to sleep there. In this way I crossed the Rocky Mountains several times.

During the Washington congress, it was Tom Ban more than anybody who taught me how to get as much information as possible and how to cope with such torrents. Nathan Kline invited me to lecture in Rockland. I spoke about the Czechoslovak antidepressant dosulepin (Dothiepin, Prothiaden),unknown in other countries at that time. Kline predicted a great future for the drug when he saw its chemical formula. There is a sulphur atom in the molecule and Kline considered that very important. In his view, it combined the advantages of phenothiazines and tricyclic antidepressants. He was right in his prediction: dothiepine became the most successful Czechoslovak drug and is still exported to many countries. But I am not sure whether it is due to the sulphur atom in the molecule.

During the congress, a dispute arose between those who saw tardive dyskinesia (TD) as a serious and frequent adverse effect of neuroleptics and those who argued that dyskinesias are simply symptoms of schizophrenia, especially of the catatonic type. Prof. Degkwitz wished to demonstrate that TD must be frequent even in American patients. A group of psychiatrists was invited to St. Elizabeths Hospital to observe. On entering the ward, Professor Degkwitz found a tall black patient with bucco-oral dyskinesia. He demonstrated him to the group and described with German thoroughness even the most minute movements of his muscles. After he had completed his lengthy description, a nurse came over to the patient and asked him to spit out his chewing gum. I think this incident postponed the general recognition of TD as a consequence of neuroleptic treatment.

The next congress in Tarragona gave me the opportunity to meet in a very friendly atmosphere Leo Hollister, Mogens Schou, Alice Leeds and Malcolm Lader. For the Czechoslovak participants, Tarragona was connected with the euphoria of the 1968 Prague Spring, a time of hope that socialism could have a human face. The 7th CINP Congress in Prague was planned in this pleasant atmosphere. I still remember the scepticism of colleagues from Eastern Germany, Poland and Hungary when I voiced my optimistic evaluation of the political evolution in Prague.

DRUG DEVELOP-MENT

The chemists in the Institute for Pharmacy and Biochemistry in Prague synthesized lysergamide and made it available for psychiatrists. I was able to confirm that chlorpromazine blocked the LSD-induced state not only when given after LSD but that it prevented the changes induced by LSD if chlorpromazine was adminis-

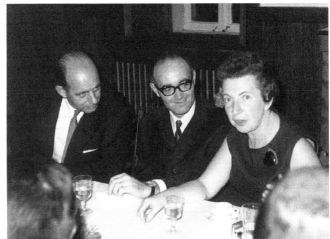

From left: Paul Kielholz, Oldrich Vinar, and Alice Leeds (right)

tered before LSD. I thought that it would be possible to test the therapeutic effects of newly-synthesized compounds in this model.

The first drug to be tested in the LSD-induced state was reserpine. Because its antipsychotic effects in patients began to show after a longer latency, the experimental subject (a nurse who volunteered after having had an experience with LSD) took reserpine before LSD. The result was terrible: she became very anxious, deeply depressed and had horrible visual illusions. It was difficult to control her behaviour as she wanted to die. A very unpleasant subjective state persisted even after she slept for twenty-eight hours. At that time *Rauwolfia* alkaloids were considered competitors of the phenothiazines and I concluded that the LSD model was not effective.

Before dropping this model I wanted to test a new sedative developed in the Soviet Union. It was chemically close to caffeine and the pharmacologists demonstrated that the chemical difference was expressed as an antagonism to caffeine. After the experiment with reserpine I did not have the nerve to accept volunteers, so I took LSD and antifeine myself. I became nearly psychotic and controlled my behaviour only with difficulty. I had to force myself to remember that I was just experiencing the effects of the drug. I had extracampine visual hallucinations. I saw a battle of two armies in my back. A lot of soldiers in the short leather trousers worn as national costumes in Swiss villages fought against an army of Russian boys with balalaikas. The psychosis-like state lasted nearly three days. I tried to dissimulate and did not speak about my "ideas of reference." Driving my car, I knew that people were watching me and someone in the car behind me was persecuting me. This was the end of my effort to use the LSD-induced state when testing new compounds for antipsychotic properties. Today, speculation about the influence of the LSD, reserpine and caffeine-antifeine combination could help to interpret these results. Nevertheless, the outcome of this experimental work turned my interest to a more clinical approach in the development of new drugs. On the other hand, it was clear to me that the war between the Swiss and Russian army in my back represented the influence of the combination of the Swiss LSD and the Russian antifeine.

Memoirs from France

CHLORPROMAZINE: A TRUE STORY OF THE PROGRESS EFFECTED BY THIS DRUG

Pierre A. Lambert

It was in the summer of 1953 that I began my thirty-year career at the Hôpital Psychiatrique de Bassens as chief of the psychiatric unit. The buildings, which had been constructed around 1850, were a classic example of the recommended architectural style for asylums in that era: a walled-in complex of structures erected to defy time, with a main central courtyard surrounded by the apartments of the director and the physicians. No one could enter or leave the premises without identifying themselves at the front gate. The hospital, in a sparsely-populated mountain zone, admits patients presenting all forms of mental pathology. It accommodates twelve hundred patients, assigned on the basis of certain characteristics of their condition to different wards, such as "agitated," "incontinent," "work therapy..."

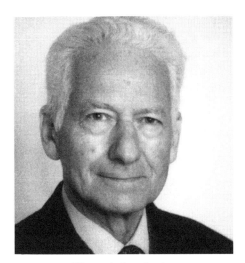

Pierre A. Lambert

Shortly after my arrival, I met Dr. C. Berthier, one of my colleagues. When I asked him if he had ever prescribed RP4560, he smiled and, as if by magic, produced a vial from his pocket. He told me that he had just returned from the Congrès de Neurologie et de Psychiatrie de

Pierre A. Lambert was trained as chemist and physician prior to becoming a psychiatrist and psychologist. He is honorary psychiatrist of the psychatric hospital at Chambéry and past president of the Comité Lyonnais de Recherches Thérapeutiques en Psychiatrie. His interest in psychopharmacology includes neuroleptics, antidepressants and mood regulators. He served on the expert advisory committee to the Ministry of Health on new drugs.

Lambert was elected a fellow of the CINP in 1958. He presented papers on "Essai de classification des neuroleptiques d'après leurs activités psycho-pharmacologiques et cliniques" (Lambert, Perrin, Revol, Achaintre, Berthier, Brousolle et Requet), on "A propos de l'action psycholéptique d'un derivé phenothiazinique l'phenothiazinyl-10 dithiocarboxylate de diethylaminoethyl ou 7,380 RP" (Lambert, Diedrichs et Charriot), on "Le 1.317 AN un medicament qui appelle une action relationelle" (Lambert, Achaintre et Brouselle), and on "Du choix d'un neuroleptique de référence. Intérêt théorique, expérimental et clinique" at the 1st, 2nd and 3rd (twice) congresses respectively; and coauthored papers on "Un nouvel antidépressif derivé de l'iminodibenzyl la trimipramine (7162 RP). Bilan clinique après utilisation depui près de trois ans" (Guyotat et Lambert), on "Appréciation des résultats cliniques et sélection [contd]

Langue Française [French-language Congress of Neurology and Psychiatry], where he had heard some papers on the promising work done with this product. Rhône-Poulenc Pharmaceutical Laboratories had supplied him with sufficient quantity to try it in a few patients, and he was quite eager to try out the injectable form of the drug that was to become known as chlorpromazine, or Largactil in France.

The patient we selected for the clinical trial with chlorpromazine was a hypomanic in a state of excitation. In preparation he was put on a special diet and moved to a room where he was easily accessible at all times to the staff. The patient responded promptly to the medication. Since four 25 mg parenteral injections of chlorpromazine administered within a day sufficed to control his excitement, we were very quickly able to confirm chlorpromazine's *sedative* effects. At this point it should be pointed out, that for many years, physicians and psychiatrists considered chlorpromazine to be essentially a sedative, a calming agent, a remarkable tranquilizer when compared to previously used medications, such as chloral, the bromides, barbiturates, and even morphine. It was its potent calming effect, in all likelihood, that had prompted the Americans to coin the term "major tranquilizer" in reference to chlorpromazine and drugs with similar sedative effects.

I observed in the schizophrenic patients I was treating right from the very first month the substantial effects of chlorpromazine in psychotic disorders. Of course, these effects had been reported by J. Delay and P. Deniker, and created enthusiasm about chlorpromazine among psychiatrists. In the course of my daily practice I encountered a sufficient number of patients, especially chronic schizophrenics whose normal contact with reality was restored in the course of treatment, to convince me that chlorpromazine could produce remission in psychotic disorders.

As early as in 1954, i.e., one year after I assumed my position in the hospital, I realized that the psychiatric profession was no longer what it had been, that the introduction of chlorpromazine forced us to review both our thinking and our treatment procedures. The advent of chlorpromazine brought an added dimension of professional satisfaction to our work, in that we could now assume the status of effective caregivers or, quite simply, full-fledged physicians. We were definitely past the stage of merely trying to interpret our patients' remarks, or fit our patients into the descriptions of the nineteenth-century alienists, and then, await the generally inevitable progression and outcome of the disease. We could now take decisive action in the serious mental pathologies. There were a number of questions regarding dosage, adverse effects, and the future prospects of patients who had undergone treatment (a question that had taken on a certain element of urgency for their families). Concerns were also expressed in an entirely different dimension by our management and nursing staff, who for the first time were seeing more patients discharged than admitted, (the operating budget had been established according to the number of hospitalization days). Although we saw ourselves as still

---

des médicaments en psychopharmacologie par l'analyse statistique" (Gayral, Lambert, Caussinus et Scheecktman), on "Le dichlorhydrate de flupheenazine (Etude des doses élevees et des traitements de longue duree)" (Gayral et Lambert), and on "La transformation de l'hôpital psychiatrique par les neuroleptiques et ses nouvelles tâches" (Balvet, Beaujard, Perrin, Berthier, Brouselle, Achaintre, Requet et revol) at the 1st, 3rd (twice) and 5th congresses respectively.

inexpert medical-practitioners who were making use of an undeniably effective therapeutic advancement, we were thrilled by the new developments.

This feeling of enthusiasm, coupled with the favorable circumstances in which we were working, led to the development of exemplary teamwork.

The new vision emerged quickly. In 1954, a pharmacist named Paul Brouillot visited the Hôpital du Vinatier in Lyons. He was sent there by Rhône-Poulenc to obtain information about their trial results, and specifically about possible adverse reactions caused by chlorpromazine. From his visits to other psychiatric centres, Brouillot was aware of the often deplorable living conditions in some of the psychiatric institutions. His trip to Vinatier proved to be a complete surprise to him. As he was shown around the hospital by a young physician, Brouillot was witnessing the renewal of interest of psychiatrists in psychiatry. It was evident from this visit that the break with the past had finally been made, and the news had to be spread. This was achieved with Brouillot's help and the financial backing of Rhône-Poulenc. Knowing that Berthier and I had had similar results with chlorpromazine, our colleague, Dr. Perrin visited us in Bassens and invited us to join forces with the medical group at Vinatier. From that time on, more than two hundred case histories of patients treated with chlorpromazine were shared between the two hospitals. An even greater step forward was taken with the decision to create a scientific association, which was named Le Comité Lyonnais de Recherches Thérapeutiques en Psychiatrie (The Lyons Committee for Therapeutic Research in Psychiatry). Professor Louis Revol, a pharmacist at the Hôpital du Vinatier who had also been appointed to the chair of pharmacy at the faculty of medicine in Lyon, was elected the first chairman.

The primary task of the twelve members of the Lyons Committee was to gather together all of the case histories of patients treated with chlorpromazine for discussion during our meetings. This process took almost a year, and it was only in October 1955 that our results were publicized in a presentation at the Colloque International sur la Chlorpromazine et les Médicaments Neuroleptiques en Thérapeutique Psychiatrique, organized in Paris by Professor Jean Delay. The results were reported by Perrin, who covered 458 cases in the Hôpital de Bassens alone. The symposium organizers were quite surprised by the number of requests for copies of the paper. One indication of the cardinal importance of the event was that psychiatrists, both in France and abroad, would thereafter refer to "neuroleptic" treatment when using chlorpromazine and reserpine.

The following year, under the direction of Prof. L. Revol, the Comité Lyonnais published an account confirming the expertise acquired through our collaborative efforts, entitled *La Thérapeutique par la Chlorpromazine en Pratique Psychiatrique* (Chlorpromazine Therapy in Psychiatric Practice) (1956). It should be noted that our "collaborative method" has been used by now for thirty years in studying new psychotropic compounds submitted by various laboratories for clinical investigations. We worked most closely, however, with Rhône-Poulenc and its representatives, Drs. Pellerat and Rives, who were responsible for explaining their new molecules to us, collecting our case histories, and writing up the summaries of our working sessions.

I would like at this time to comment briefly on the period from 1956 to 1960. Our group was characterized by the members' mutual trust and willingness to discuss collaboratively each individual case history. This ensured the adherence to an implicit code of ethics right from the very beginning.

During the very first year of the trial, one member of our group had discovered that the administration of chlorpromazine in doses of 500 mg per day produced more clear-cut results than with lower doses, especially in cases of chronic schizophrenia. Although the administration of higher doses was recommended to the group, we continued to administer much lower dosages. It was only after our contact with Prof. Labardt from Basel, who confirmed the satisfactory tolerance of this dosage, that the group decided to adopt higher doses. This change in the dosage of the therapy was, in all probability, the reason for the higher number of remissions observed subsequently. These remissions were not of long duration. This, however, was attributable not to a progressively diminishing effectiveness of the medications, but rather to a lack of the resources needed to follow up patients in remission after their discharge from hospital. During a presentation at the World Congress of Psychiatry, held in Zurich in 1957, I reported that 50 percent of schizophrenic patients with chronic delusions were readmitted to the hospital less than a year after their discharge.

It was primarily two factors, the substantial effects of chlorpromazine on mental disorders, coupled with the necessity for maintenance therapy, that prompted me to create a special area in the Hôpital de Bassens for patients being treated with chlorpromazine. In 1957 a specific section of the building was assigned to a single hospital unit that served both out-patients and in-patients in the catchment area. When discharged from hospital, patients were followed up either in the health centre or through home visits. Such a regional health policy was recommended by the French Ministry of Health in 1960. It was extended to the entire country in 1970, and later sanctioned by the World Health Organization. The implementation of this system with the introduction of chlorpromazine made it possible to mitigate prejudice and bring about changes in public reaction to the mentally ill. Of particular note is the fact that through this home-based monitoring system, I was able to follow up, in both the family and social milieux, patients who had undergone extended periods of treatment with new compounds.

Many phenothiazine derivatives have been synthesized. After being tested in the laboratory, some of these derivatives were referred to the Comité Lyonnais for clinical studies. As a result, mopazine, although similar to chlorpromazine, was shown to be less effective, and levomepromazine proved to have a stronger sedative effect. The most notable discovery was the one reported by P. Broussolle at the Congrès de Neurologie et de Psychiatrie, held in Bordeaux in 1966. Broussolle presented results obtained using prochlorperazine, a new phenothiazine with a piperazine side chain. The action of the new agent was described as "disinhibiting," a term that was later adopted by clinicians to describe a neuroleptic which, among other properties, stimulates the often passive behaviour of chronic schizophrenics. This discovery guided researchers toward the synthesis of other piperazines, and subsequently piperidine, phenothiazine neuroleptics which had more marked antipsychotic (and parkinsonism-inducing) properties. Since the daily therapeutic doses of these new compounds were much lower than for chlorpromazine, we conducted further trials, out of which came, in the 1960s, a prolonged-action injectable neuroleptic which was referred to as "slow release neuroleptic."

As early as 1956, after clinicians had compared reserpine and chlorpromazine (comparisons that proved favorable to chlorpromazine), it became evident that the properties and indications of neuroleptics varied. Furthermore, the launching in 1958 of haloperidol, a product with a significantly different chemical formula, created a need for comparative classification of the classification of the various compounds. The classification we developed was presented at the first congress of the CINP held in Rome in 1958. The title of the paper summarized its fundamental points: *La Classification psychopharmacologique et clinique des différents neuroleptiques. Indications thérapeutiques générales dans les psychoses* (The Psychopharmacologic and Clinical Classification of Neuroleptics: General Therapeutic Indications in the Treatment of Psychoses). The creation of this classification system served to establish the reputation of the Comité Lyonnais, both in France and, most notably, in certain West European countries. The classification was reprinted in a 1960 issue of *La Presse médicale* and subsequently became known as the Lambert-Revol Classification System. At the left end of the classification were listed sedative-type neuroleptics such as levomepromazine, and at the right end, "incisive-type" neuroleptics such as haloperidol. The system has continued to serve as a reference guide and basis for the classification of most new neuroleptics. In addition, it has been used by teaching professionals, prescribers of psychiatric therapies, and, judging from its widespread use in the advertising of new products, for clinical trial by pharmaceutical laboratories. Chlorpromazine occupies a relatively central position in this classification system.

One of my colleagues at the Hôpital de Bassens had the idea of setting up a large thirty-bed dormitory for female bedridden patients treated with chlorpromazine. The room was dark and silent, the curtains were drawn, and the patients watched by a sister from the convent. From time to time, more often in the morning, one of the women would get up and express herself somewhat timorously, but in terms of reality. As of that moment, the direction of the patient's life was changed, to the great surprise of the families, who were sometimes recalcitrant: They told us her condition was incurable.

About that time I developed a procedure of my own, based on Sakel's insulin coma therapy, which until the introduction of neuroleptics was the only treatment available for schizophrenia. It involved the induction of hypoglycemic comas through insulin injection, while maintaining the patient on chlorpromazine. In looking back today, the results appeared to have been satisfactory. The procedure was subsequently abandoned for two reasons: the depletion of the pool of chronic cases and the progress made in the development of psychotropic drug treatments. Yet while it was in effect, this therapy enjoyed the full support of our nursing staff. A new type of relationship with the patients was emerging, which went beyond the mere administration of medication to gain insight and hope for improvement. In short, although the medication remained appreciated, its therapeutic effects were recognized as often inadequate and in need of being complemented. Whether the patients were treated with chlorpromazine or with another neuroleptic, their newfound interest in reality, as evidenced by their participation in occupational therapy, sports, and therapeutic games, took on an added value. As an example, the Hôpital de Bassens was able to form a soccer team, which included more than 50% of our patients on neuroleptics, who participated in matches against teams from other psychiatric hospitals.

For over twenty years a certain spirit of competition existed between the École Parisienne (the College of Sainte-Anne) and the École Lyonnaise (the Comité Lyonnais de Recherches Thérapeutiques en Psychiatrie). This spirit of competition, provided a forum for general debate, an opportunity to organize congresses or symposia and to write papers, as well as for publishing articles and books. On behalf of the Comité Lyonnais, I was able to compile a series of articles, contributed by various authors, entitled *Actualités de Thérapeutique Psychiatrique* [New Developments in Psychiatric Therapy] into three volumes, which were published respectively in 1963, 1967, and 1972. At the Committee's invitation, a number of researchers and clinicians, including Glowinski, Laborit, and Julou, presented their theories and reported on the progress of their work. The Committee also established some international contacts, through events such as the 1959 meeting held in Lyons with a group of German psychiatrists, who reciprocated with an invitation to attend their meeting in Berlin the following year.

We were moving in a new direction, a direction that had never been called into question by the Committee: patients were being recognized as clinical trial subjects and their situations considered within the context of their personal histories. A number of us were involved in fields

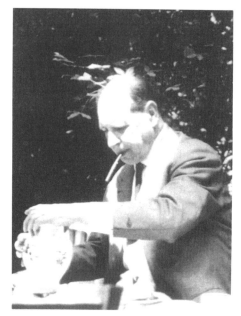

Henry Ey

like psychoanalysis and conducted in-depth investigations. Our concern for both the psychological and social aspects of a person was made explicit in the very first book published by the Committee in 1956. In his introduction, Henry Ey wrote that there is nothing more dangerous than representing mental illness in simplistic terms. He also found the notion inconceivable that chlorpromazine's physical action on the fundamental processes of mental illness could preclude the need for psychotherapy. In 1964, an important symposium, perhaps the first one on the subject, was held by the Committee in Lyons. The various papers presented, which covered approaches used by both psychiatrists and psychoanalysts, were published in a reference work entitled *La Relation Médecin-Malade au Cours des Chimiothérapies Psychiatriques* [Doctor-Patient Relationships and the Administration of Psychiatric Chemotherapy] (Lambert, 1965).

I have already mentioned the first congress of the CINP, held in Rome in 1958. This event has remained a memorable experience for both organizers and participants. The setting of the Villa d'Este is forever associated in our memories with the moment of universal recognition, by an international forum, the concept of psychopharmacology, the discovery of antidepressants. We realized that the significance of chlorpromazine would be soon surpassed by the numerous further discoveries it had triggered.

Psychiatrists of my generation have witnessed great changes over the last fifty years. In the Hôpital de Bassens, we now have a maximum of four hundred adult patients, most of them in-patients who are not institutionalized and are usually admitted only for a short time. The outer walls have been partially demolished, and the entrance to the hospital has been replaced by a reception area. An even greater number of people are treated on an outpatient basis, and the regional health policy has made both the quality of care and the staff-patient ratio more humane.

We are undoubtedly still faced with problems in therapeutic methods, not to mention a great deal of human suffering. We have also had to complement the action of neuroleptics and other psychotropic agents, whose role was unique in revolutionizing the practice of psychiatry. But where would we be today, some fifty years later, without the introduction of chlorpromazine?

PSYCHOTROPIC DRUGS AND PSYCHOTHERAPY

Jean Guyotat

It was in 1964 that I became the head of the department of psychiatry of Hôpital du Vinatier in Lyon, France, but prior to this I had become a member of the Comité Lyonnais de Recherches Thérapeutiques en Psychiatrie (CLRTP). The CLRTP provided me with an opportunity to compare my own clinical experience with psychotropic drugs to that of my colleagues. In those days, we did not use rating scales to evaluate the changes quantitatively, i.e., in terms of scores in the course of treatment with psychotropic drugs, but described the changes we encountered in patients' psychopathological symptoms and the observations reported by the nurses on patients' behaviour. It was on the basis of these observations and descriptions that we decided whether to use a particular psychotropic drug. Our task was easier than it is today in that there were not many drugs to compare and the results with the new drugs were very different from what we would have obtained using conventional treatments. That was the state of affairs at the time I became interested in participating in clinical drug trials with different types of phenothiazines and with the first antidepressants.

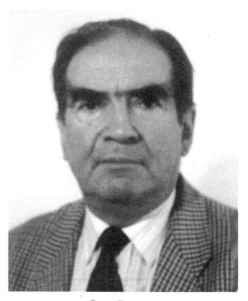

Jean Guyotat

Jean Guyotat is emeritus professor of psychiatry at the University of Lyon. He was chief of the psychiatric service of the university at Hôpital Vinatier and his primary activities included pharmacotherapy, psychotherapy and liasion psychiatry. He was co-editor with P. Deniker and T.H. Lemperiere of the *Manuel de Psychiatrie Clinique* (1990) and authored *Étude Cliniques d'Anthropologie Psychiatrique* and *Filitation et Puerperalité*, published in 1991 and 1995 respectively.

Jean Guyotat was elected a fellow of CINP in 1958. He presented papers on "Evaluation psychometrique des effets d'un psychotonique (8.228 R.P.): considerations méthodologiques" (Guyotat, Beaujard et Guillamin), on "Un nouvel antidepressif derivé de l'iminodibenzyle: la trimeprimine (7162 R.P.). Bilan clinique après utilisation depuis près de trois ans" (Guyotat et Lambert), on "Une méthode d'étude des effets psychodynamiques de certaines substances psychotropes (thymoanaleptiques)" (Guyotat), and on "Les effets des médicaments antidépresseurs dans les psychoses. Incidence de la structure, de la personalité et de l'environment" (Guyotat, Favre-Tissot et Marie-Cardine) at the 2nd, 3rd, 4th and 5th Congresses respectively. He also participated as a formal discussant of Working Group 6 (Dynamics and Significance of Psychopharmacological Intervention in Psychiatry) at the 4th Congress.

Prior to "Vinatier" I was in private practice and worked part-time as a psychotherapist at the Unité de Soins de Psychiatrie à l'Hôpital Général. I started to use chlorpromazine in 1954 in hospitalized patients with an acute psychotic episode, and as a practitioner I was in a position to follow the patients stabilized on chlorpromazine over a number of years – one patient over twenty years – after discharge from the hospital. My experience provided evidence that it was possible for a practicing psychiatrist to treat psychotic patients outside of hospital. The treatment of psychotic patients without removing them from their family environment was an important new development, that resulted mainly from the introduction of chlorpromazine and other neuroleptics.

An even more specific aspect of my practice resulted from my interest in psychoanalysis and from starting psychoanalytic training in Geneva. Since I had to attend my training sessions in Switzerland where imipramine was already available, I was able to bring back regularly a supply of the drug to France, where it was not available as yet. Because of my psychoanalytic training, which at the time was unique in Lyon, many colleagues referred to me patients with obsessive compulsive disorders. Since fifteen or so of these patients responded favourably to imipramine, I reported on the therapeutic effects of imipramine in obsessive neuroses in a paper published in 1960.

I subsequently extended the use of imipramine to a number of disorders labelled as "functional," which were to be called few years later "masked depression." Since I followed these patients for well over a year, I had information to share with my colleagues in the CLRTP on the effects of imipramine in "masked depression."

About the same time I realized that general practitioners were becoming increasingly interested in the use of psychotropic drugs. I also noted that because of their limited knowledge in the field they were inclined to prescribe meprobamate or a benzodiazepine instead of an antidepressant. To get some information on psychotropic drug use, I conducted in 1960 a survey on prescribing practices with the participation of 200 medical practitioners from our region.

My interest in psychopharmacology and psychoanalysis led me to the study of the psychodynamics of psychotropic drug action. Similar research to ours in France had been conducted by our colleagues in Germany and Canada. We reviewed our findings of this research in a round table discussion at the Third World Congress of Psychiatry in Montreal in 1961. Participants of the round table were Roland Kuhn, Gerard Sarwer-Foner, and Hassan Azima, among others. Five years later I was invited to report at the Fourth World Congress of Psychiatry, held in Madrid in 1966, on the effect of treatment with antidepressants on interpersonal relationships. Lastly, in collaboration with my colleagues from the CLRTP, I published a book on the doctor-patient relationship during pharmacotherapy with psychotropic drugs. In this book we reviewed the results of a double-blind, placebo-controlled study with pharmacotherapy and psychotherapy.

I would like to conclude this memoir by stating that I'm in agreement with P.-A. Lambert on many issues, but my practice led me to use neuroleptics in a different context from his. In variance with him, however, my primary interest has been to gain more insight into the links between psychotherapy and chemotherapy, which, as we all know, remains a concern for many of our colleagues.

FORTY YEARS IN THE PSYCHIATRY OF HOPE

Jean-Claude Scotto

I appeared in psychiatry at the same time as the antidepressants. Some of you may not see these two events as equally important, but I do. All joking aside, however, I know that I would not have gone into psychiatry if I hadn't believed in the potential of this specialty for developing fast, efficacious methods of care.

The past forty years have gone by so quickly that only a few milestones stand out. I remember working as a ward supervisor, under the direction of Professor Jean Sutter, in the psychiatry teaching centre, at the Hôpital de Mustapha in Algiers. One day in 1958, Yves Pelicier entered, holding a small glass flask in his right hand, while saying, "Here is something that will make our sulky little schizophrenic smile." The pills were iproniazid, and they did in fact elicit a smile from our young patient.

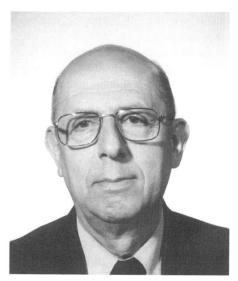

Jean-Claude Scotto

In 1961, while fulfilling my military duties in the psychiatric ward of the Hôpital d'Instruction des Armées d'Alger (Algiers Army Teaching Hospital) I gave haloperidol, which was to become one of the most extensively used neuroleptics, to a patient for the first time. To my surprise, a single intramuscular injection of this new neuroleptic almost instantaneously resulted in rigidity with complete immobilization of the patient. Later on we had another surprise in that, without any change to the product or mode of administration, the drug did not produce similar manifestations as promptly as when it was first administered.

In 1963, I travelled to Paris with Professor Jean Sutter, where we attended the meeting of the Société de Psychopharmacologie de Langue Française [Psychopharmacological Society of French-Speaking Psychiatrists]. There I met, for the first time, some of the great represen-

Jean-Claude Scotto is professor of psychiatry at the Université d'Aix-Marseille II, Director of the Department of General Psychiatry at CHU Sainte Marguerite in Marseille, and a founding member of the Association Française de Psychiatrie Biologique. He is the president of the Association Française de Psychiatrie et de Psychologie Sociales.

Jean-Claude Scotto was elected a fellow of the CINP in 1970. He coauthored a paper on "Recherches préliminaires sur le métabolisme de la fluphenazine chez l'homme" (Viala, Sutter, Scotto et Cano) presented at the 6th Congress.

tatives of French psychiatry. I still have memories of the smiling authoritativeness of Pierre Deniker and the consummate charm of Jean Delay. Later, I met Henri Ey, whose captivating speech was only matched by his fascinating writing style.

In 1965, in the old, dilapidated ward of the Hôpital de la Timone in Marseilles – where Professor Jean Sutter had found refuge following our exodus from Algiers – we conducted clinical trials with fluphenazine, a new neuroleptic at the time. A small group of patients seemed to tolerate the product very poorly and we observed six consecutive cases of what we believed to be neuroleptic malignant syndrome. We published the results as such. However, with the passing of time it appears that this was actually a minor epidemic of encephalitis.

Research with antidepressants was pursued at the time on both sides of the Atlantic. In view of the activating effect of these drugs, Jean Sutter suggested comparing, in a double-blind study, treatment with an antidepressant alone and in combination with a psychostimulant.

With the invaluable collaboration of Henri Luccioni, we developed our own assessment scales around the time that the methodology of the placebo-controlled, double-blind design was adopted. There has been an ongoing discussion over the past thirty years between those who are for and those against this methodology. Personally, I am in favour of "pilot projects," which, in my opinion, despite their subjectivity, will reliably identify the characteristics of new drugs.

I remember well the introduction of lithium, the long-acting neuroleptics, the substituted benzamides, and the new generation of antidepressants. And I especially remember my experiences with metapramine, a selective noradrenergic drug. It was as effective (or almost as effective) as clomipramine and it did not present any iatrogenic risks for patients. We administered it successfully by the intravenous route to an eighty-year-old patient (in the presence of a cardiologist with electrocardiographic monitoring). Everything went well and the patient recovered. Many other depressed patients also benefitted from this drug. Unfortunately its manufacturer decided to render it into a widely prescribed drug, used by general practitioners, and had therefore chosen to lower the dosage below the effective one. As a consequence of this decision, the drug was eventually taken off the market, leaving a number of patients who were successfully treated with it "up in the air." This entire affair, which was certainly not a unique event, posed an ethical dilemma for the pharmaceutical industry. The problem was never resolved, or at least not in France.

Indalpine offered a similar story. Its launching sparked such a rapid infatuation that, four years later, when the product was taken off the market due to undesirable hematologic side effects, many of us protested. Even today, many regret that this remarkable antidepressant could not be "saved" by ensuring safe prescription, as would later be the case for the clozapine.

Clozapine, also rejected in its time due to its blood toxicity, later returned to use with all the necessary precautions and became the prototype drug of what are now referred to as the atypical neuroleptics. I successfully treated many patients with this drug who were refractory to typical neuroleptics. Since then, many other new atypical neuroleptics have enriched our pharmacopoeia for the treatment of "schizophrenic deficit states."

In the much more common field of anxiety and sleep disorders, improvements with tranquilizers and non-benzodiazepine hypnotics have raised hopes that perhaps one day we will no longer have to resort to products which were abused at an increasingly alarming rate.

At the same time, however, the gap has continued to grow between the remarkable progress made in the neurosciences and the clinical use of psychotropic drugs by the many therapists who have not yet mastered prescribing psychotropics. Today, we still see patients in our departments who are not receiving adequate pharmacological treatment. Many psychiatrists fail to recognize that mental illness has a biological component. Yet in a seminar for students held in the 1960s, Henri Ey said that "psychiatry could never be anencephalic."

The steadily increasing number of meetings, and even of new associations, helped to channel psychiatric research in the right direction. The Collegium Internationale Neuro-Psychopharmacologicum has played a significant role in this regard. I personally still retain rich and vivid memories of the various conferences I attended, and especially of the congresses in Tarrogona in 1968 and Copenhagen in 1972. By the same token, the Association pour la Méthodologie de la Recherche en Psychiatrie [Association for Methodology in Psychiatric Research], founded in 1971 by Henri Luccioni at the Clinique Universitaire de Psychiatrie de Marseille [Marseilles Psychiatric Teaching Clinic] continues in its efforts to promote improved research techniques in psychiatry, and particularly in pharmacopsychiatry. However, much work still remains to be done in order to bring to the psychiatric profession a much needed eclecticism, along with a harmonious integration of biogenesis and psychogenesis, pharmacology and psychotherapy.

Since the discovery of chlorpromazine in psychiatry, the results obtained in the ensuing forty-five years have been so impressive that our present era can only be seen as a transition period, a period characterized not by its lack of new discoveries, but rather by its potential for building on the incredibly rapid progress already made. There is no cause for harboring any doubts regarding the future of pharmacopsychiatry, provided of course that expectations do not extend to the eradication of mental illness.

THE BOOM OF RESEARCH IN THE 1960s

Daniel Ginestet

I was a member of Jean Delay and Pierre Deniker's team in the early 1950s at the time chlorpromazine was introduced in the treatment of psychiatric patients. There were great expectations and excitement which continued for years throughout the subsequent introduction of a number of therapeutically effective drugs which were to find their place in Delay and Deniker's comprehensive classification of psychotropics in the category of neuroleptics (antipsychotics), thymoanaleptics (antidepressants) and anxiolytic sedatives (minor tranquilizers).

There was a close collaboration in those years between a small group of pharmacologists in Paris, which included J.-R. Boissier, P. Simon, and H. Nakajima (who was to become about 30 years later, the Director General of the World Health Organization). And there was also increasing awareness of developments in the United States and Canada. To get first-hand information on what was taking place in the United States, I became a visiting scientist at the National Institute of Mental Health (NIMH) and spent

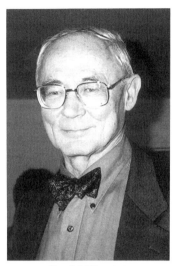

Daniel Ginestet

about 5 years there, from 1962 to 1967. Since I was in the United States at the time of the 5th CINP Congress in 1966, I was asked to report at the meeting some of our findings in pilot studies at Sainte-Anne Hospital in Paris. Deniker also agreed that with some regularity, I present our findings to American and Canadian colleagues at the NIMH and other places. I have wonderful memories of Heinz Lehmann's friendly cordiality, of Max Fink's and Turan Itil's provocative dynamism, and of Thomas Ban's charming authority.

The research I was involved with during those years included clinical studies with long-acting neuroleptics and with several new dibenzothiazepine, dibenzoxazepine, and dibenzodiazepine drugs. From the dibenzodiazepines I worked with, clozapine was to become the prototype of atypical neuroleptics. I recall that our study with clozapine was prematurely

Daniel Ginestet trained under Jean Delay and Pierre Deniker between 1951 and 1959 and became *chef de clinique* in 1960. His research in pharmacology spans the years 1962 to 1972. After being professor of psychiatry in the Faculté de Paris from 1973 to 1995 and *chef de service* at the Hôpital Paul Brousse from 1983 to 1995, Ginestet is now a consulting professor.

Daniel Ginestet was elected a fellow of CINP in 1964. He authored a paper on "Différences entre neuroleptiques, tranquillisants et hypno-sédatifs dans leurs applications et leur éfficacité pour le traitement des désordres psychiatriques" presented at the 5th Congress, and coauthored a paper on "Intérêt des controles cliniques et polygraphiques simultanés pour l'évaluation précoce de l'activité de certaines drogues chez l'homme" (Delay, Deniker, Verdeux, Ginestet et Peron) presented at the 3rd Congress.

terminated because of the marked sedation, seizures and thermoregulatory disturbances with the drug. Nevertheless, clozapine remained at the heart of many heated discussions between Pierre Deniker and Hanns Hippius, the main proponent of clozapine, who maintained that he discovered the antipsychotic which is free of extrapyramidal effects. Another controversy during those years, but in this case between us and our American colleagues, was about the disinhibitory effect of pipothiazine that we noted with Pierre Peron-Magnan, in low doses.

I was also involved with Wirz-Justice, Boissier, and Simon in research which was focused broadly on the relationships between biochemistry and mental illness. We were trying to replicate Arnold Friedhoff's finding of a "pink spot" in the urine of schizophrenics, but of course without success. With Peron-Magnan I was studying the model psychosis induced by Ditran and its instant antidote, tetrahydroaminoacridine, to be introduced under the brand name, Cognex. Furthermore, with the help of Gerald Klerman we had the opportunity to work with flurothyl (Indoklon), a substance which could induce covulsions by inhalation. We found Indoklon effective in treating melancholic patients.

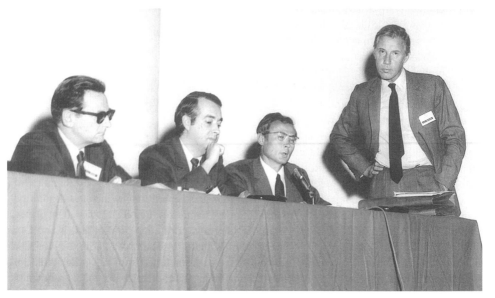

International Symposium on hallucinogens at Laval University (Québec 1968). From left: Theodore L. Sourkes, André Villeneuve, Daniel Ginestet and Jacques Boissier (right)

Finally, I would like to mention the several months I spent with my friend André Villeneuve at Saint-Michel Archange in Québec City (Canada). It was during my training with him that I learned that research and clinical practice are not mutually exclusive of each other.

In closing I would like to add that during the 1960s many clinical trials were conducted with a steadily increasing number of drugs, almost as if we had to compensate for the years of neglect of developing drugs for the treatment of mental illness and especially for the tretament of schizophrenia. Whether the three decades which followed have produced treatments with a better therapeutic ratio than that of the prototype psychotropics is outside the scope of this presentation. Regardless, the 1960s will remain one of the most important periods in the development of psychopharmacology.

Memoirs from Italy

PSYCHOPHARMACOLOGY AND PSYCHOPATHOLOGY

Antonio Balestrieri

After my graduation from medical school I worked for a short time in the Institute of Pharmacology at the University of Padova. Becoming a psychiatrist, I had therefore great expectations from the new drugs which appeared in the early 1950s.

I had been involved in studying the anticonvulsive effect of phenothiazines in animals (1) and exploring the possible antiparkinson effect of chlorpromazine in patients. By the late 1950s, however, because of my growing interest in psychiatry and psychopathology, I became involved in research with hallucinogenic drugs. It was in the course of this research that I discovered the cross-tolerance between hallucinogenic drugs (2, 3, 4).

It was a commonly-held belief in the early 1960s that there is a relationship between mental disease and the phenomena induced by hallucinogens. Since our findings indicated that

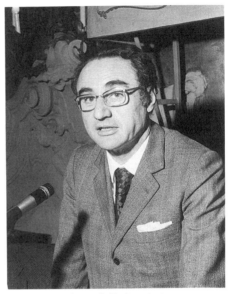

Antonio Balestrieri

the hallucinations induced by hallucinogens are similar to those seen in psychomotor epilepsy, I raised the possibility that the underlying pathology of the hallucinations encountered in psychomotor epilepsy and in schizophrenia might be the same (5, 6).

As early as 1961 I tried to synthesize the findings of my psychopharmacological research in a monograph entitled, *Patologia Mentale e Farmacologia* (7). I dealt in this monograph

Antonio Balestrieri, born in 1926 is a past president of the Italian Psychiatric Association. He is director of the university psychiatric clinic at the University of Verona. His different fields of interest and publications (in addition to psychopharmacology) include anthropology, ethology and the biology of behaviour.

Balestrieri was elected a fellow of the CINP in 1964. He presented papers on "Acquired and crossed tolerance to mescaline, LSD-25 and BOL-148" (Balestrieri and Fontanari), on "Some aspects of the sensitivity to hallucinogenic drugs" (Balestrieri and Balestrieri), on "Hallucinatory mechanisms and the content of drug-induced hallucinations" and on "Problèmes théoretiques sur la tolérance aux médicaments psychotropes" (Balestrieri et Tansella) at the 1st, 2nd and 5th Congresses respectively. Balestrieri was a formal discussant of the 3rd Working Group (Experimental and clinical neurophysiology) at the 4th Congress; and a discussant (from the floor) of the First Symposium (The problems of antagonists of psychotropic drugs) at the 2nd Congress.

with the use of drugs in the study and treatment of mental illness. Seven years later, in a publication on nervous integration and clinical problems I reviewed the findings of my researches (8).

My primary interest through the years has been the use of drugs as a means for studying psychopathology and especially the relationship between drive, consciousness, delusions and hallucinations.

I regret that only the therapeutic effects of psychotropic drugs are explored these days and that the possibility of using drugs for gaining a better understanding of mental health and disease is virtually ignored.

Psychopathology, biological psychiatry and psychopharmacology still remain to be linked in the most fruitful way.

REFERENCES

1. Balestrieri, A. (1955). Le azioni di alcuni derivati della Fenotiazina nei confronti di agenti convulsivanti. Arch. Int. Pharmacodyn., 100: 301-373.

2. Balestrieri, A. (1960). Studies on cross-tolerance with LSD-25, UML-491 and JB 336. Psychopharmacologia, 1: 257-259.

3. Balestrieri, A. (1961). Some aspects of the sensitivity to hallucinogenic drugs. Neuro-Psychopharmacology, 2: 44-47.

4. Balestrieri, A. (1961). Patologia Mentale e Farmacologia. Padova: CEDAM.

5. Balestrieri, A. (1964). Hallucinatory mecanisms and the content of drug induced hallucinations. Neuropsychopharmacology. 3: 388-390.

6. Balestrieri, A. (1968). Nervous integration and clinical problems. International Pharmacopsychiatry, 1: 159-167.

7. Balestrieri, A., and Fontanari, D. (1959). Acquired and crossed tolerance to mescaline, LSD-25, and BOL-148. Archives of General Psychiatry, 1: 279-282.

8. Balestrieri, A., and Tansella, M. (1969). Problèmes théoriques sur la tolérance aux médicaments psychotropes. In A. Cerletti and F.J. Bove (eds.). The Present Status of Psychotropic Drugs: Proceedings of the 6th International Congress of the Collegium Internationale Neuro-Psychopharmacologium,(pp 373-375). Amsterdam: Excerpta Medica Foundation.

FROM THE LACTATE-PYRUVATE RATIO IN SCHIZOPHRENIA TO TRYPTOPHAN PYRROLASE ACTIVITY IN DEPRESSION

Alfonso Mangoni

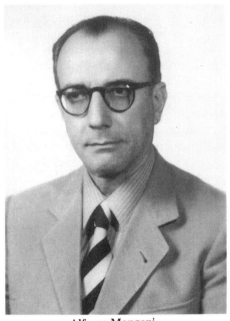

Alfonso Mangoni

When I received the invitation from the History Committee of the CINP to contribute to this volume, I thought that it would be difficult to reconstruct my experience of many years ago. However, I began with zeal, and because I am a meticulous person, I was able to find the protocols and correspondence relating to my experiments, which I have dusted off for posterity.

To begin, I would like to say that my scientific and academic life has been rather atypical, in the sense that most of my colleagues who dedicated themselves to the neurosciences have directed their activity either to basic biological or clinical research, and those who have cultivated both these fields over a substantial period of time have been few. As a university student, I had a particular interest in diseases of the nervous system. However, when I graduated in medicine from the University of Rome in 1952, I was advised to apply myself to the basic sciences before specialising in nervous and mental diseases. Having to decide about the discipline, I chose biochemistry, a field that was really a frontier in those years. I remember that in my student years in the Italian universities, biochemistry was not a required course but was partly taught in the physiology program. I

Alfonso Mangoni received his medical degree in Rome in 1952. After a research appointment, residency at Harvard Medical School, and serving as scientific officer and registrar at the Carshalton Medical Research Council, he returned to Italy in 1962 to head the Biochemical Laboratory in the Institute of Psychiatry at the University of Milan (until 1970). From 1972 until 1980 he was professor and head of the Institute of Nervous and Mental Diseases at the University of Cagliari. Since then he has been professor and head of the First Department of Neurology of the University of Milan.

Alfonso Mangoni was elected a fellow of CINP in 1966. He coauthored papers on the "Effect of chlorpromazine and haloperidol on tryptophan metabolism in schizophrenia" (Cazzullo and Mangoni) and on "Sleep patterns in depressed patients treated with a MAO inhibitor. Correlates between EEG and metabolites of tryptophan" (Cazzullo, Penati, Bozzi and Mangoni), presented at the 5th and 6th Congresses respectively.

therefore became a "voluntary assistant" (that is, without pay) in the Institute of General Physiology of the Faculty of Mathematical, Physical, and Natural Sciences at the University of Rome.

My first project at the Institute was a study of the permeability of the blood-brain barrier to amino acids in dogs using paper chromatography. I subsequently studied two adaptive enzymes, xanthine oxidase and tryptophan peroxidase (pyrrolase), under a number of different experimental conditions.

In 1957 I moved to the United States to become a research associate at the Institute of Living in Hartford, Connecticut, where I continued my basic research. My intention by that time was to dedicate myself to clinical neurochemical research. Since in those days most advanced neurochemical research was carried out in laboratories of psychiatric hospitals, I had to become a psychiatrist to be able to do the work I was interested in.

In 1959 I became a resident in the Department of Psychiatry at the Massachusetts General Hospital in Boston. My first exposure to neuropsychopharmacology took place early in my residency when, during the presentation of a case of depression, one of my colleagues suggested treatment with imipramine, a new drug at the time. The proposal did not receive much support. There was considerable reservation, a cautious attitude even in centres of excellence, towards psychoactive drugs in the United States in those years. They had been introduced just a few years earlier and were only slowly entering clinical practice. Paraldehyde was still the leading sedative used in the control of agitation, status epilepticus, and delirium tremens. We were at the dawn of neuropsychopharmacology.

At the end of 1960 I transferred to the Medical Research Council at Carshalton (UK). As a scientific officer and registrar I had the responsibility for the laboratory and the metabolic ward. It was during my tenure at Carshalton that I designed an experiment to study oxidative mechanisms in schizophrenia which had just been demonstrated to be altered. Although I used the methodology employed in the original experiments, i.e., measured the lactate-pyruvate ratio in "schizophrenic plasma" incubated in nucleated chicken erythrocytes, I was not able to confirm the findings in the original report.

At the end of 1962, I transferred to the Psychiatric Clinic of the University of Milan to become the head of the clinical biochemical laboratory. It was in Milan that I began to study some of the metabolic aspects of depression. The generally accepted view at the time was that depressed patients, because of their assumedly low brain concentration of serotonin, benefited from the administration of monoamine oxidase inhibitor drugs. With this premise in mind, I decided to study in depressed patients the terminal metabolites of the indole and kynurenine pathways of tryptophan metabolism, i.e., 5-hydroxy-indoleacetic acid and xanthurenic acid, respectively. What I found was that depressed patients had increased xanthurenic acid levels compared to control subjects. There was no difference in 5-hydroxyindole-acetic acid levels between patients and controls. Based on these findings I formulated the hypothesis that, as a result of an increase in hepatic tryptophan pyrrolase activity, in depressed patients there is a shift in the conversion of tryptophan towards the kynurenine pathway, to the detriment of the indole pathway. My assumption proved to be correct. Subsequent research by other investigators indicated an increase in tryptophan pyrrolase activity in depression. In view of this I designed a series of studies to find out whether tryptophan pyrrolase activity can be influenced by the administration of antidepressant drugs. In the course of these studies I was able to demonstrate that both imipramine and tranylcypromine decreased tryptophan pyrrolase activity and thereby increased the availability of tryptophan for serotonin formation. The reported increase of plasma cortisol, a well-known inducer of tryptophan pyrrolase activity, provided further support for my hypothesis.

In the early 1970s, I was appointed professor, first in Cagliari and subsequently in Milan. I also moved from the department of psychiatry, first to the Nervous and Mental Diseases Clinic and later to the Neurology Clinic.

One of my first neurological studies was concerned with metoclopramide, a compound widely used in the treatment of gastrointestinal disorders of the "dyskinetic type." The question I was trying to find an answer for was whether metoclopramide, a substance with a somewhat similar pharmacological profile to butyrophenone neuroleptics, has an effect on the metabolism of dopamine in the brain. What I found was that in the rat, metoclopramide increased homovanillic acid levels in the brain. Dopamine, norepinephrine and 5-hydroxyindoleacetic acid levels remained unchanged.

During the same period, I became interested in the therapeutic effect of some dopamine-agonist drugs, and especially of apomorphine, in extrapyramidal disease. Apomorphine's therapeutic action in Parkinson's disease was already known, but the drug was not of practical value because of its significant emetic effect. However, by antagonizing its emetic effect with metoclopramide or sulpiride, a single 10 mg dose of apomorphine reduced rigidity and tremor in Parkinson's disease without causing nausea or vomiting. In doses of 1-4 mg, i.e., below the emetic dose, apomorphine was shown to have beneficial effects on involuntary movements in Huntington's chorea as well (perhaps by acting on autoinhibitor presynaptic receptors rather than on postsynaptic dopaminergic receptors).

In an open study I was able to demonstrate the therapeutic effect of clonidine on essential tremor. In a controlled study I found that both clonidine and propranolol, given as intravenous infusion, significantly reduced tremor.

During the last decade, my primary objective has been finding an effective pharmacological treatment for Alzheimer's disease. In a multicentre clinical trial I studied the short-term efficacy of selegiline, a selective monoamine oxidase inhibitor, and our findings clearly indicated that the drug has favourable effects on cognitive function as well as on activities of daily living. In other words, improvement was observed with regard to self-sufficiency and overall functioning. I also noted that selegiline might be effective in slowing the progress of Alzheimer's disease.

To conclude my autobiographical account, I would like to put on record how pleased I am about the merger of psychopharmacology with neuropharmacology. Clinical experience indicates that it is not always possible to distinguish psychic from neurological symptoms and that in psychiatric and neurological disorders the same regions of the central nervous system might be involved. I hope that a better understanding about the functional relationships between all the different components of the nervous system will yield a better understanding of psychiatric and neurological diseases, which in turn will enable us to develop better treatments for both.

THE RISE OF PSYCHOPHARMACOLOGY IN MY LIFE

Carlo L. Cazzullo

My personal enthusiasm for psychopharmacology comes from my conviction about the importance of biological mechanisms (genetic, metabolic, etc.) in mental pathology. I was trained in neurology and psychiatry by Carlo Besta, a famous professor in the 1930s at the University of Milan, with a special interest in the biology and histology of nervous and mental diseases; and my first interest relevant to psychopharmacology was the role of vitamins in physiological and pathological brain functioning. The results of my original research on vitamin C (ascorbic acid) and B3 (nicotinic acid) in the cerebrospinal fluid of neurological and psychiatric patients, were published in the journal *Vitamin und Hormone* (Munich) in 1943.

My first encounter with neurotransmitters took place in 1947 at the Rockefeller Institute in New York, where, as a visiting scientist (investigator), I was studying, under the direction of Nobel laureate Herbert Gasser, with R. Lorente De No, the role of electrical nervous transmission. As early as the late 1940s I had been hoping for the utilization of drugs in the treatment of mental disease. I greeted with great expectations the introduction of new psychotropic drugs in the early 1950s.

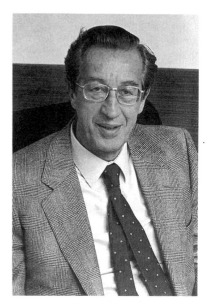

Carlo L. Cazzullo

Carlo Lorenzo Cazzullo was chairman of the Department of Psychiatry and the Postgraduate School in Psychiatry at the University of Milan from 1959 to 1991. He is now emeritus professor of neuropsychiatry. The author of twenty-two books, a three-volume textbook in psychiatry, and more than six hundred scientific papers in different languages, he served as president of the Italian Psychiatric Association from 1968 to 1991 (in 1991 he became the first honourary president of the association). He is also the founder of the Association for Research on Schizophrenia, established in 1982.

Cazzullo was elected a fellow of the CINP in 1958. He presented papers on "Ten years of psychopharmacology: Critical assessment of experimental and clinical data"; on "Sleep patterns in depressed patients treated with a MAO inhibitor. Correlation between EEG and metabolites of tryptophan" (Cazzullo, Penati, Bozzi and Mangoni); on "Pharmacological and clinical differences in the actions of sedative-hypnotic tranquillizers and neuroleptic drugs. Differences in neuropathology"; and on "Effects of psychotropic drugs on motor, autonomic and verbal conditioning in man" (Cazzullo and Goldwurm) at the third, fifth (twice) and sixth Congresses respectively. He was also a discussant from the floor at the First Symposium (The problem of antagonists to psychotropic drugs) at the second Congress.

In 1958, after my return to Italy from the United States, I became professor of neurology and psychiatry at the University of Milan and chairman of the first department of psychiatry in the country. As chairman of a department I was able to embark on basic and clinical research in neuropsychopharmacology. For some time I had been interested in the effects of reserpine on the brain. One of our first projects was directed to the study of the central nervous system effects of the drug in rabbits, using for the first time (with Terranova) histochemical and histological techniques. We presented our findings in Lyon in 1957, at the fifty-fifth Congrès des Médecins Aliénistes et Neurologistes de Langue Française. About the same time we also carried out research with chlorpromazine, using the same techniques. In these studies we were able to show the effect of chlorpromazine in high doses on the nerve cells.

Bernard Brodie's work suggested to us that changes in drug metabolism might account for the toxicity of psychotropics. We also learned from Brodie that psychotropic drug metabolism might be an excellent tool for the study of biochemical mechanisms in the brain. It was with consideration of Brodie's teachings that we started our systematic studies (in collaboration with Borgna) on the effects of chlorpromazine in schizophrenic patients. Our objective was the detection of toxicity as well as the delineation of changes in psychopathology in schizophrenic patients treated with the drug. The mechanism of side effects and the efficacy of the drug on the acute symptoms of psychosis were also examined.

Professor Emilio Trabucchi was first to appreciate our research with psychotropic drugs. As an expression of his appreciation he invited me to the 1st International Congress of the CINP, organized in Rome in 1958. It was at this congress that I was elected a fellow of the

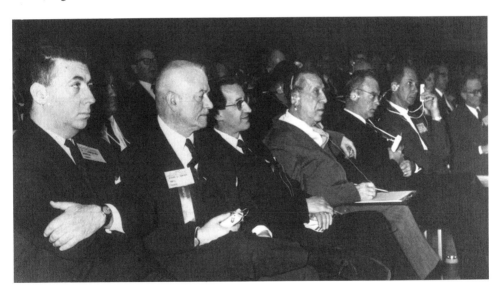

Listening to Jean Delay's Presidential Address at the 5th Congress in Washington, in the first row from left are: Gerald J. Sarwer-Foner, Pierre Deniker, Carlo L. Cazzullo, Max Rinkel, Vernon Kinross Wright and Leo Hollister (right)

organization. Subsequently, six years later in 1964, I founded with Professor Trabucchi in Milan, the Italian Society of Neuropsychopharmacology.

Our work with reserpine and chlorpromazine led to a comprehensive research program which included all psychotropic drugs released for clinical use. In this research program we used histological and histochemical analyses of the "cerebral parenchyma," and especially that of the "neurons," after the administration of low, medium and high doses of the drugs; and correlated the dose-effect relationships obtained in histological and histochemical findings with the dose-effect relationships in clinical practice. We presented our findings in three papers: the first, delivered at the third CINP Congress in Munich in 1962, the second, at the fourth World Congress of Psychiatry in Madrid in 1966, and the third, at a conference held at the Pasteur Institute in Paris in 1968.

Our histological and histochemical studies with psychotropic drugs were complemented with electrophysiological studies (in collaboration with A. Guareschi). We employed electro-encephalography to study the effects of chlorpromazine and haloperidol on brain potentials. It was on the basis of the collected information in these studies that we proposed in 1968 the following neurodynamic classification of psychotropic drugs:

- drugs with deep neuronal activity that modify the neurobiochemical substrate and the morphology of nuclei of nerve cells, e.g., reserpine, phenothiazines, thioxanthenes, butyro-phenones, and MAO-inhibitors;
- drugs with superficial neuronal activity that act on the surface of the cells without modifying their morphology, e.g., meprobamate and benzodiazepines;
- drugs with intermediate activity that act in a reversible manner at the cellular membrane level and on the cytoplasm, e.g., tricyclic antidepressants.

Our series of systematically conducted studies contributed to knowledge about the mechanisms and sites of action of psychotropic drugs, as well as to the early detection of their potential toxicity (especially of the potential toxicity of the monoamine oxidase inhibitors). It also indicated that combined administration of imipramine and a monoamine oxidase inhibitor might be toxic. The imipramine-induced brain edema, by modifying the permeability of the neuronal membrane, facilitates the penetration of monoamineoxidase inhibitors into the cell, producing changes in the cell nucleus.

The same studies brought to the attention the importance of protecting the CNS with neurotropic substances in case of chronic treatment with psychotropics, and especially of chronic treatment with substances with deep neuronal activity; and that pretreatment with "adenosine triphosphate" could prevent structural modifications of nerve cells by chlorproma-zine, a substance with deep neuronal activity. Our results in this area of research were referred to by Deniker at the second CINP Congress, held in Basel in 1960 and the American Psychiatric Association meeting in Atlantic City in 1962.

Starting in the early 1960s (in collaboration with Dr. Goldwurm), we also pursued research, on changes in conditional reflex variables and behavioural measures in pharmacotherapy of schizophrenia and depression. We presented our findings on the effect of antipsychotics on the behaviour of schizophrenic patients at the fifth CINP congress, held in Washington in 1966, and the effect of antidepressants on the behaviour of depressed patients at the seventh CINP congress, held in Prague in 1970. At the Washington congress I also presented findings on the effect of chlorpromazine and haloperidol on tryptophan metabolism in schizophrenia. At the 6th CINP congress, held in Tarragona two years later (in 1968), I presented (in collaboration with Penati) our findings on the effect of tryptophan metabolites on the sleep pattern (as detected by EEG} of depressed patients treated with a monoamine oxidase inhibitor. In the same year (1968), with consideration of prior communications of G.J. Sarwer-Foner, H. Denber and the late H. Azima, in collaboration with De Martis we introduced a combined method of treatment, i.e., psychotherapy and pharmacotherapy, in anxious-depressed patients.

By the mid-1970s there were three main lines of psychopharmacological research pursued under my direction in the Department of Psychiatry at the University of Milan. The first line consisted of studies of new molecules with psychotropic properties, emphasizing safety profile of the drugs. It included preclinical research in animals with histopathological assays after acute and chronic drug administration. The second line of research entailed the determination of the presence and concentration of the psychotropic drug and its metabolites in "biological fluids." Finally the third line of research was directed at correlating biological measures (neurochemical and immunological) with pharmacokinetic data.

We also had a neuropsychopharmacology laboratory with gas chromatographs which allowed for the generation of some early pioneering information on possible correlations between the plasma levels of some antidepressants and antipsychotics, and the therapeutic and side effects of the drugs. We were also able to generate in our laboratory some preliminary information on drug metabolism and bioequivalence.

We studied drug-drug interactions, age-related changes in the bioavailability of antidepressants and the "kinetic profile" of long-acting antipsychotics. Our findings indicated that older patients should be "managed pharmacologically" differently from younger patients.

In addition to research, my department was also involved in the dissemination of information on psychopharmacology. We held "International Monothematic Meetings on Psychiatry and Psychopharmacology" with some regularity.

I enjoyed my participation in CINP activities. The Collegium has played an important role in psychiatric education in psychopharmacology. The congresses of the organization provided opportunities to meet some fascinating people. I would like to mention some of those I have established a warm friendship with, based on mutual respect and esteem. My close relationship with Herman Denber, the "strict" secretary of the first and second executives, started actually prior to the founding of CINP, during my stay in New York when I was at the Psychiatric Institute of Columbia University. It was also during that time that I attended the extraordinary lectures of Paul Hoch, president of the third executive. But my friendship with Pierre Deniker started in 1960 at the Basel Congress after his endorsement of my proposal to use adenosine triphosphate for the protection of the CNS from the toxic effects of reserpine and chlorpromazine. Deniker introduced me to Jean Delay, his teacher, with whom I often discussed French literature. Pierre and I used to refer to him as *L'Immortel* after he became a member of the Academie Française.

I would also like to mention several other good friends, like Max Hamilton. Clever and lovable, he used to say, "Would you like to know something about English psychiatry? Well, Fish's schizophrenia, Hamilton's rating scale, Stengel's suicide!" His death was a great loss to me personally. Another good friend was the late Nenad Bohacek from Zagreb.

Thomas Ban is a special friend whom I met for the first time at the inaugural meeting of the Collegium Activitatis Nervosae Superioris, a collegium inspired by the late Professor Horsley Gantt. I was one of the founders. We became friends when we met first in the 1960s and since that time we have been in close contact.

Finally, I am happy to recall my dear friend Nancy Andreasen, who dedicated her book to me with the following words: "To C.L. Cazzullo, 'il Papa' of Italian psychiatry."

MY MEMOIRS AND EMOTIONS ON THE BIRTH OF PSYCHOPHARMACOLOGY

Rosalba Terranova-Cecchini

I had always been fascinated by the morphology of the neuron, by the incredible connectedness of the neuronal network and how endogenous biochemical substances affect the cellular membrane and synaptic connections. As a medical student I studied the histology of the central nervous system, and since the early 1950s I have been involved in studying the nerve cell and especially the relationship between the biochemical changes in the nerve cell and the electrophysiological changes in the brain.

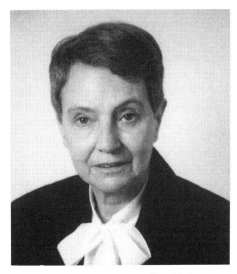

Rosalba Terranova-Cecchini

My research collaboration with Professor Carlo Cazzullo began in the 1950s. First we studied brain metabolism in experimental hibernation and experimentally induced encephalomyelitis, a subject in which he had been involved during his stay in the United States. Later on, with the emergence of psychopharmacology, the focus of our research shifted to clinical problems relevant to treatment with psychotropic drugs.

The shift in the focus of my research was intimately linked to the fact that patients were developing neurological side effects, while dramatically improving with drugs that would later on be referred to as neuroleptics. At the time we still were trying to answer the question whether the new drugs have therapeutic effects. Our clinical-research team therefore had heated discussions regarding the need for therapeutic doses which caused neurological side effects. Another interrelated question was whether the "Parkinsonian-type pathologies" were transitory or permanent; and a third, whether chronic administration of dosages which caused neurological side effects would lead to irreversible nervous tissue damage.

Rosalba Terranova-Cecchini was born in La Spezia, Italy, in 1929. She graduated from the University of Milan in 1953 and became professor of neurology and psychiatry in 1961. Since 1993 she has been president of the Transcultural Health Institute Foundation Cecchini Pace.

Rosalba Terranova-Cecchini was elected a fellow of CINP in 1962. She presented papers on "The effect of non-guidance on the pharmacological treatment of mental disorders" and on "Considérations clinico-expérimentales sur l'action spécifique des inhibiteurs des monoamine oxydases" at the 2nd and 5th Congresses respectively.

With the increasing use of chlorpromazine and reserpine in the treatment of schizophrenia, more and more patients were afflicted with "Parkinson-like symptoms." Because of this I decided to the study the pathomechanism of drug-induced extrapyramidal manifestations with the idea of developing a method for preventing it. It was in the course of this research that I hypothesized – with consideration of the role of adenosine triphosphate (ATP) in cellular metabolism – that ATP can prevent the neuronal damage caused by neuroleptics. Our findings in clinical studies were supportive of my hypothesis and indicated that ATP provided a "real protective shield" for the nervous tissue.

Professor Cazzullo and I presented our findings with ATP at the first CINP Congress in Rome in 1958. Two years later we were pleased to receive from Jean Delay and Pierre Deniker one of their publications on the protective effect of ATP against neurological syndromes in pharmacotherapy with neuroleptics. They presented their findings on 25 July 1960 at a meeting of the Société de Biologie, and sent us a copy of their paper with the following dedication: "Cordial hommage des auteurs à les initiateurs de cette recherche."

After the introduction of tricyclic and monoamine oxidase inhibitor antidepressants I was rapidly able to find a method of protecting cellular metabolism from the effects of these drugs. The results of our studies were presented at the second CINP congress in Basel in 1960.

The 1960s were stimulating years. There was an intense effort to treat mental illness and also to understand the role of the "cerebral biochemical system" in the transmission of information in the neuronal network. Among the different neurotransmitters there was an especially great interest in serotonin in Italy because of the work done by Erspamer, a pharmacologist in Rome.

I remember the unforgettable encounter I had with Wooley at the Rockefeller Institute in New York. Wooley was quite old at the time, but still very enthusiastic and full of curiosity. He was known as the Great Blind, and I realized, after speaking to him, that the nickname fitted him perfectly.

By then I was involved in studying the effects of hallucinogens in animals. Perhaps I had gone too far in this area of research. I was reminded that animals (rabbits in this case) could not tell me about their hallucinations. But by studying their behaviour after the administration of hallucinogens I learned that they became tense, frightened, and intent upon escaping. The manifestations were not the kind that could be tied to neurotoxicity but rather resulted from a perceptual change. In my opinion even the rabbit can develop a model psychosis.

While pharmacotherapy may not cure mental illness, it facilitates social interactions. Patients treated with the new drugs can engage in a dialogue that allows the psychiatrist to penetrate the diverse world of their mind. I was determined to understand the diversity of thinking in human beings. In my search I went to the Psychiatric Hospital in Ambohidiatrimo in Madagascar, where I met a transcultural psychiatrist who taught me to see what I could not see by restricting myself to microscopic studies of the neuronal cytoplasm. He also taught me about medicinal plants, and by studying these plants, including *Rauwolfia serpentina,* my knowledge about the biology of the mind was increased.

I would like to conclude this memoir by saying that my studies in psychopharmacology and neurology provided me with the essentials that identify me as a doctor and an interactive researcher.

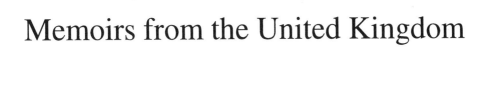

Memoirs from the United Kingdom

AN UNORTHODOX PSYCHOPHARMACOLOGIST REMEMBERS

Hannah Steinberg

The sixties were, of course, a wonderful time for drug development and for the growth of the CINP. How the CINP first came to my notice, or I to its, I cannot exactly remember.

I was a young psychopharmacologist, with a first degree (BA 1st Class Hons.) in Psychology and a PhD in what today would be called "psychopharmacology" on impairment by low concentrations of nitrous oxide of cognitive behaviours of varying complexity (1). In those days nitrous oxide was not of much interest. It is today, however, because of its relevance to problems of consciousness, as well as its unusual speed of induction and waning (less than five minutes at either end), which makes it into an elegant tool for experiments.

I had become a lecturer in Pharmacology at my original and distinguished college, University College London, and by the time of the first official meeting of the CINP in Rome in 1958 I had also published further work with Summerfield and Russell on memory and stress (recall could be improved by

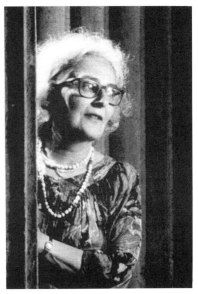

Hannah Steinberg

nitrous oxide on interference theory principles, and the disruption caused by the laboratory stress of an insoluble problem could similarly be reduced) (2, 3). Somehow people got to hear of me and I was invited to Rome in 1958.

Rome was very exciting. We met in a vast, albeit unfinished, conference centre, with few slide projectors and lots of speakers who needed them. We soon learnt that by following a man who carried projectors between auditoria, we could achieve properly illustrated presentations.

In 1970 Hannah Steinberg became the first Professor of Psychopharmacology in Europe, and probably in the world: she has a PhD in Psychopharmacology from University College London. She is an Honorary Member of the British Association for Psychopharmacology and a Distinguished Affiliate of the APA Psychopharmacology Section. She is probably best known for pioneering research, with colleagues, on special effects of drug combinations, and scientific models for predicting them. For the last ten years she has also been involved in demonstrating psychological benefits, such as creativity, of physical exercise and endorphins, and of hazards such as exercise addiction which have turned out exceptionally topical.

Steinberg was elected a fellow of the CINP in 1958. She served as Vice-President on the 7th and 9th Executives and presented papers on "Effect of drugs on weight loss induced by mild daily stress" (Steinberg and Watson) and on "Drug induced changes in visual perception" (Steinberg, Legge, [contd.]

My clearest memory is of a symposium comparing drug-induced abnormal states in animals and men, at the end of which a large number of "discussants" were seated on the platform to make communication easier. Alas, most took the opportunity to present work of their own, and before it came to my turn, I received a note from the chairman, Joel Elkes, entreating me to really try and discuss other peoples' papers that had gone before. So I did and was rewarded with good arguments and the compliment of "wonderful girl" from Sir Aubrey Lewis, the doyen of the Maudsley Institute of Psychiatry, who had the reputation of not praising lightly.

The contents of that meeting, as of most subsequent ones, well reflected the broad sweep of problems that scientists and clinicians were busy with at the time: methodology, phenothiazines and schizophrenia, "tranquilizers," LSD and psychoses, sleep, biochemistry and other basic mechanisms, the beginnings of antidepressants, you name it... In retrospect it is really impressive how broad the coverage was, and the Rome meeting could be said to have more or less launched internationally the new era in the treatment of mental disorders by drugs.

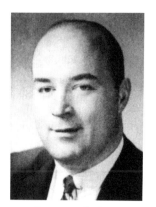

I also met many new colleagues who became firm friends, including Jonathan Cole who was said to have vast money bags available from the U.S. Public Health Service for distribution to promising investigators. I remember being greatly impressed when he treated me to lunch out of a well-used and clearly private leather purse. Some time later we did actually get generous grants through the NIH Psychopharmacology Service Centre, of which he was the chief.

Basel in 1960 represented an important meeting, with a session on antagonists introduced by J. H. Gaddum, one of the foremost pharmacologists of his generation. He had also been greatly encouraging to my colleagues and me in our drug-behaviour interactions research which at the time was fairly unique and therefore rather lonely. Several times we were tempted to give up, but he persuaded us to continue. He said

Jonathan O. Cole

that the work dealt with the most important unsolved problem in biology: how the brain worked. Basel also saw the beginnings of operant conditioning experiments with psychoactive drugs, which became so influential, especially in the United States. I found them interesting, but somewhat limited and too dependent on elaborate apparatus (which in those days often went wrong, at least in London) and "schedules." I also believed that these methods, which depended heavily on learning, were less sensitive to small doses of drugs than more spontaneous and natural ones (4).

---

and Summerfield) at the 1st and 2nd Congresses respectively. She coauthored papers on "Effects of drugs on hypoglycemia induced by stress in rats" (Watson and Steinberg) and on "Using drugs to alter memory experimentally in man" (Summerfield and Steinberg), on "Experiments with amphetamine-barbiturate mixtures" (Rushton and Steinberg), on "Early experience and adult reactions to drugs" (Rushton and Steinberg), and on "Drug combinations and their analyses by measuring exploratory activity in rats" (Rushton and Watson) at the 1st, 2nd, 3rd, 4th, and 5th Congresses respectively. She also was a formal discussant of the 3rd Symposium (Comparison of abnormal behavioural states induced by psychotropic drugs in animals and man) at the 1st Congress, of the 1st Symposium (Methods of comparison of behaviour changes in animals and man) at the 3rd Congress, and of Working Group 3 (Psychology and experimental psychopathology) at the 4th Congress.

In Munich, 1962, the first symposium began with a paper by the late Hans Eysenck in which he suggested how psychological theory, especially dimensions of personality, could systematize one's approach to the classification of drugs. Though ingenious, I doubted whether this umbrella approach would help one subsume the multifarious effects of psychoactive drugs, and said so.

In 1962 I had also been promoted to the new post of Reader in Psychopharmacology by the University of London. The quaint title of "Reader" had to be explained to my colleagues abroad; the nearest I could think of was "associate professor" in the U.S. But mine was the first university title in psychopharmacology in the Western World, as far as I knew, and this did a lot for my self-confidence, making me feel that we had "arrived." Altogether it gave us what is nowadays called a higher profile, and our essentially non-mainstream research was taken more seriously.

In 1964 we met in Birmingham, U.K, with Philip Bradley as host. It was a pleasure that a growing number of British investigators were able to come and contribute. In Birmingham my collaborator Ruth Rushton and I gave our first communication on amphetamine–barbiturate combinations (massive increases in the spontaneous locomotor activity of rodents which could not be obtained with any dose of the separate constituent drugs). This was an unusual and unexpected, at least by us, potentiation of two opposite drugs. The reasons for this, as far as we know, are still not fully understood. The combination also improved test performance in people.

The meeting I remember most clearly was held in Washington in 1966. It gave me my first experience of the U.S. Hard work though it was, I loved every moment of it, including our superior and largely paid-for guest accommodation at the Mayflower Hotel, as well as the small diner next door where the impecunious Brits met most mornings for breakfast. They included such luminaries as Horace Barlow, Philip Bradley, Michael Shepherd, Arthur Summerfield, Larry Weiskrantz, and so on.

It was in Washington that we gave our first long paper on drug combinations (again, massive mutual potentiation of dexamphetamine and amylobarbitone on rodents' locomotor activity, even when ataxic) and on using footprint analysis to measure ataxic gait in rats – and later in man (4, 5). Because we were poor, we had to use simple semi-natural methods in mice and man, and I think that this rather appealed to the more electronically-minded Americans. We were also very pleased that Professor (now Sir) Arnold Burgen of Cambridge did some mathematics for us, to back up our own isobols (two-dimensional diagrams of equi-active dose combinations). During the meeting I received my first American job offer, which was very tempting. But on balance I decided that, having been a child refugee from Austria, I needed the security of staying in the U.K., my host country. By the time the CINP met in Prague 1970, it was quite clear that psychopharmacology was properly established and that many of both the older and the newer drugs really worked.

In Copenhagen, 1972, there was increasing evidence for refinements of approaches, and cannabis and CNS stimulant drugs were much discussed. It was a big program, consisting of four plenary sessions, 13 symposia and 167 free communications of which 90 were posters. I had my own symposium to look after, on long-term effects of psychotropic drugs, in which a colleague and I gave the first paper. Long-term effects are best known as flashbacks from LSD-25, but they can be detected with many other drugs, often when there is no reason to suppose that a drug or its active metabolites are still present in the organism. We are slowly getting a greater understanding of how this can occur. I was also involved in a symposium on new approaches to the discovery of psychoactive drugs, a subject I continue to find fascinating, and which was introduced with handsome slides by Professor Pletscher. Often I ruefully found that others had many more means than we did for translating new ideas into action.

Overall, the benefits of CINP have been enormous. For example, I had learnt very early that American research workers tended not to know or quote British or other foreign work. By getting us to meet each other in person, CINP did much to redress this balance, and for that alone the organization merits full marks. Membership also opened doors to collaborators all over the world and to the support of pharmaceutical companies, which was and still is a priceless asset. Most valuable, perhaps, was the growing stream of information (or the gaps in it) and of opinion which swirled through CINP meetings and publications over the years.

REFERENCES
1. Steinberg, H. (1954). Selective effects of an anaesthetic drug on cognitive behaviour. Quart. J. Exp. Psychol. 6: 170-180.
2. Russell, R.W. and Steinberg, H. (1955). Effects of nitrous oxide on reactions to stress. Quarterly J. Exp. Psychol. 7: 67-73.
3. Steinberg, H. and Summerfield, A. (1957) Reducing interference in forgetting. Quart. J. Exp. Psychol. 9: 146-154.
4. Rushton, R. and Steinberg, H. (1963). Mutual potentiation of amphetamine and amylobarbitone measured by activity in rats. Brit. J. Pharmacol. 21: 295-305.
5. Rushton, R. Steinberg, H. and Tinson, C. (1963). Effects of a single experience on subsequent reactions to drugs. Brit. J. Pharmacol. 20: 99-105.

THE FIRST STEPS OF A PSYCHOPHARMACOLOGIST

Malcolm Lader

The 1960s were a decade of consolidation. The major advances had been made in the 1950s with the introduction of lithium, the antipsychotic (neuroleptic) drugs, imipramine, and the MAOIs. Meprobamate held out the promise that safer drugs than the barbiturates could be used to treat anxiety. I was a medical student in the 1950s when those innovations occurred. The teaching of psychiatry in my medical school – let it remain nameless – consisted of ten visits to the local mental hospital. We were shown how the locks on the wards worked and how the hospital was almost self-sufficient for vegetables (relying on patient labour). The medical superintendent had more absolute power in his little fiefdom than did Louis XIV in seventeenth-century France. As an aside, we were shown a few cases of such rarity that I have only occasionally encountered them since.

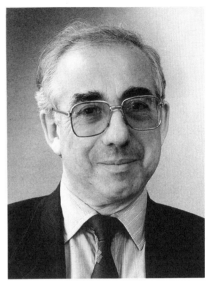

Malcolm Lader

Despite this unsatisfactory beginning, I was not alienated from psychiatry forever, but harboured the hope that somewhere rationality lurked both in the topic and in the patients. Meanwhile, I qualified in medicine but had a particular interest in pharmacology. I also had an interest in experimental psychology after reading the handbook edited by S.S. Stevens. All these interests were going to coalesce in an unforeseen way.

Towards the end of my internship, a job was advertised for research in human psychopharmacology. The post was funded by the extramural section of the National Institute of Mental Health (under the aegis of Jonathan Cole). The grant was given to Heinz Schild, Michael

Malcolm Lader trained in physiology, medicine, pharmacology, and psychiatry and has formal qualifications in each of these disciplines. He is an external member of the scientific staff of the Medical Research Council and professor of clinical psychopharmacology at the Institute of Psychiatry, University of London. He is also an honorary consultant at the Bethlem Royal and Maudsley Hospital, and conducts and supervises clinics dealing with anxiety, sleep and depressive disorders, and drug treatment problems. His thirty years' experience in psychiatry and clinical pharmacology and his research into drugs used in psychiatry have resulted in 15 books and about 680 scientific articles.

Lader was elected a fellow of the CINP in 1964; he served as vice-president on the 11th and 12th Executives, and as councillor on the 13th. He presented a paper on "A comparative bioassay of amphetamine and caffeine in man" and on "Pharmacology of anxiolytic drugs in patients" at the 6th Congress and 7th Congresses, respectively.

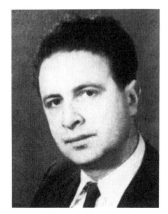

Michael Shepherd

Shepherd, and Hannah Steinberg. Schild was a basic pharmacologist of international reputation, Shepherd a well-known academic psychiatrist, and Steinberg a leading psychopharmacologist. Shepherd was also a founding member of the CINP. Eventually, I was recruited as the most junior member of the team, together with J.D. Montagu and Lorna Wing.

I asked Heinz Schild what I should do. He was a world expert on bits of guinea-pig ileum suspended in fluid baths. He professed to see no fundamental difference between his preparations and the ones that I was supposed to work on: namely, the intact human. He told me, "Develop techniques like Pavlovian conditioning and bioassay sedatives." I was too jejune to realize that this was an impossible task, so I attempted it. First, I ascertained that conditioning – linking a "to-be-conditioned" stimulus with an unconditioned one – was little used in pharmacological experiments in humans. Furthermore, little was known about how the unconditioned response behaved to repeated applications. I told Schild that I would like to sort that question out first, and in a few weeks I would move on to his suggestion of conditioning.

I never did. Habituation of autonomic responses, such as sweating, heart rate, and EMG, kept me busy for the rest of my PhD and for years thereafter. Indeed, we bought a Grass polygraph in 1960 which was finally scrapped in full working order in 1990! I then decided on a clinical training in psychiatry and completed this at the Maudsley Hospital under the legendary Sir Aubrey Lewis. I returned to clinical research in 1966 and have beavered away quietly ever since.

My research was originally with the benzodiazepines, and these have always been an interest of mine. However, this interest has waned over the past ten years, and I think that their clinical importance is less than it was, although their basic pharmacology is crucial in giving us insights into psychotropic drug mechanisms. But in the years after their introduction, the empirical approach had to suffice. We were concerned with quantifying both their efficacy and their unwanted effects. Sedation was measured as an acceleration in habituation of autonomic responses as a correlate of a therapeutic effect, and psychological impairment as a correlate of unwanted effects. Our techniques were sufficiently precise to allow assays. For example, our research culminated with a comparison of two doses of chlordiazepoxide, two of amylobarbitone sodium, and a placebo. This is a 2+2+1 assay, just like Heinz Schild's guinea-pig ileum. These researches were documented in a Maudsley Monograph (Lader and Wing, 1966) which has become a citation classic.

We were really optimistic about the benzodiazepines. In view of the cloud that these drugs subsequently fell under (and to which process I contributed), I have looked over my views in the 1960s. I found the idea perhaps most representative of my thinking in one of the earliest textbooks of psychopharmacology (Shepherd, Lader and Rodnight, 1969). Thus: "Chlordiazepoxide can produce physical dependence." And: "In conclusion, although there are interesting pharmacological differences between chlordiazepoxide and the barbiturates, the clinical differences are minimal." It was but nine years until I wrote a paper entitled "The benzodiazepines the opium of the masses," and the pendulum began to swing against the benzodiazepines. Short term, they are excellent drugs; long term, the risks of adverse effects, including dependence, outweigh the advantages: the problem is preventing short-term use from becoming long-term.

I was under the tutelage of CINP members right from the start of my research career. My first congress was the third in Munich in September 1962. It was also my first international meeting. I met up with Jonathan Cole and thanked him for the NIMH support. I also made the acquaintance of a number of men and women hitherto just great names but now quite real. They included Hanns Hippius, Karl Rickels, Pierre Pichot, J.J. Lopez-Ibor, Martin Roth, Nathan Kline, Herman Denber, Phil May, David Wheatley, Philip Bradley, Paul Janssen, Donald Klein, Mogens Schou, Harris Isbell, Carlo Cazzullo, Paul Kielholz, Frank Ayd, and Fritz Freyhan. Most are still alive and are still attending CINP congresses thirty-five years on.

However, the highlight of the meeting was a wine tasting: 1959 was a great year for German wines, and we were given some super ones to try – Trockenbeerenauleses, Eisweins, and even some excellent reds. Unfortunately, my wife and I were neophyte oenophiles, so most of the wines were dispatched with haste, to the detriment of my attendance at the congress the next day.

I missed Birmingham and Washington but gave my first paper in 1968 at Tarragona. By then I had been a member for four years. In 1970 the congress was in Prague, but this was a rather sad occasion because of political complications at that time. In the later 1970s I was vice-president for four years. During that period the decision was taken to make all congresses "open," instead of alternating open meetings with closed ones restricted to members. I miss those smaller gatherings but recognize their financial vulnerability. Hopefully, the smaller and regional CINP meetings will fill that need.

Looking back over nearly forty years of psychopharmacology, I can discern three phases: 1955-70, the years of introduction and innovation, usually on an empirical basis; 1970-85, a period of consolidation (for the optimists) or stagnation (for the pessimists); and 1985 onwards, which saw the rationalization of psychopharmacology, reflecting the rapid development of the neurosciences. In conclusion, I have been privileged to live through interesting times. I hope that others have found psychopharmacology as interesting as I have, lying as it does across the boundaries of so many disciplines.

PSYCHOPHARMACOLOGY – THE ROLE OF CLINICAL BIOCHEMISTRY IN THE 1960s
Fragments of a Story Line

Merton Sandler

As far as psychopharmacology is concerned, the clinical biochemistry of the 1960s actually began in 1955. Nature had conveniently provided an elegant human model, the malignant carcinoid syndrome, with which to study the metabolism of the newly discovered endogenous monoamine, 5-hydroxytryptamine (5-HT). Never mind that the origin of the associated flush was obscure, so that, in retrospect, we were dealing with a poly-pharmacological situation; we were dazzled by the fact that a substantial proportion of the body's tryptophan reserves were siphoned off into 5-HT production, and Sid Udenfriend, Al Sjoerdsma, and their colleagues at Bethesda exploited this model to the hilt. The main clinical spin-off was a robust method of measuring the major 5-HT metabolite, 5-hydroxyindoleacetic acid (5-HIAA), in human urine which could be performed in any cottage hospital laboratory.

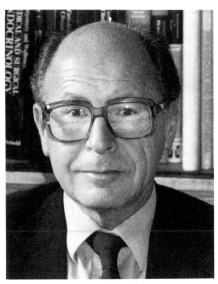

Merton Sandler

More important for psychopharmacology, however, they also invented the spectrophoto-fluorimeter, originally used for measuring 5-HT in a variety of human and animal body sites – such as brain, gut and platelets – but later employed for a multiplicity of small molecules, both endogenous and xenobiotic, in minute concentration in health and disease. Mike Pare and I applied these new Bethesda techniques assiduously and descended on the first CINP congress in Rome to display our wares. Although our findings of a 5-HT *deficit* in phenylketonuria but a *plethora* in certain other varieties of mental handicap failed to win us the Nobel prize, they have at least held up over the years.

Merton Sandler is emeritus professor of chemical pathology at the University of London. He has worked on monoamine metabolism in humans for forty-five years and has been the recipient of many international prizes and awards. Although he really wanted a quiet life, he still travels extensively and has been called by some the Woody Allen of the international monoamine circuit.

Sandler was elected a fellow of the CINP in 1974. He was a Councillor of the 14th, 15th, 16th and 17th Executives and coauthored papers on "A trial of iproniazid in the treatment of depression" (Pare and Sandler) and on "5-Hydroxytryptamine deficiency in phenylketonuria: its relation to the abnormalities of phenylalanine metabolism and to the associated mental defect" (Pare, Sandler and Stacey), both presented at the 1st Congress.

In retrospect, the great bonus for me at that congress was meeting the shy, self-effacing Julie Axelrod, another Bethesda man, who did win the Nobel prize for his work on catecholamine metabolism. In those days, the metabolic disposition of the catecholamines, noradrenaline and adrenaline, was an almost complete mystery. Although they were known to be substrates for monoamine oxidase (MAO), very little of any direct oxidatively deaminated metabolite could be detected in urine. The big breakthrough had been provided by Marvin Armstrong of Salt Lake City – I remember his seminal abstract in the 1957 *Federation Proceedings* so well – who first identified the O-methylated oxidatively deaminated catecholamine metabolite, vanilmandelic acid (VMA), in the urine of patients with pheochromocytoma. Julie was to build on this platform and identify the crucial O-methylation and allied mechanisms, making sense of events occurring at the adrenergic synapse for the first time.

It was actually Colin Ruthven and I who devised the first clinical assay procedure for urinary VMA and went on to develop one for 4-hydroxy-3-methoxyphenylglycol (MHPG) and for homovanillic acid (HVA), the major metabolite of dopamine. Because of a mail strike, I delivered our VMA paper by hand to the *Lancet* offices, which at that time were quaint and Dickensian; I remember old men with stiff, winged collars standing at high desks to mark up manuscripts. Although we failed to establish any striking catecholamine output variations in human mental illness, the tests found a ready usefulness in the diagnosis of catecholamine-secreting tumours. There was a similar reciprocal relationship in the field of 5-HT studies. Mike Pare and I, who were the first to administer 5-hydroxytryptophan (and, for the record, dopa) in humans, noted a new and characteristic urinary metabolite pattern in subjects so treated. Thus the 5-hydroxytryptophan-secreting carcinoid tumour was first identified because of the similarity of its urinary indole chromatogram to that derived from our volunteers.

John Jepson, who devised the paper chromatographic system we were using to sort out our problems, died early. He and Gerald Curzon both made major contributions to determining the indole excretion pattern. Small molecules were the order of the day, and in the clinical field at least, little attention had been paid to the enzymes responsible for their formation and degradation. Even so, Davison and I wrote our first paper on MAO in 1956 (using the Warburg apparatus), but it was another ten years before Youdim and I produced early laboratory evidence of its multiplicity. The advent of the selective inhibitor, clorgyline, enabled Johnston to separate the two forms, MAO-A and B, pharmacologically, but it took another twenty years for Jean Shih and her colleagues, using molecular biological techniques, to prove that we were all dealing with two separate, but similar enzymes.

Another selective inhibitor, deprenyl (selegiline), this time of MAO-B, emerged in the mid-1960s as a result of the drive and ingenuity of Joseph Knoll and his colleagues in Budapest. Both selective inhibitors were invaluable for the study of human pathological material. Glover and I were able to demonstrate unequivocally that dopamine is largely metabolized by MAO-B in the human brain, unlike the rat, where its degradation is effected by MAO-A. Human endometrial MAO-A also proved to be powerfully potentiated by progesterone.

In the early 1960s, MAO inhibitor therapy for depressive illness was in its high summer, and the test to quantify the degree of inhibition by measuring any reduction in 5-HIAA output after 5-HT ingestion enjoyed a transitory vogue. Even before the cheese effect was identified, bringing this therapeutic approach to its virtual close, Herman van Praag in Groningen had smartly observed that the MAO inhibitor he employed caused a decrease in 5-HIAA output when 5-HIAA itself was ingested.

In the late 1960s, Farouk Karoum and I turned to gas chromatography and gas chromatography/mass spectrometry for the clinical biochemical assay of small molecule monoamine metabolites. We were fortunate. This new methodology had emerged just in time for the L-dopa revolution in Parkinson's disease. Thus we helped to disentangle the myriad metabolites of L-dopa and its adjuvant drugs with their possible therapeutic roles – and a great many papers were written.

Although this brief account of an exciting decade has been, of necessity, somewhat Anglocentric, it would be even less complete if I failed to mention the ingenious contributions of Irv Kopin to the quantification of catecholamine metabolites, or of Dennis Murphy for his research on biochemical aspects of clinical pharmacology. Both still work at Bethesda, which remains the epicentre of the monoamine upheaval of the past forty-five years. After the sixties, the seventies were perhaps years of consolidation. But that is another story.

EARLY DAYS IN BIOLOGICAL PSYCHIATRY

Alec Coppen

When I started my studies in biological psychiatry in the late 1950s, the field was pretty open since there had been very little work in the area, apart from studies in the genetics of psychiatric illness carried out in the 1920s and 1930s. So if one chose one's subject wisely, one was a bit like Lewis and Clarke in their exploration of the United States – wherever one went, one was certain to come across new and interesting discoveries.

When I started with the Medical Research Council (MRC) of the United Kingdom in 1960, I had certain principles in mind. I had selected the area of affective disorders as my field, and I was determined to concentrate on the biochemical abnormalities found in patients showing this condition. I decided that the basic requirement was a clinical research ward, where systematic and accurate measurements could be undertaken on rigorously selected patients under controlled con-

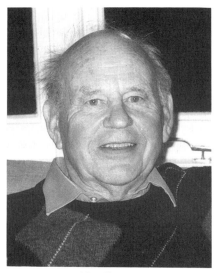

Alec Coppen

ditions. This approach was rapidly agreed upon between the MRC and the National Health Service with the minimum of delay and bureaucracy. I also determined that patients selected for study should lose nothing by being admitted to our ward, so that they would have the best treatment and be followed up very carefully.

Our general plan of investigation was to study patients when they were depressed (or manic) and at various intervals after recovery. This basic facility is essential to biological studies in patients, and a close everyday interaction with them is a great stimulus to achieve what I consider the end point of all these studies: a reduction of their morbidity and mortality. Attached to the ward was a laboratory in which we were able to perform a wide range of investigations.

Another important approach was to collaborate with other specialist units. For example, when measuring whole-body electrolytes, we worked with the Radiological Protection Unit

Alec Coppen qualified in medicine after army service during the Second World War and then went on to Maudsley Hospital. He entered the MRC Unit for Neuropsychiatric Research where he pioneered the 5HT theory of depression and numerous other biological aspects of mood disorders. He was head of the UK Centre for Biological Research in the WHO network and president of the British Association of Psychopharmacology (1976-1978).

Coppen was elected a fellow of the CINP in 1968. He was a Councillor of the 12th, and served as President of the 16th Executive.

in Sutton, where they measured the K40 in our patients in a whole-body counter. We were also able to observe in our patients the fallout from the various nuclear bombs that were being exploded at that time by the USSR and the United States.

We identified three main areas of interest: electrolytes, monoamines, and endocrine changes. Our interest in endocrine changes was initially in the area of adrenal cortical activity, and we showed, even after allowing for admission to hospital (which has a marked effect on cortisol secretion), that there was increased activity both during and after recovery from an episode of depression, although it slowly subsided to normality after some weeks.

Our interest in the endocrinology of mood extended to changes that had been observed around the time of the menstrual period. About 1960, when Neil Kessell and I became interested in this subject, there were almost no systematic studies. Dalton had published her well-known observations on schoolgirls' performance, and Linford Rees had also published observations in this area, but in general there was little awareness of mood changes around the menstrual period.

Kessell and I therefore devised a systematic investigation of the problem by sending a questionnaire to sample patients randomly selected from general practitioners' lists. Working at this time had many advantages. Menstruation was still an amazingly taboo topic, and little had been written in the popular press, so that our subjects were being questioned about mood changes around the menstrual cycle for the first time. Secondly, this was before the introduction of the contraceptive pill, which in itself could have effects on the premenstrual syndrome. The results of this investigation were really quite dramatic. There was a syndrome of mood changes before the period severely affecting at least 10 percent of the population. Curiously enough, it took some time for news of our work to reach the general population because, hard as it is to believe now, newspapers were very coy about publishing anything on the subject of menstruation. I think that, in general, it was a great relief to many women to learn that they were not alone with regard to their symptoms, although at the time we could not suggest any very effective treatment.

Another interest of ours was in monoamines. This work received a great boost in 1963 when we were able to show that, in a double-blind trial, tryptophan very significantly improved the antidepressant action of MAOIs and tryptophan augmentation compared favourably to placebo augmentation. This action was so marked that for many years, it was a powerful instrument in treating patients who responded poorly to standard antidepressants. The reason that the practice was discontinued was that tryptophan was taken off the market because of problems with its production (which did not actually affect the tryptophan available in this country). It is interesting that these observations on tryptophan supplementation have recently been paralleled by studies on depressive patients subject to tryptophan depletion, which can cause a worsening of their symptoms. Our tryptophan and MAOI studies were the first positive evidence of a link between serotonin (5HT) and depression and led many groups to undertake a series of investigations into 5HT and its metabolite, 5-hydroxy-indole acetic acid (5HIAA) in depressive patients. We looked at CSF and brain concentrations, at blood concentration of total and free tryptophan, and at 5HT platelet transport. Our interest in 5HT was taken up by other European centres, but curiously enough, it was met by hostility in the United States. There was a rather absurd, but fruitful rivalry between the noradrenaline and 5HT theories of depression. Of course, there is no simple theory of depression, but evidence has accumulated over the years that 5HT does have a fairly central place in the disorder.

One of the great developments during the 1960s was the realization that mood disorders were not single episodes, but were largely a recurrent and chronic condition that required long-term treatment. Jules Angst was very influential in showing this fact, and careful evaluation of the outcome of our own patients brought it home to us. My own interest in lithium resulted from my early work in electrolytes, where we showed an increase in residual (mainly intracellular) sodium in patients when they were depressed.

This topic brought me into contact with Mogens Schou about 1960, and we met many times to discuss the best way of testing long-term treatment in mood-disorder patients. We did not find any effect of lithium on the abnormality of sodium distribution, but we did find subsequently that lithium normalized the decreased 5HT transport in depressive patients. However, these results stimulated our interest in the long-term treatment of mood-disorder patients, which has been the most important development in this area in the last fifty years. Schou's early trials were rather convincing, but were flawed in terms of modern standards of testing treatments. But it should be recalled that randomized, placebo-controlled retrials were a relatively new development at the time when the first observations were made by Schou and his co-workers.

I saw the importance of carrying out a prospective double-blind trial of prophylactic lithium in the late 1960s. This we did with three other centres, and we were able to show two things: both unipolar and bipolar illnesses without long-term treatment have a very poor outcome; and long-term maintenance treatment can considerably improve these patients' long-term outlook. Later on, we carried out a second randomized, double-blind trial on the continuation treatment by lithium of patients who had received ECT. The results were striking. ECT is the most effective treatment for depression: its onset of improvement is rapid, and it is useful in a very broad spectrum of patients. Its main drawback is that there is a very frequent occurrence of relapse: over 60 percent of patients relapse within one year if they receive a placebo. On the other hand, patients who receive maintenance/prophylactic treatment with lithium show a very low relapse rate during this time. In fact, ECT and maintenance/prophylactic treatment with lithium together represent by far the most effective treatment of the condition. Studying the mode of action of antidepressant drugs has led to many hypotheses about the pathology of depression. It is tantalizing that we have so little information about the mode of action of ECT.

We had set up a mood-disorder clinic for administering lithium and other long-term treatments. One lesson we learned is that simply prescribing treatment is not effective. Patients must be informed about the nature of their illness. They must be seen at regular intervals and their compliance ensured by, if possible, plasma monitoring. As the patient becomes accusomed to the regime, the follow-up intervals can be lengthened or the patient devolved to the general practitioner. By now we must have known about the recurrent nature of unipolar depression for thirty years, but I would be surprised if the number of patients who receive adequate maintenance treatment represents more than 2 or 3 percent. The most common cause of suicide is depressive illness, and we have shown that maintenance treatment can reduce suicide by 70 percent. Not to treat recurrent depression is a serious medical mistake.

During the early years of drug development, we came across the problem of dosage. We found, for example, that patients metabolized drugs at very different rates so that a standardized dosage could produce a fourteen-fold difference in the steady state of plasma concentration. The question arose whether there was a plasma concentration of a tricyclic drug that was optimum – the so-called therapeutic window. The existence of such a "window" was alleged for nortriptyline. We examined the position for amitriptyline, and after a lot of work, including an international investigation that I organized for the World Health Organization, we concluded that 150 mg of amitriptyline was adequate for most adult Europeans. However, in other ethnic groups, such as the Japanese, the rates of metabolism are so different from those in people of European origin that we cannot extrapolate results from one group to another. After a lot of experience in this area, we carried out what I feel was the definitive investigation on lithium dosage. This, I can say, is the dose, on a once-a-day regimen, that would produce a twelve-hour plasma level of 0.5-0.7 mmol/l. More than this is counter-productive. The investigation showed that higher levels produced poorer response, probably because of the effect on the thyroid. Lithium now is one of the best established of all the psychotropic compounds. John Davis has reported twenty-six randomized, double-blind trials on lithium prophylaxis, all showing a very marked effect on the course of mood disorder.

Neurochemistry and psychopharmacology have become elaborate and complex, and the number of publications on any one topic increases year by year. Because of this development, I feel that we are in a similar position to the one outlined by John Maddox in an editorial published in *Nature* entitled "Finding the Wood among the Trees." Maddox was commenting on molecular biology, but his remarks are also highly appropriate to our field. "Is there a danger," he asked, "where there are grants for producing data but hardly any for standing back in contemplation ... [that] the accumulation of data will get so far ahead of its assimilation into a conceptual framework that the data will eventually prove an encumbrance?" It seems to me that, in general in psychopharmacology, the treatment of mood disorders has not improved very much overall in the last twenty years, in spite of an explosion of new data.

RESEARCH IN GENERAL PRACTICE

David Wheatley

My real introduction to psychopharmacology was at the third CINP congress, held in Munich in September 1962.

I had founded the General Practitioner Research Group three years earlier to undertake clinical trials of new drugs of all kinds with patients treated in their home milieu (1) by family doctors. Since each clinical trial was performed by several general practitioners in collaboration, our studies with psychotropic drugs were

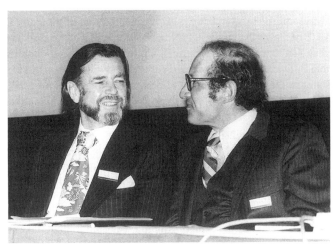

David Wheatley (left) with Carl Rickels

among the first multicenter clinical trials in the psychiatric literature. It was sometime in early 1962, just about the time that we completed one of our multicenter studies with a psychotropic drug, that I saw a notice in the medical press about the Munich meeting and decided to submit a paper. To my chagrin, the secretary, Philip Bradley, rejected it because it exceeded the limit of four quarto pages. But I found that by retyping it on American quarto paper (rather larger than the English equivalent), I could accommodate the full text within the requisite four pages. It was accepted without further comment.

I was hooked! Then I was given an introduction to Jonathan Cole, at the time the Director of the Psychpharmacology Service Center of the National Institute of Mental Health (NIMH)

David Wheatley started professional life in general practice, developing an early interest in psychopharmacological research. He has been head of the General Practitioner Research Group (Psychopharmacology Research Group) since 1958. He has published or edited several books and journals, and established the Maudsley Hospital Stress Clinic in 1985, acting as director until 1992. In 1985 he developed the widely-used Wheatley Stress Profile (WSP). He was the founder and first president of the International Society for the Investigation of Stress (1988-1992). Currently he is consultant psychiatrist to the Royal Masonic Hospital in London and consultant to San Diego's Feighner Research Institute (London branch).

Wheatley was elected a fellow of the CINP in 1966. He presented papers on "Evaluation of psychotherapeutic drugs in general practice," "Some problems in collating multi-participant research results," and on "Drug insufficiencies in the treatment of neurotic illness," at the 3rd, 5th, and 6th Congresses, respectively.

of the USA, and after visiting the NIMH, I applied for and was awarded a research grant from NIMH to investigate the use of psychotropic drugs in general practice. It was difficult to undertake this type of work in the United States in those years, but it was quite easy in the United Kingdom with my ready-made General Practitioner Research Group. It was with the support of my NIMH grant that the Psychopharmacology Research Group was developed – "the group within the group" – consisting of members with a special interest in psychotropic drug trials. After that, I never looked back, and the grants continued for the next twelve years. I was required to attend two meetings a year: that of the Early Clinical Drug Evaluation Unit (ECDEU, now the NCDEU, "New" having replaced "Early" in its name) held in the spring or early summer, and the American College of Neuropsychopharmacology (ACNP) meeting, held in December. So I regularly travelled twice a year to agreeable locations in the United States in the most stimulating of company. The group originally consisted of those who had received NIMH grants, and there were only some twenty-six of us, I being the single representative from Europe. I can truly say this was the major turning point in my life. We psychopharmacologists were then a small – and, we liked to think, elite – band, and we felt privileged to be in the vanguard of this newly developing speciality. In addition, I was afforded the opportunity to meet many congenial colleagues, with whom I have spent happy and intellectually stimulating hours. Space will not allow me to name them all, but they especially included Ron Fieve, Marty Katz, Turan Itil, Jerry Levine, Tom Ban, Subit Gabay, and many others.

With the aid of the NIMH grants, I was able to undertake many general-practice studies, mostly in anxiety and depression, and these culminated in my first book, *Psychopharmacology in Family Practice,* which was published in 1973 (2). Methodology was relatively unsophisticated in those days, and I could write the whole book myself, although the project took some six months to complete. Between 1960 and 1990 I attended all the CINP meetings, with the exception of Jerusalem in 1982, and presented papers at many of them. It was at the Prague meeting in 1970 that I first suggested to Alec Coppen that we ought to start a national organization in England similar to the ACNP in the United States. With the cooperation of Anthony Hordern and advice from Frank Ayd, the British Association for Psychopharmacology (BAP) was founded in 1974, Max Hamilton becoming its first president and myself the first secretary. It was not designated a "college" because of confusion that might have ensued with the English Royal Colleges, which also award higher specialized degrees. The subsequent history of the BAP has been documented elsewhere (3). During this time I also published three books in the BAP "Psychopharmacology of" series, based on symposia that I had organized for the association, concerned respectively with sleep, old age, and sexual disorders.

THE EARLY YEARS

It can truly be said that, over the years of the NIMH grants, our group "rode the crest of the wave" with adequate support to pursue independent research projects that covered the whole field of psychotropic drug use, with the exception of psychoses that would have been difficult to assess in the community setting. In the early days we were still using the amphetamines to treat depression (effective as "instant antidepressants") and barbiturates to treat anxiety. This research resulted in one of our first papers on placebo comparisons of phenobarbitone in anxiety, dexamphetamine in depression, and a combination of the two in mixed anxiety-depression (4). Many other publications followed, and I mention only a few of which I feel particularly proud: "Influence of doctors' and patients' attitudes in the treatment of neurotic illness (5)," "Potentiation of amitriptyline by thyroid hormone" (which confirmed Arthur Prange's original observations) (6), and "Zopiclone: a non-benzodiazepine hypnotic: Controlled comparison to temazepam in insomnia," the first clinical report on this new type of hypnotic (7).

It was in 1984 that I developed my interest in stress, and I became the first editor of the journal *Stress Medicine*, an appointment that I held until 1992. At the same time I established the Stress Clinic at the Maudsley hospital in London, which I directed for the following seven years; I then transferred the clinic to the Royal Masonic Hospital, also in London. In order to assess the medical and psychiatric effects of stress, I designed the Wheatley Stress Profile (WSP) (8), which has subsequently been translated into Chinese, Japanese, Russian, Spanish, Italian, and Rumanian and is in regular use in those countries (9). At that time I also founded the International Society for the Investigation of Stress (ISIS) and served as its first president. From this interest in stress came my second book, *Stress and the Heart*, with contributions from a number of international experts, the introductory chapter being written by Hans Selye himself. This publication later appeared in a second English edition and in Spanish translation. Of the many conferences that I was able to attend, I particularly remember a World Health Organization meeting in Belgrade in 1968, at which photographs of some well-known psychopharmacologists of the time were taken. These individuals look surprisingly youthful, and many of them remain active today, a testament to the satisfaction that the pursuit of psychopharmacology surely brings.

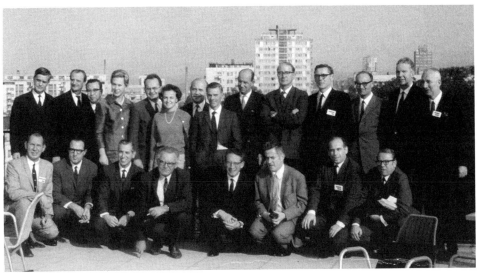

WHO Psychopharmacology Group meeting in Belgrade (1968).
First row, from left: Leo E. Hollister, unidentified, Jerry Levine, unidentified, Max Hamilton, Walter Pöldinger, Thomas Ban and Turan Itil.
Standing row, from left: first five unidentified, Boris Lebedev, unidentified, Pierre Pichot, John Wing, Paul Kielholz, James Klett, Oldrich Vinar, unidentified, and Andrzej Jus.

AND THE FUTURE?

I now come to what I consider the most exciting recent development in our field of research. I refer to the realization that phytomedicine may provide many profitable fields for scientific discovery. The outstanding example has been the development of Taxol, a highly effective treatment for breast cancer. Substances and mixtures of substances, with stimulant or depressive effects on the central nervous system, are produced by the plant world in particular abundance. Ginkgo, hypericum, piper, valerian, lavendula, humulus, passiflora, and mellisa are typical examples, and their effects are now being determined using modern EEG investigative measures and controlled clinical trials. For example, when I first started in practice, the British pharmacopoeia contained a number of preparations derived from plant extracts, and I particularly remember tincture of valerian, which was advocated for anxiety and insomnia. But with the advent of the barbiturates and then the benzodiazepines (BZDs), it quickly sank into oblivion. In view of the demise of the BZDs, it is interesting to know that a placebo-controlled trial of valerian using sleep EEGs has shown that it prolongs sleep at slow wave sleep (SWS) and shortens SWS latencies.

I was sceptical when I was asked to participate in a double-blind, amitriptyline-controlled trial of hypericum (St John's wort) in depression, until I learned that the compound had been in use in Germany for over ten years. Not only was it approved for prescription under the German health service, it was also available over the counter, where it outsold Prozac, the most widely prescribed antidepressant worldwide. I was impressed enough to agree to take part, and the results showed the two drugs to exert equivalent antidepressant effects in the cases of mild to moderate depression, for which the trial had been designed (10). "Phytomedicine and Stress" is the title of a symposium to be held at the Second World Congress on Stress at Melbourne, Australia, in October 1998.

So I can truly say that I have dined at the high tables of psychopharmacologia, and I am immeasurably the richer for the abundance of gourmet fare that I have enjoyed for the greater span of my creative life. I am glad that my appetite remains healthy for the many more delights that I am sure await me in the future.

REFERENCES

1. Wheatley, D. (1960). The General Practitioner Research Group. *Practitioner* 184: 542-547.
2. Wheatley, D. (1973). *Psychopharmacology in Family Practice*. London: W. Heinemann.
3. Wheatley, D., and Healy, D. (1994). The foundation of the British Association for Psychopharmacology. *J. Psychopharmacology* 8: 268-278.
4. Wheatley, D. (1967). Influence of doctors' and patients' attitudes in the treatment of neurotic illness. *Lancet* 2: 1133-1135.
5. Wheatley, D. (1962). Evaluation of psychotherapeutic drugs in general practice. *Psychopharmacology Service Center Bulletin* 2: 25-31.
6. Wheatley, D. (1972). Potentiation of amitriptyline by thyroid hormone. *Arch. Gen. Psych.* 62: 229-233.
7. Wheatley, D. (1985). Zopiclone: a non-benzodiazepine hypnotic: Controlled comparison to temazepam in insomnia. *Brit. J. Psychiat.* 146: 312-314.
8. Wheatley, D. (1990). The stress profile. *Brit. J. Psychiat.* 156: 685-688.
9. Wheatley, D., Golden, L., and Jianlin, J. (1995). Stress across three cultures: Great Britain, the United States and China. *Ann. NY Acad. Sci.* 771: 609-616.
10. Wheatley, D. (1997). LI 160, an extract of St John's wort, versus amitriptyline in mild to moderately depressed outpatients a controlled 6-week trial. *Pharmacopsychiatry* suppl. 30: 77-80.

PSYCHOPHARMACOLOGY IN THE 1960s

Trevor Silverstone

The 1960s were years of promise and excitement in the world of psychopharmacology. For the first time, we had at our disposal a range of effective drugs with which to address many of the major clinical problems in psychiatry: imipramine for the treatment of depression, chlorpromazine for schizophrenia, and chlordiazepoxide for anxiety. It is no exaggeration to say that these drugs, all of which had been introduced only a short time before the decade began, truly revolutionized clinical practice. Also, by dramatically ameliorating the condition of patients who had hitherto required long periods of hospitalization, they ushered in the modern era of community-based psychiatry.

When I began my residency at the Maudsley Hospital in 1961, the questions were: Are these drugs really as effective as the initial reports suggested? And, if they are, how do they work?

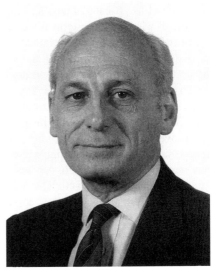

Trevor Silverstone

(Work, that is, in neurochemical terms.) It was hoped that the answer to this latter question would lead inevitably to an understanding of the biological mechanisms underlying the psychopathological processes we were observing in our patients' delusions, hallucinations, suicidal despair, mania, and crippling anxiety. This understanding would, in turn, allow even more effective compounds to be developed on sound scientific principles rather than the largely serendipitous observations that had led to the first wave of psychotropic agents.

Not everyone believed that the new drugs were as good as the early, uncontrolled observations indicated. In Britain, claims of efficacy met with considerable scepticism. It was

Trevor Silverstone obtained his medical education at the University of Oxford and at St Bartholomew's Hospital, including a year as a Fulbright scholar at the University of California, Los Angeles. After completing his psychiatric residency at the Institute of Psychiatry and the Maudsley Hospital, London, he spent a year in the Department of Psychiatry at the University of Pennsylvania. He was then appointed to the teaching staff of the Medical College of St. Bartholomew's Hospital, which carried with it an honorary consultant appointment to the Hospital. He subsequently became head of the Department of Psychological Medicine in the Medical College, part of the University of London. In 1992 he emigrated to New Zealand to become a professorial research fellow and director of the Psychopharmacological Research Group in the Department of Psychological Medicine, Dunedin School of Medicine, at the University of Otago. For many years he has maintained a research interest in affective disorder, particularly bipolar disorder, and has published widely on this topic. His *Drug Treatment in Psychiatry*, coauthored with the late Paul Turner, has gone through five editions.
Silverstone was elected a fellow of the CINP in 1970.

not until they had been subjected to the rigorous scrutiny of controlled clinical trials that the the new drugs became generally accepted. I sometimes think that the contrast in the way in which chlorpromazine became integrated into clinical practice in France, compared to what happened in the United Kingdom, reflected national characteristics as much as the weight of scientific evidence. Jean Delay and Pierre Deniker had reported to the French Psychiatric Association in the 1950s that, on the basis of their clinical experience with the drug, they were convinced of its efficacy in ameliorating psychosis: "Et voilà! it works!" This was an early example of what has been termed the French Impressionist school of psychopharmacology. The British, on the other hand, wanted firmer evidence. A husband-and-wife team of pharmacologists in Birmingham, the Elkes, were able to confirm these impressions in a controlled clinical trial (one of the first such trials undertaken in any medical specialty). "By Jove, these French chappies were right!" The Americans, also conforming to their stereotype, went on to undertake multicentre studies of a range of neuroleptics in much larger numbers of patients.

Clinical trials require reliable measures of outcome by which to judge the degree and rate of improvement. The problem of how to measure the effects of psychotropic drugs in human subjects was attracting considerable research attention in those years. In the field of depression, Max Hamilton's rating scale of depression had been introduced in 1959 and was assuming the primacy that it still holds in clinical trials of antidepressant drugs. Max himself was a frequent attender of meetings related to psychopharmacology. He could always be counted on to make trenchant and provocative comments and was a refreshingly candid debunker of overvalued ideas. Malcolm Lader, in his comparative assessment of the effects of benzodiazepines and barbiturates in relieving anxiety, went one step further. He combined the assessment of psychological state, using visual analogue scales, with the direct measurement of physiological arousal, using skin conductance. This work had considerable influence in getting barbiturates replaced by benzodiazepine compounds. In the treatment of anxiety the benzodiazepines were much safer and were non-addictive (or so it seemed at the time, despite Leo Hollister's significant, but largely ignored, observation that withdrawal of chlordiazepoxide in large doses led to clear-cut withdrawal symptoms). *Sic transit gloria mundi.*

While we were not able to reach our goal of obtaining a comprehensive understanding of the biological mechanisms underlying the major psychiatric syndromes, several major scientific advances took place that have moved us closer to it. Two of the most significant contributions were made by one man, the Swedish pharmacologist Arvid Carlsson, who, in my opinion, has not been given the credit he deserves. The first of his two seminal contributions was the finding that in animal preparations the neuroleptic drugs chlorpromazine and haloperidol both led to a preferential increase in the metabolites of dopamine in the synaptic cleft with an increase of homovanillic acid, the metabolic end product of dopamine in the urine. He argued that the increase of dopamine was a consequence of the drug's dopamine-receptor blocking effect in the postsynaptic neuron. He was right, and his findings provided the basis of the dopaminergic hypothesis of schizophrenia, which in turn led to the introduction of increasingly more selective dopamine antagonists for the treatment of schizophrenia.

The second of Carlsson's two contributions was the demonstration that amphetamine releases noradrenaline from noradrenergic neurons and dopamine from dopaminergic neurons and that the release of these catecholamines is responsible for the different actions of amphetamine. Amphetamine is a compound of considerable interest to psychiatrists in that its actions impinge on the pathophysiology of affective disorders and schizophrenia. In modest doses it can elevate mood and reduce hunger, actions with obvious relevance to the phenomenology of affective disorders. In higher doses it can produce a paranoid psychosis indistinguishable from that seen in some patients with paranoid schizophrenia. I have never understood why these properties of amphetamine have not been used to a greater extent in studies of the pathological mechanisms of bipolar disorder and paranoid schizophrenia. I would think think that an examination of the changes of mRNA in dopaminergic neurons exposed to amphetamine would shed considerable light on the processes involved in mood regulation and perhaps also on the genesis of paranoid delusions.

The neurochemistry of mood and the pharmacology of antidepressant drugs were the targets of much research in the 1960s. It was uncertain whether the antidepressant effects of drugs such as imipramine and amitriptyline were due primarily to their action on noradrenergic or serotonergic pathways. While not necessarily viewing the question as an either/or situation, many authorities in those days seemed to take a position favouring one neurotransmitter over the other. Among those in the serotonin camp, as it were, was Alec Coppen, while others believed that the catecholamines, particularly noradrenaline, were of greater significance. Still others, such as Herman van Praag, suggested that there might be two types of depressive syndrome: one in which the primary disturbance was a relative insufficiency of serotonin and another in which it was a lack of noradrenaline. As there were no pharmacologically selective antidepressants available at that time, it was not possible to resolve the argument one way or the other. We now know that these neurotransmitter systems interact with each other and with many others, and that it is not appropriate to regard any one as holding primacy over the others. These facts were not clear in the 1960s. Arguments in favour of one or the other neurotransmitter took up a lot of space in the journals and were the subjects of heated debates at scientific meetings.

Another contentious issue in the area of affective disorders was the value of lithium in prophylaxis. During the 1960s Mogens Schou and his colleagues in Denmark suggested on the basis of clinical evidence that lithium, as Cade had originally implied, was effective in preventing recurrences of both manic and depressive episodes in patients with bipolar disorder. (It should be remembered that only in 1960 had this disorder been recognized as separate from unipolar depression, following the confirmation by Jules Angst in Switzerland and Carlo Perris in Sweden of Leonhardt's contention that the family history of depressed patients who had had a previous episode of mania [bipolar depression] differed from that of depressed patients who had not experienced a previous episode of mania [unipolar depression].) However, some were unconvinced. Writing from the Olympian heights of the Institute of Psychiatry in London, Barry Blackwell and Michael Shepherd airily dismissed Schou's evidence, suggesting, in a celebrated article published in the prestigious *The Lancet*, that the suggested value of lithium in bipolar disorder was likely to be yet another "therapeutic myth." Their comments led to one of the more notable public rows yet seen in psychopharmacological circles. Nathan Kline, a somewhat larger-than-life figure in American psychopharmacology, galloped out like a knight in shining armour to defend the honour of lithium in the august pages of the *American Journal of Psychiatry*. There followed a knock-about correspondence between Kline and Blackwell which is still well worth reading, if only for its amusement value. Interestingly enough, the question of the efficacy of lithium in the prophylaxis of bipolar disorder has still not been fully resolved, with recent articles appearing which again question the scientific validity of the evidence on which the original claims were made. *Plus ça change ...*

Gerald Russell and I adopted an approach similar to that of Malcolm Lader in our simultaneous measurements of hunger and fasting gastric motility in young women suffering from anorexia nervosa. When I went to the United States in 1954 to work with "Micky" Stunkard at the University of Pennsylvania, I turned my attention to amphetamine-induced anorexia. By developing a reliable and simple method for measuring food intake, I was able to begin what turned out to be a long series of studies on the mechanisms of action of anorectic compounds. I tried to replicate in human subjects what pharmacologists, such as Silvio Garattini at the Mario Negri Institute in Milan, were finding in animal models.

In contrast to the United Kingdom, in the United States the academic climate of the 1960s in most university departments of psychiatry was dominated by those holding a psychodynamic (mainly Freudian) viewpoint. Psychotropic drugs were considered a second-best treatment option, reserved largely for those unable (usually for financial reasons) to undertake the lengthy process of analytically-oriented psychotherapy. However, it was about that time that stirrings of change could be detected. Influential bodies such as the National Institute of Mental Health – and enlightened pioneers such as Jonathan Cole, Leo Hollister, Karl Rickels, Frank Ayd, and the late George Winokur – were undertaking important research in psychopharmacology and promoting the view that drug treatment was more effective than psychodynamic therapy in reducing the sufferings of patients with schizophrenia, major depression, and anxiety. I was fortunate enough, during my time in the United States and subsequently, to meet many of these leading figures in psychopharmacology.

On my return to the United Kingdom, I was appointed to the faculty of the Medical College of St Bartholomew's Hospital (Bart's). Michael Pare, a senior colleague of mine at Bart's, produced one of the first papers on what has later come to be called pharmacogenetics. He asked patients presenting a depressive disorder whether they had first-degree relatives who had suffered from a similar illness and, if so, to which drug they had responded. From an admittedly small sample, it looked as if the families of his patients bred true not only for illness experience, but also for specificity of treatment response; there were families who responded preferentially to tricyclic antidepressants and others who responded better to monoamine oxidase inhibitors. In my view, this important observation has never really received the attention it deserves. The head of the Department of Psychological Medicine at Bart's at that time was Linford Rees, one of the leading figures in psychopharmacological circles. He strongly supported psychopharmacology research in his department and did all that he could to promote my career in the field. I personally have a lot to thank him for.

As is often the case when one looks back to times past, the earlier era appears bathed in a golden glow of simple innocence as less complicated and less demanding. After all, in the 1960s we knew of only two noradrenergic receptors and two serotonin receptors (there are now at least seventeen). There were very few journals devoted to psychopharmacology, the only one of any note being *Psychopharmacologia*, with its first issue published in 1959. Now there are at least a score. And, of particular relevance to this article, commissioned as it was to mark the CINP meeting in Glasgow in 1998, there was really only one significant international forum devoted to the promulgation of new research in psychopharmacology, the Collegium Internationale Neuro-Psychopharmacologicum, held every two years. Now many countries have their own national organizations, and a meeting devoted to psychopharmacology is held somewhere in the world almost every other week. If nothing else, the full name of our association is redolent of a bygone age: who nowadays would saddle a scientific forum devoted to advances in the pharmacological approach to psychiatric disorders with a tongue-twisting, grandiloquent title in a dead language? Some things were different then.

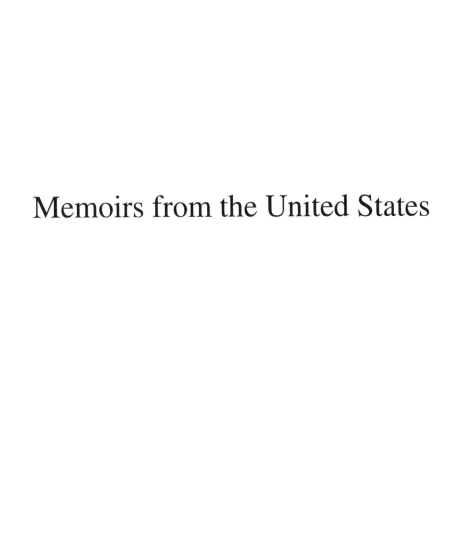

Memoirs from the United States

MY INVOLVEMENT WITH KETAMINE
Dissociative Anesthetic, Model Schizophrenia
Edward F. Domino

Ketamine is still a useful drug thirty-four years after its first administration to human volunteers. One day in 1964, Alex Lane, head of clinical pharmacology at Parke Davis, called to ask if I was interested in testing a short-acting phencyclidine (PCP) analogue called CI-581 in humans. He knew of my interest in PCP as an anesthetic and, in low doses, as a psychotomimetic. Although human clinical research with PCP had stopped in 1961, many of us were still impressed that it produced the best chemical model of schizophrenia (1). I told Lane that I would be interested in setting up a clinical study with CI-581 on the condition that I first study it in animals. Since PCP caused marked canine delirium, I injected various doses of CI-581 in dogs. Although I observed canine delirium, it was less pronounced and of shorter duration than that caused by PCP. Larger doses of PCP produced seizures, but increased doses of CI-581 did not produce such

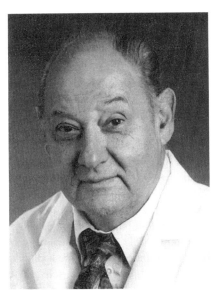

Edward F. Domino

marked convulsions. In monkeys, CI-581 was an excellent short-acting anesthetic agent. There was no emergence delirium as in dogs.

The chemical was thoroughly tested by Parke Davis for toxicity and found to be safe; the firm wanted to initiate clinical trials quickly. Since I am a clinical pharmacologist and not a clinical anesthesiologist, I contacted Gunter Corssen, one of my colleagues at the University of Michigan, who was interested in intravenous anesthetic agents. When I showed him CI-581's effects in monkeys, he was also convinced that we should test it in humans. I would be responsible for its initial human clinical pharmacology, and he for its use in clinical anesthesia. This was the beginning of several very exciting years of clinical research. We wrote up a protocol, which was approved by the Human Use Committee for the Parke Davis clinical

Edward F. Domino is professor of pharmacology at the University of Michigan in Ann Arbor and a board-certified clinical pharmacologist. Since graduation from medical school and clinical training in general medicine, anesthesia, and psychiatry, he has been interested in neuropsychopharmacology at both the experimental and the clinical levels.

Domino was elected a fellow of the CINP in 1966. He presented papers on the "Role of the central cholinergic system in wakefulness, fast wave sleep and 'no-go' behaviour," and on "Behavioural and electrophysiological aspects of antianxiety agents" at the 6th and 7th Congresses, respectively.

research unit at the State of Michigan prison in Jackson, a high-security facility. Visiting this place is quite an experience. In the days after the Second World War, ethical criteria were established to study prisoner volunteers in an approved manner. There were elaborate precautions to ensure that anyone volunteering for such experiments would be free to withdraw from further research should he desire to do so.

Our initial study involved adult males who were physically healthy and appeared emotionally stable. After all the ethical and clinical issues were settled, we began our work in the summer of 1964. The first human was given CI-581 on the third of August. The volunteers' responses to anesthetic doses of the compound were identical to what we had seen in monkeys. The subjects did comment on peculiar dreams that occurred during recovery from anesthesia, but the degree of emergence delirium was not great. We concluded that CI-581, like PCP, produced general anesthesia, but it was shorter acting and resulted in much less delirium. General anesthesia with CI-581 was very strange, in that the subjects were profoundly analgesic and "trance-like." They did not appear to be asleep or anesthetized, but rather were disconnected from their surroundings. After discussing this strange zombie-like state with my wife, I decided to use the term "dissociative anesthesia" to describe it. The overall incidence of mental side effects during emergence from anesthesia was about 30 percent. Many of our volunteers stated that they had very strange experiences, including feelings of floating, being in outer space, without their arms or legs, feeling dead, and so on.

We requested psychiatric consultation as to whether CI-581 produced a psychotic state similar to that occurring with PCP. Elliot Luby of the Lafayette Clinic was my choice for psychiatrist, but Parke Davis felt that he was too closely identified with the schizophrenomimetic actions of PCP. The clinical psychiatrist hired by the company interviewed our subjects during their emergence from anesthesia. He concluded that the mental effects during emergence from CI-581 were not schizophrenomimetic, but resembled those caused by general anesthesics such as diethyl ether. A major issue was whether the subjects hallucinated. Were they seeing objects or hearing sounds that were not present, or were these distortions of sensory input and illusions? Some Parke Davis personnel were extremely upset at the suggestion that the drug produced hallucinations. In our first publication on CI-581, we used the compromise terms "dream-like" states, "dream" reactions, and so on.

After we published our first clinical pharmacological experience with CI-581 in 1965 (2), the drug was given the generic name ketamine. In collaboration with Corssen we carried out additional studies with ketamine in patient volunteers, the results of which were reported in 1966, 1968 and 1969 (3, 4, 5). Later my interest in ketamine and PCP focused on their use as general anesthetics in infrahuman primates. In collaboration with Lau, we also developed a gas chromatographic/mass spectrometric assay for ketamine and its metabolites and studied its pharmacokinetics with Zsigmond (6). Elemer Zsigmond, who replaced Gunter Corssen as professor of anesthesiology at Michigan, was impressed that surgical patients given diazepam seemed to have less emergence delirium following ketamine. As a result, we initiated another study in volunteers in an attempt to tame the ketamine "tiger" of emergence reactions using diazepam as a pre-medication. With Zsigmond we found that diazepam in adequate intravenous doses about ten minutes prior to ketamine markedly reduced its psychic sequelae.

To my amazement, in the 1970s PCP emerged as a drug of abuse in the United States. This prompted me to organize a scientific workshop on PCP under the auspices of the American College of Neuropsychopharmacology in San Juan, Puerto Rico, on December 13, 1979. The proceedings were subsequently published in 1981. At that meeting, I met Jean-Marc Kamenka, a medicinal chemist at the École Nationale Supérieure de Chimie in Montpellier, France. We decided to hold joint French-American seminars on various arylcyclohexylamines, of which PCP and ketamine were prototypes. The first meeting was held in La Grande Motte in Montpellier on September 22-24, 1982. David Lodge from London contacted us before the meeting. He had found something exciting about PCP and ketamine, and wanted to make a presentation at our seminar. We invited him to do so, and at the meeting he made a monumental announcement. He and his colleagues had found that various arylcyclohexylamines selectively reduced excitation of mammalian neurons by aspartate-like amino acids (7). This was very important news in basic science! Finally, we had a mechanism of action that explained the profound actions of PCP, ketamine, and related arylcyclohexylamines on the brain.

As neuroscientists learned more about glutamic acid and its multiple receptors as excitatory neurotransmitters, interest increased in the possible role of glutamate in schizophrenia (8). There has been a resurgence of interest in re-examining the psychological effects of low doses of ketamine because it is a non-competitive agent acting on the N-methyl-D-aspartate (NMDA receptors). Ketamine is a good model of schizophrenia in normal volunteers, it exacerbates psychiatric symptoms in schizophrenics, and it induces mental symptoms in patients with Huntington's disease.

In contrast to PCP, ketamine never represented a serious drug-abuse problem. I assume that this was because it is more difficult to synthesize in illicit laboratories; it is also less potent and shorter acting than PCP. It is not scheduled as a drug of abuse by the U.S. Drug Enforcement Agency, but that situation may be changing. In some parts of the United States, ketamine is abused, and eight states have scheduled it to control its availability. In the U.S. drug culture, ketamine is called K, Special K, or Vitamin K (9). It is remarkable that some humans find the dissociative state produced by ketamine and its predecessor, PCP – chemical models of schizophrenia – reinforcing. Only time will tell whether ketamine abuse will become more prevalent.

The wild tiger in ketamine emergence delirium from anesthesia was always a problem. The pros and cons of ketamine were reviewed by many experts on the occasion of its twenty-fifth anniversary as an anesthetic agent (10). What changes will its fiftieth anniversary bring? Will ketamine become an obsolete anesthetic? Will it really help in our understanding of schizophrenia? How much of a drug-abuse problem will it become? I would like to know the answers since, after all, with many others I helped in its delivery.

REFERENCES

1. Luby, E.D., Cohan, B.D., Rosenbaum, F., Gottlieb, J., and Kelley, R. (1959). Study of a new schizophrenomimetic drug, Sernyl. Arch. Neurol. Psychiat. 81: 363-369.
2. Domino, E.F., Chodoff, P., and Corssen, G. (1965). Pharmacologic effects of CI-581, a new dissociative anesthetic, in man. Clin. Pharmacol. Ther. 6: 279-291.
3. Corssen, G., and Domino, E.F. (1966). Dissociative anesthesia: further pharmacologic studies and first clinical experience with the phencyclidine derivative CI-581. Anesth. Analg., 45: 29-40.
4. Corssen, G., Domino, E.F., and Bree, R.L. (1969). Electroencephalographic effects of ketamine anesthesia in children. Anesth. Analg. 48: 141-147.
5. Corssen, G., Miyasaka, M., and Domino, E.F. (1968). Changing concepts in pain control during surgery: dissociative anesthesia with CI-581 – a progress report. Anesth. Analg. 47: 746-759.
6. Domino, E.F., Zsigmond, E.K., Domino, L.E., Domino, K.E., Kothary, S.P., and Domino, S.E. (1982). Plasma levels of ketamine and two of its metabolites in surgical patients using a gas chromatography/mass fragmentography assay. Anesth. Analg. 61: 87-92.
7. Lodge, D., Anis, N.A., Berry, S.C., and Burt, N.R. (1983). Arylcyclohexylamines selectively reduce excitation of mammalian neurons by aspartate-like amino acids. In J.M. Kamenka, E.F. Domino, and P. Geneste (eds.) Phencyclidine and Related Arylcyclohexylamines: Present and Future Applications (pp.595-616). Ann Arbor: NPP Books.
8. Bunney, B.G., Bunney Jr, W.E., and Carlsson, A. (1995). Schizophrenia and glutamate. In F.E. Bloom and D.K. Kupfer (eds.), The Fourth Generation of Progress (pp.1205-1214). New York: Raven Press Ltd.
9. Cloud, J. (1997). Is your kid on K? Time 20 October (pp.90-91).
10. Domino, E.F. (ed.) (1990). Status of Ketamine in Anesthesiology. Ann Arbor: NPP Books.

WHEN NEUROPSYCHOPHARMACOLOGY WAS NEWS TO ME AND THEREAFTER
Comments of a "Cholinergiker"

Alexander G. Karczmar

My early work would not have predicted my becoming a neuropsychopharmacologist, and once I came into what might be considered the vicinity of that field, my path was multi-forked. Altogether, my several lives, including those as a neuropsychopharmacologist and a *Cholinergiker*, took many detours.

I came to the United States in September 1940, having escaped from Poland, where before the war I had studied biology and medicine in a somewhat desultory fashion at the Joseph Pilsudski University (now Warsaw University). In New York I became a graduate student at Columbia University. My PhD mentor was Selig Hecht, professor of biophysics, who was the first investigator to tread the quantal territory when he demonstrated in 1941 that retinal cells respond to a few photons. I could possibly have followed Hecht's approach to mentalization, as done in the 1990s by Roger Penrose and the late John Eccles, but I took a wrong turn in this road to neuropsychopharmacology since my thesis concerned regeneration and the trophic action of nerves in urodele (salamander) larvae.

After I graduated from Columbia in 1946, David Nachmansohn offered me a research position in his laboratory, probably not because of any merit on my part but because he was a great admirer of Hecht. If I had accepted his offer, I would have embarked directly into cholinergic neuropsychopharmacology. However, since I was tempted by an offer from the late Theodore Koppanyi of an academic position in his pharmacology department at Georgetown University in Washington, DC, I went there via a different route.

Koppanyi's history in scientific research had been quite varied. He had started as a *Wunderkind* (he was referred to that way by Arthur Koestler in his book *Midwife Toad*), studying eye regeneration and transplantation in the rat and the frog in Vienna. In his early twenties, he published papers on the subject with no less a luminary than Paul Weiss. Koppanyi appeared to be successful in his work, and a Nobel Prize was thought to be a certainty until at a congress he was unable to demonstrate his findings in public. (This anecdote is apocryphal and one of the myriad stories told about Koppanyi.) In the late twenties he emigrated to the United States, where he first worked at the University of Chicago. It was only later, after he moved to Cornell University Medical College, that under the guidance of R. Hatcher he finally

Alexander G. Karczmar was born in Warsaw, Poland, in 1917. After studying medicine and biology in his native city, he earned a PhD at Columbia University in 1946. He subsequently held research and teaching positions at various American institutions. Since 1956 he has been associated with Loyola University, of which he is now professor emeritus, and Hines Veterans Administration Hospital in Illinois, where he is still active as co-director of treatment initiative.

Karczmar was elected a fellow of the CINP in 1970. He presented on "Neurophysiological, behavioral and neurochemical correlates of the central cholinergic synapses" at the 7th CINP Congress.

embraced pharmacology, particularly that of emesis and defecation. And then, as chair of pharmacology at Georgetown University, he embarked on his lifelong studies of barbiturates, the autonomic nervous system, and anticholinesterases (as well as development, aging, and comparative pharmacology).

My work with Koppanyi mainly concerned anticholinesterases (antiChEs), their toxicity, and their role in the autonomic and somatic nervous systems. It was already at a time when the effects of cholinergic drugs on behaviour and conditioning was well known.

At one time Koppanyi watched me as I continued my work on regeneration with the salamander larvae. Intrigued with what he saw, he suggested that centrally acting lipid-soluble drugs, when dissolved in the water of the salamander pond, should penetrate through the skin of salamander larvae and act on the CNS. So we embarked on the study of the "overt behaviour" of the salamander larvae, including behavioural development and reflexogeny, as well as exploratory, social, and feeding functions. We described the effects of antiChEs such as physostigmine and di-isopropylfluorophosphate (DFP), atropine, and nicotine on these parameters of the larvae (1). Stimulated by the work of Hofmann, Hoffer, Osmond, and others, we studied the effects of LSD-25 on the same parameters. In these studies we were able to show the depressant action of atropine on exploration and general overt behaviour, and the antagonism of these effects by antiChEs. We were also able to show that the action of antiChEs on the CNS was direct, i.e., independent of ChEs inhibition. As for LSD-25 we found that it caused the larvae to swim in an erratic way, a behaviour perhaps analogous to the erratic net

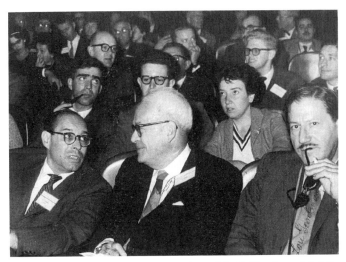

From left: **A. Karczmar, C. D. Leake and L. S. Goodman (right)**

building by spiders exposed to the substance.

So my cholinergic and neuropsychopharmacological pathways – at least with regard to salamander psychology – converged. In fact, when I moved in 1953 from Georgetown to the Sterling-Winthrop Research Institute (SWRI) in Rensselaer, New York, I still continued to use the larvae to demonstrate the difference in the "overt behavioural" effect of quaternary versus tertiary "neuromyally" active antiChEs.

At SWRI my activity involved the development of clinically useful drugs, e.g., ambenonium, an antimyasthenic drug, Myordil, an antiarrhythmic agent. This was not exactly neuropsychopharmacology.

The situation changed only in the early fifties, after the Rhône-Poulenc company developed chlorpromazine and Frank Berger developed meprobamate (Miltown), a prototype of the muscle relaxants subsequently referred to as anxiolytics or minor tranquilizers. (One of the early muscle relaxants was called Soma after the drug used in Aldous Huxley's *Brave New World.*) At SWRI we had a patent on a flat nucleus developed by the firm's chemist, Bernie Zenitz, and we proceeded to attach certain side chains to the nucleus and test the resulting compounds for their chlorpromazine-like properties. We followed a similar process with respect to prospective meprobamate-like drugs.

We screened the compounds in question using tests employed by the Rhône-Poulenc investigators in the development of chlorpromazine, including assessment of their hypothermic effect, their capacity to potentiate the anesthetic effects of pentobarbital, and so on. When we visited Karl Pribram, at that time the director of the Hartford Life Institute, to consult him on these matters, he told us bluntly: "I would not dignify these measurements with the term *tests.*" Well, a screening process is a friend of an investigator working for a pharmaceutical company, and a micro in-depth analysis makes the director of the company his enemy.

We, however, employed a test that was developed by Joseph Brady in the early fifties and consisted of an automated conditioning system for measuring the conditioned emotional response (CER) of rats. It was essentially a nocturnal test, and many drug companies loved it, since it converted the working day into a twenty-four-hour affair. The rats worked through the night for some food, and the technicians could arrive in the morning and find the records ready for them. I prodded SWRI to become the first company to acquire a few Brady systems.

Another test expanded my studies of overt behaviour from salamanders to monkeys; a third consisted of monitoring motor and related activities; and a fourth was the study of facial expressions, taking advantage of Charles Darwin's book on the facial expressions of monkeys and apes. Altogether, I exposed drugged and control macaca monkeys to standardized challenges – including my presence in the monkey cage – and recorded their coded behaviour and expressions using a shorthand processor. Maurice Tainter, the director of SWRI at the time, thought that this was a crazy test. He was more impressed with the effects on overt behaviour of large, rather than small doses of the drugs in question, e.g., large doses of meprobamate-like agents caused a characteristic flaccid paralysis.

Ultimately, we developed a few promising drugs in animal tests. While it was difficult to compete with a drug such as chlorpromazine, we hoped that a milder tranquillizer we had developed, which seemed to be similar to promazine (Sparine), would have a good chance for clinical use. Unfortunately, SWRI was not able to hold onto clinical investigators capable of carrying out phase 3 research with the compounds in question. So not much, in terms of psychopharmacology, came out of my effort at SWRI.

In 1956 I moved to the Loyola University Medical Center as chair of the Department of Pharmacology and Therapeutics. At Loyola, with several friends and departmental colleagues who were, and are, very prominent electrophysiologists – Syogoro Nishi, Kyo Koketsu, Alan North, Les Blaber, and later Nae Dun – and with my friend Vincenzo Longo, an EEG expert at the time at the Istituto Superiore di Sanità of Rome, I embarked on a neurophysiological and neuropharmacological study of the central and peripheral cholinergic systems. At the same time I continued my work on the effect of drugs on conditioned, as well as overt, behaviour.

It was in the area of drugs and conditioned behaviours that I was helped and inspired by my connection with the CINP, formed in 1957, and the American College of Neuropsychopharmacology (ACNP), founded three years later. I became a participant in the CINP through my friendship and contacts with Corneille and Simone Radouco-Thomas, Jacques Boissier, Steve Brodie, Tom Ban, Silvio Garattini, Emilio Trabucchi, Oldrich Vinar, Zdenek Votava, and others. In fact, while Corneille likes to reminisce about the formation of the collegium at a gathering in a Milan trattoria that included himself and the Italian mafia of Emilio and Silvio, I remember the initiation of the ACNP at a gathering in a Geneva bar, which included Steve Brody, Corneille, and myself. That social event also led to the founding of the *International Journal of Neuropharmacology*, now called simply *Neurpharmacology*. (I served for many years on the editorial board.)

At Loyola, the late Charles Scudder and I used mice of various strains in the study of overt behaviour. We developed in the 1960s a pseudo-natural habitat to study the ethology of these strains, my great friend George Koelle called, "Mouse City" and we could measure social, parental, aggressive, feeding, sexual, exploratory, cognitive, emotional, and learning behaviour. We combined this study with that of learning as we employed a pentalever avoidance conditioning climbing screen (2), and we demonstrated the facilitatory effects of cholinergic agonists on Mouse City exploratory behaviour and on learning.

During those years we also studied the significant analgetic effect of cholinergic agonists, which we showed to be independent of cholinergic-endogenous opioids interaction (3); and we established that – compared to catecholaminergic and antiserotonergic drugs, which facilitate aggression in the case of certain, but not all, paradigms – the cholinergic agonists increase or evoke aggression under all circumstances. Altogether, studies concerning this and other behaviours led us to posit the theory that the cholinergic system has a general alerting and cognitive effect which seems to underlie the teleological interaction between an organism and its environment. I called this behaviour "cholinergic alert non-mobile behaviour" (since it induced a certain degree of muscle relaxation and attenuation of locomotion), or CANMB. In fact, since Longo, Scotti di Carolis, and I (4) established that the cholinergic system predominantly – even after depletion of catecholaminergic neurotransmitters – induces REM sleep, I compared the CANMB to an awakened REM-sleep behaviour (5).

With Charles Scudder and Alfred Kahn, we employed a site preference paradigm to measure alcohol "addiction," as "addicted" rats or mice overcame the site preference – and also a punishment paradigm – to enjoy a bottle of alcohol, which sometimes contained concentrated liquor. We also tried to relate compulsive and addictive behaviour to attenuation of acetylcholine release and depression of the cholinergic muscarinic system.

As for relating our behavioural and conditioning studies to cholinergic neuronal electrophysiology, our work and that of others emphasizes the multiple excitatory, inhibitory, and modulatory effects of the cholinergic system. Furthermore, these effects are widespread in view of the strategic multiplicity of central cholinergic pathways. Thus the long-lasting muscarinic potential facilitates the neuronal effects of other transmitter systems effects, as stressed by Chris Krnjevic and ourselves, and similar cholinergic-noncholinergic interactions underlie neuronal modes of learning. Altogether, these neuronal cholinergic phenomena seem to be relevant for cognitive and related cholinergic effects, although the specific causal relationship may be posited only speculatively at this time. Some of these views were expressed and combined with those of philosophers of cognition, such as Steve Toulmin, at a symposium that the late Jack Eccles and I organized at the Loyola University Medical Center (6). This symposium was famous for the presence of three Nobel Prize winners (Eccles, Bovet, and Granit) and other luminaries, such as Jean Piaget, Mortimer Mishkin, Holger Hyden, and Seymour Kety.

These and related experiences led me in two directions. First, although, as a devoted *Cholinergiker,* I have no desire to deprecate the role of the cholinergic system in behaviour and cognition, I cannot fail to realize that the brain acts as an orchestra of its transmitter and modulatory systems. Today this may appear to be a trite notion, but not so long ago catecholamine, serotonin, peptidergic, and cholinergic investigators did not speak to one another. I am glad that I was one of the first researchers to press for a mending of our ways, as I helped to organize multi-transmitter sessions at the tenth CINP congress and the seventh International Cholinergic Congress.

Secondly, and in conclusion, the cholinergic system has so many cognitive implications that unavoidably the studies of this system have led me, as it did my friends the late John Eccles and Ben Libet, to consider the Cartesian problem and other problems of consciousness and creativity. Furthermore, when one can no longer work in the laboratory, why not ratiocinate? I broached these subjects in a few recent reviews (7), and health permitting, I may treat them more extensively in the book on the cholinergic system on which I have been working for the last few years.

REFERENCES
1. Karczmar, A.G., and Koppanyi, T. (1953). Central effects of di-isopropyl-fluorophosphate in urodele larvae. *Schmiedebergs Arch. f. Path.* 219: 261-270.
2. Karczmar, A.G., and Scudder, C.L. (1969). Learning and effect of drugs on learning of related mice genera and strains. In A.G. Karczmar and W.P. Koella (eds.), *Neurophysiological and Behavioral Aspects of Psychotropic Drugs* (pp. 133-160). Springfield, Ill.: Charles C. Thomas Publ.
3. Koehn, G.L., Henderson, G., and Karczmar, A.G. (1980). Di-isopropyl phosphofluoridate-induced antinociception: possible role of endogenous opioids. *Europ. Pharmacol.* 61: 167-173.
4. Karczmar, A.G., Longo, V.G., and Scotti de Carolis, A. (1970). A pharmacological model of paradoxical sleep: the role of cholinergic and monamine systems. *Physiol. & Behav.* 5: 175-182.
5. Karczmar, A.G. (1993). Brief presentation of the story and the present status of the vertebrate cholinergic system. *Neuropsychopharmacol.* 9: 181-199.
6. Karczmar, A.G., and Eccles, J.C. (eds.) (1972). *Brain and Human Behavior.* Berlin: Springer-Verlag.
7. Karczmar, A.G. (1996). Loewi's discovery and the XXI Century. In J. Klein and K. Loffelholz (eds.), *Cholinergic Mechanisms: From Molecular Biology to Clinical Significance* (pp. 1-27). Amsterdam: Elsevier.

THE RISE OF PSYCHOPHARMACOLOGY IN THE 1960s
A Memoir

Allan F. Mirsky

My first exposure to research with centrally acting drugs occurred during my graduate student years at Yale between 1950 and 1954. I was a small part of a large team of investigators, led by the eminent John Fulton, who were studying frontal lobe functions in primates, including humans. The interest in this brain structure was stimulated by the fact that many of the veterans of the Second World War had developed or were developing severe neuropsychiatric disorders, and the Veterans Administration of the United States was anxious to develop effective methods for treating them. It was believed at that time that prefrontal lobotomy was an effective treatment for schizophrenia; consequently, the VA was supporting fundamental research that would illuminate the functions of the frontal lobe and the reasons for the therapeutic effects of prefrontal lobotomy. This was, of course, several years before the introduction into the United States of the compound chlorpromazine, whose therapeutic effects in schizophrenia had been described by Delay and Deniker in a congress publication in 1952.

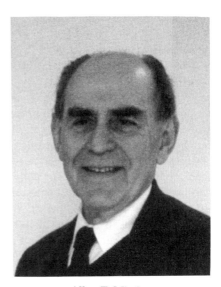

Allan F. Mirsky

We were particularly interested in the deficit shown by monkeys with prefrontal cortical lesions: they were impaired in the performance of delayed-response-type tasks. Among the hypotheses to account for the deficit was that they were inattentive to the stimuli. The lesioned animals were hyperactive, pacing continuously in their cages, and scarcely looking at the task stimuli. To slow down their perpetual pacing, we administered a short-acting barbiturate to

Allan F. Mirsky received a BS degree from the City College of New York in 1950 and a PhD in clinical and physiological psychology from Yale University four years later. From 1961 to 1980 he was on the faculties of the departments of psychiatry, psychology, and neurology at Boston University. Between 1954 and 1961 and since 1980 he has been a research scientist in the Intramural Research Program of the National Institute of Mental Health in Bethesda, Maryland. He is also an adjunct professor at Johns Hopkins University and chair of the neuropsychology advisory committee of the World Health Organization.

Allan F. Mirsky was elected a fellow of the CINP in 1966. He presented a paper on "The relationship between EEG and impaired attention following administration of centrally acting drugs" (Mirsky and Tecce) at the 5th Congress.

prefrontally lesioned monkeys just before testing their delayed alternation performance. The result of the experiment was positive, in that there was a modest, but significant improvement in performance as a result of the sedative effects of the drug. Thus the barbiturate apparently slowed down the animals long enough to allow them to look at the task stimuli. As I think about that experiment now, I believe that the prefrontal lesions might be a possible model mechanism for Attention Deficit Hyperactivity Disorder (ADHD), and that the study should be replicated with methylphenidate, which was not available in 1952. If early experiences are critical for determining one's later behaviour, then my first exposure to such research was to see drugs as research tools to modify behaviour – attention, specifically – in reversible fashion. This has characterized most of my work with centrally acting drugs, and I said as much in a paper that Rosvold and I wrote in 1960 (1).

The first seven years after I received my PhD (1954-61) were spent in the Intramural Research Program of the National Institute of Mental Health (USA). I was a member of the section on animal behaviour, whose chief was Haldor (Hal) E. Rosvold. We were part of the newly established Laboratory of Psychology, headed by David Shakow. Conan Kornetsky, who was then in Seymour Kety's Laboratory of Clinical Science, and I collaborated on a number of studies aimed at specifying the behavioural effects of a variety of fascinating and important psychoactive compounds, some new and some old. Among these were chlorproma-zine and its close phenothiazine derivative, perphenazine; LSD; the barbiturates, including secobarbital, phenobarbital, and pentobarbital; and ethanol (2). All these drugs had profound effects on behaviour, none of which were well understood. I was also curious about the extent to which the effects of some of these compounds resembled those of sleep deprivation. However, my overarching goal was to use the drugs (and sleep deprivation, as well) to model the central effects of an equally mysterious phenomenon, the alterations in consciousness seen in petit mal epilepsy – the "absence attack."

Petit mal (absence) epilepsy is also known as centrencephalic and, more recently, cortico-reticular epilepsy. I was one of a group of investigators, including Michael Myslobodsky of Tel Aviv University, who believed that understanding the central events occurring during an absence attack was the key to illuminating the whole basis of consciousness. And centrally acting drugs provided a powerful tool in that endeavour because they produced exquisitely titratable, reversible effects on consciousness and alertness. In the 1950s Penfield and Jasper had explicated their theory of the alteration of consciousness seen in petit mal attacks. It was, for them, a disturbance in the functioning of the "centrencephalic" system, a deep subcortical organizing system with widespread connections to all parts of the forebrain. I was struck by the fact that both epileptologists Penfield and Jasper and neuropharmacologists Bradley and Elkes had implicated brainstem (reticular activating system) structures in their exciting theoretical accounts. For Penfield and Jasper, this was the "focus" of petit mal epilepsy; for Bradley and Elkes, the afferents to this system constituted the site of action of chlorpromazine. I hoped that studying the central effects of drugs such as chlorpromazine would unlock the secrets of the petit mal absence attack.

Kornetsky and I wrote several theoretical papers in the 1960s in which we attempted to integrate some of our findings. In one (3) we presented a model to explain why some drugs had one behavioural effect, whereas other drugs had the opposite effect. For example, chlorpromazine produced more impairment of sustained attention (as assessed by the incinti-nous performance test, or CPT) than of focused attention (as assessed by the digit symbol substitution test, or DSST). Other drugs (e.g., the barbiturates and LSD) had the reverse effect, producing more impairment of focused attention (on the DSST) than of sustained attention (on the CPT). I well remember the helpful advice provided by Abraham Wikler, who was then the editor of *Psychopharmacologia*. He urged us to delve more deeply into the then-sparse neuropharmacological (and related) literature on these compounds in order to add depth to our theory. It was one of the first and only times I can recall that an editor had actually requested a longer, rather than a shorter, paper. In a second paper (4) we extended the model to explain why patients with schizophrenia and normal controls responded differently to chlorpromazine. In this account we relied heavily on the inverted-U hypothesis, relating arousal level to performance. The seminal research of Bradley and Elkes among the first important neuropsychopharmacology papers was extremely influential in our thinking in both articles.

After leaving the NIMH in 1961, I went to the Division of Psychiatry at Boston University Medical School. The division chair was Bernard Bandler, who was later succeeded by Sanford Cohen. I went on, with wonderful assistance from colleagues Eva Bakay Pragay and Susana Bloch, to develop monkey models of the behaviour we had been studying in humans. This entailed creating analogues of sustained attention (i.e., a CPT for monkeys) and focused attention (i.e., a DSST for monkeys). We used these models extensively, first to see if the dissociation we saw in humans with chlorpromazine and secobarbital could be replicated with monkeys (it could) and later to investigate brain electrical activity during administration of chlorpromazine and secobarbital (5, 6, 7, 8). We were impressed that the action of chlorpromazine seemed to resemble more closely than did secobarbital the behavioural state we saw in patients with absence attacks. Secobarbital produced a period of erroneous, disinhibited responding, followed by a gradual induction of a somnolent state; during this time, responses gradually and incrementally slowed in our monkey subjects that were performing the CPT. Finally, there was a complete absence of responsiveness. As the drug wore off, the slow responding recurred, followed by the reappearance of disinhibited responding, before normal task behaviour was restored. In contrast, chlorpromazine produced a long-lasting effect, in which periodic lapses in responding to task stimuli were interspersed with near-normal responses. Disinhibited responding was virtually never seen with chlorpromazine. Thus it provided a more accurate model than the barbiturates of the behavioural effects we saw in patients with absence epilepsy.

The problem with chlorpromazine, however, was that its effects on brain electrical activity, either at the cortical surface or in the depths, bore little or no resemblance to the EEG patterns observed in absence epilepsy (9). The classic signature of absence seizures – the three-per-second, symmetrical, and synchronous spike-wave pattern – was never seen with chlorpromazine. In order to reproduce the spike-wave pattern convincingly, we had to use the drug chlorambucil (10) and later conjugated estrogen (11).

The last of the studies I did during the era of the 1960s and early 1970s involved examining the behaviour of single precentral cortical neurons as influenced by secobarbital and chlorpromazine (12). This was the first study I carried out, with colleague Suso Otero, using the single neuron recording techniques learned in Ed Evarts' laboratory at the NIMH during my sabbatical year in 1972-73.

My studies in psychopharmacology have been both personally and professionally rewarding. I am grateful that I had the opportunity to work in this area of research, and I trust that some of my publications conveyed the excitement of exploring what was then, and to a large extent still is, the *terra incognita* of the effects of drugs on the brain.

REFERENCES

1. Mirsky, A.F., and Rosvold, H.E. (1960). The use of psychoactive drugs as a neuropsychological tool in studies of attention in man. In J.G. Miller and L. Uhr (eds.), *Drugs and Behavior.* New York: Wiley.

2. Mirsky, A.F., and Kornetsky, C. (1969). The effects of centrally acting drugs on attention. In D.E. Efron (ed.), *Psychopharmacology: A Review of Progress 1957-1967.* (pp. 91-104). Washington, DC: U.S. Government Printing Office.

3. Mirsky, A.F., and Kornetsky, C. (1964). On the dissimilar effects of drugs on the digit symbol substitution and continuous performance tests. *Psychopharmacologia,* 5: 161-177.

4. Kornetsky, C., and Mirsky, A.F. (1966). On certain psychopharmacological and physiological differences between schizophrenic and normal persons. *Psychopharmacologia,* 8: 309-318.

5. Mirsky, A.F., and Bakay Pragay, E. (1970). EEG characteristics of impaired attention accompanying secobarbital and chlorpromazine administration in monkeys. In D. Mostofsky (ed.), *Attention: Contemporary Theory and Analysis* (pp.403-417). New York: Appleton-Century Crofts.

6. Bakay Pragay, E., and Mirsky, A.F. (1973). The nature of performance deficit under secobarbital and chlor-promazine in the monkey: a behavioral and EEG study. *Psychopharmacologia,* 28: 73-85.

7. Bloch, S., Bakay Pragay, E., and Mirsky, A.F. (1973). Heart rate and respiratory rate changes during drug-induced impairment in a conditioned avoidance task in monkeys. *Pharmacology, Biochemistry and Behavior,* 1: 29-34.

8. Bakay Pragay, E., and Mirsky, A.F. (1977). Effect of secobarbital and chlorpromazine on cortical and subcortical visual evoked potentials in the monkey. *Psychopharmacology Bulletin* 13: 61-64.

9. Mirsky, A.F., Tecce, J.J., Harman, N., and Oshima, H. (1975). EEG correlates of impaired attention performance under secobarbital and chlorpromazine in the monkey. *Psychopharmacologia* 41: 35-41.

10. Mirsky, A.F., Bloch, S., and McNary, W.F. (1966). Experimental "petit mal" epilepsy produced with chlorambucil. *Acta Biologiae Experimentalis* 26: 55-69.

11. Mirsky, A.F., Bloch, S., Tecce, J.J., Lessell, S., and Marcus, E. (1973). Visual evoked potentials during experimentally induced spike-wave activity in monkeys. *Electroencephalography and Clinical Neurophysiology* 35: 25-37.

12. Otero, J., and Mirsky, A.F. (1976). Influence of secobarbital and chlorpromazine on precentral neuron activity during attentive behavior in monkeys. *Psychopharmacologia* 49: 1-9.

SCHIZOPHRENIA AND THE CONTINUOUS PERFORMANCE TEST

Conan Kornetsky

The decade of the 1960s was a period of change for me. In June 1959 I had moved from the Laboratory of Clinical Sciences at the National Institute of Mental Health in Bethesda, Maryland, to become associate research professor in the Department of Pharmacology at Boston University School of Medicine. And four years later I was promoted to the rank of professor in the Departments of Psychiatry and Pharmacology. The years I had spent at the NIMH, 1954-59, were exciting ones; this was just after the discovery of the effectiveness of chlorpromazine in the treatment of schizophrenic patients. In addition, during this short period the first of the antidepressant and anxiolytic drugs had become available. Although psychoanalytic thinking was especially strong during the decades immediately after the Second World War, the new discoveries in pharmacology and neuroscience opened the door for experiments that tested neurobiological hypotheses of the etiology of mental illness.

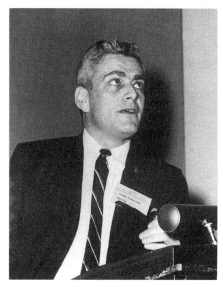

Conan Kornetsky

Much of my research at Bethesda was directed towards the elucidation of the behavioural effects of these newer, as well as the older, psychoactive drugs in normal and schizophrenic subjects. Among the findings was that the schizophrenics' response to acute doses of chlorpromazine was different from that of the normal control subjects. A colleague at the NIMH, Allan F. Mirsky, was studying the *absence* in petit mal epilepsy. The behavioural test that he

Conan Kornetsky was born in Portland, Maine, in 1926. He received his PhD in psychology from the University of Kentucky in 1952, when he worked in the Laboratory of Clinical Science at the NIMH, Bethesda, Maryland. In 1959 he went to Boston University, where he is a professor of psychiatry and pharmacology. He has received a Career Scientist Award from NIMH for his career at Boston University. Currently his research is directed toward elucidating the neurobiology of the rewarding effects of abused substances.

Kornetsky was elected a fellow of the CINP in 1962. He presented on "Attention dysfunction and drugs in schizophrenia" at the 5th Congress and coauthored a paper on "Changes in conditioned behavior under chlorpromazine and d-amphetamine as a function of the motivational characteristics and parametric values of the tests" (Latz, Kornetsky and Bain) at the same Congress. Kornetsky was a formal discussant in Working Group 3 (Psychology and Experimental Psychopathology) at the 4th Congress.

used in his experiments was the continuous performance test (CPT). He was among the authors of the classic paper that first described in 1956 this simple, but powerful instrument for measuring sustained attention (1). Because it often seemed that schizophrenic patients had difficulty in attending, we thought that the CPT might be a useful tool for the study of drug effects in normal subjects and schizophrenic patients. This collaboration led to the publication of several papers in which we defined the effects of some centrally active drugs in normal subjects based on the relative dissociation that they had on cognitive versus attention tests. Our work was summarized in a 1964 paper (2). In a paper two years later (3) we wrote the following: "The hypothesis states that the schizophrenic patients are in a state of chronic hyperarousal. This results from dysfunction in those areas of the brain concerned with the maintenance of arousal and attention, i.e. the brain stem reticular activating system." I presented the evidence for this theory in 1966 at the 5th CINP Congress in Washington, DC.

Among the critical findings was that schizophrenic patients, as compared to normal control subjects, had an attenuated response to acute doses of chlorpromazine on tests that measured sustained attention. The relative lack of response of schizophrenic patients to acute doses of chlorpromazine was not limited to behaviour. At a meeting of the American Society of Pharmacology and Experimental Therapeutics in 1958, we reported the results of an experiment in which we gave 200 mg of chlorpromazine to normal volunteers and to schizophrenic subjects at 7:00 p.m. Once the subjects went to bed, they were kept supine until 7:00 a.m. the next morning. After we had recorded their supine blood pressure (BP), they were instructed to stand for sixty seconds and their BP was once again recorded. In the normal subjects there was a marked drop in BP upon standing that was absent in the schizophrenic patients.(4) Because none of the patients had been chronically treated with antipsychotic medications, this lack of response to a single dose of chlorpromazine could not be attributed to previous exposure to the drug.

During the 1960s and into the 1970s we published a number of papers using the CPT based on the overarousal hypothesis of schizophrenia. Among the significant findings was that chronic schizophrenics, when compared to alcoholics (one week post-withdrawal), showed significant impairment on the CPT but not on the digit symbol substitution test (DSST), a simple test of cognitive functioning; while the alcoholics had no difficulty with the CPT, they showed significant loss of function on the DSST. The subjects were matched for both age and educational ability (5).

Because not all schizophrenic patients performed poorly on the CPT, we decided to compare "good" and "poor" attenders on a variety of clinical and familial characteristics. Also, because we had found that phenothiazine therapy improved the performance of patients on the CPT (6), we decided to compare these characteristics in patients maintained on medication and in non-medicated patients (7). In order to carry out this study we tested every schizophrenic patient at Medfield State Hospital in Medfield, Massachusetts, who was willing and could perform a simple psychological test, and who had been hospitalized for a minimum of two years. Our final sample was sixty-nine patients. Of these, twenty-seven were not receiving medication, while the remaining forty-two were on chronic treatment with phenothiazines or a combination of phenothiazines and antiparkinson drugs. Because we rarely found a non-schizophrenic control subject who made more than two errors of omission on the CPT, only patients with three or more errors were defined as poor attenders.

One of our hypotheses was that there would be more mental illness in the families of the poor attenders than of the good attenders. Although the total number of subjects not on medication was small, the hypothesis was supported by a stepwise multiple regression analysis and by Fisher's exact test. As far as I am aware, this was the first study suggesting a relationship between CPT performance in schizophrenic patients and familial psychiatric states. Although we predicted that poor attenders would have an earlier onset of illness, longer hospitalization, and more pathology as determined by psychiatric ratings, these predictions were not borne out. There was, as hypothesized, a lack of significant difference on the DSST. On the other hand, there were differences between patients maintained on medication and those not on medication on these same variables with the off-medication group having a greater incidence of psychopathology than the on-medication group, as measured by the Lorr and Venables scales, as well as poorer performance on the CPT.

At the end of the 1960s a young psychiatrist, Gerald W. Wohlberg, became a postdoctoral fellow in my laboratory. Gerry was interested in the question of whether or not the attentional impairment in some schizophrenic patients was a "trait" or "state" deficit. If it were a trait deficit, it would be present in remitted schizophrenic patients who were functioning well without antipsychotic medication. Finding such patients was not an easy task. Gerry examined individually 700 records of formerly hospitalized patients in Boston-area hospitals and found 16 remitted schizophrenics who met our criterion, along with 20 normal volunteers. Somewhat unique was the use of female subjects only. The remitted schizophrenics made significantly more errors on the CPT than the control subjects, confirming the presence of a trait deficit in the remitted schizophrenic patients (8). My excitement over these findings was soon overwhelmed by a terrible tragedy. Gerry, upon completing his postdoctoral fellowship with me, was appointed to the faculty of Boston University School of Medicine. Among his duties was the supervision of residents at Boston State Hospital. A paranoid schizophrenic, previously discharged against medical advice, returned to the hospital and held his treating resident at gunpoint. Gerry intervened, and just as it seemed that the patient was about to give up the gun, he fired. Gerry was hit in the head, and after a month in coma he died.

In 1976 I published my last paper on the hyperarousal hypothesis of schizophrenia. It described the lack of response of schizophrenic patients to d-amphetamine. The research, however, had been conducted at Medfield State Hospital between 1960 and 1963. Because the results were primarily negative, I did not submit the paper for publication until 1976, when it became evident that the negative results were important (9). My previous experiments with d-amphetamine in normal subjects suggested that if this drug improved performance, it did so primarily by focusing attention. In 1963 I had the naive idea, based on the inverted-U hypothesis of schizophrenia arousal, that chronic d-amphetamine treatment in schizophrenics would have positive effects. We had done some experiments in which we found that schizophrenics did not respond to a large single dose of d-amphetamine. Because of the lack of effect, I thought that if we placed these chronic schizophrenics on daily administration of d-amphetamine, it would have a positive effect on their disease state.

I wrote a protocol for such an experiment and presented it to the committee on human experimentation at Medfield State Hospital. The committee members believed that the chronic use of d-amphetamine in this population would result in the patients not sleeping at night and becoming difficult to manage. They therefore allowed me to carry out a brief two-week pilot experiment that focused on the patients' sleep behaviour. The results were basically negative; that is, the patients' sleep behaviour was hardly affected, despite the oral administration of 20 mg of d-amphetamine every night at 8:00 p.m. for a week. Unfortunately, I did not follow up this lack of response in the patients with the originally proposed chronic amphetamine experiment. But because a number of papers indicated that amphetamine or methylphenidate exacerbated schizophrenic symptoms and these findings were used to support the dopamine theory of schizophrenia, I decided that my conflicting results were important. The major difference was that all my subjects were chronic schizophrenics. It is of interest that there have been some reports of improvement in schizophrenic symptoms in some patients treated with d-amphetamine (10,11).

In addition to experiments carried out in human subjects, I was also involved in animal experimentation. Most of my work of this type in the 1960s was directed towards the development of an animal model of the attention deficit seen in the schizophrenic patient. Not without some difficulty, we developed a homologous model of the CPT. The next task was to determine if we could manipulate the performance of the rat on the CPT by altering its central arousal level. The work of Bradley (12) and Keith and Eva Killam (13) had implicated the mesencephalic reticular formation in the action of chlorpromazine. Our hypothesis was that at least some schizophrenic patients were in a state of central excitation or overarousal. We therefore decided to see if we could reproduce this state in the rat by low-level electrical stimulation of the reticular formation. We hypothesized that, as we increased the level of stimulation in the rat, performance on the CPT would improve. After reaching a maximum level, further increase in stimulation would result in impairment in CPT performance. The levels of stimulation used caused no apparent increase in motor behaviour, but we did find that we could produce an inverted-U curve, with errors of omission being a function of stimulus intensity.

The critical test was to combine a dose of chlorpromazine that by itself impaired the performance of the rat with reticular stimulation. We were under no illusion that stimulating the reticular formation was a model for schizophrenia, but we did believe that we might be modelling the basis for the attention dysfunction in schizophrenic patients. In a series of experiments (14, 15) we found, as predicted, that combining a level of stimulation which increased errors of omission on the CPT with a dose of chlorpromazine that also increased omission errors resulted in a performance level indistinguishable from that seen when both stimulation and chlorpromazine were absent. We continued doing experiments using this model and found that similar results to those of electrical stimulation of the reticular formation could be obtained by using a push-pull cannula and exposing the reticular formation to various levels of norepinephrine. This resulted in errors in CPT performance that could be reversed by chlorpromazine as well as by a number of other antipsychotic medications that were available at the time (16, 17).

These early experiments with the CPT used instrumentation that was quite crude by modern standards; however, I believe that much of what we achieved has stood the test of time. Although the reticular formation has, for the most part, ceased to be a major focus in studies of schizophrenia, a recent anatomical study of the brains of schizophrenics by Garcia-Rill and colleagues (18) states that their results "implicate the brain stem reticular formation as a pathophysiological site in at least some patients with schizophrenia." Further, they suggest that the findings account "for sensory gating abnormalities, sleep-wake disturbances and, perhaps, hallucinations." Also, the CPT is still a frequently used instrument in the study of schizophrenia, Cornblatt and Keilp (19), in a review of research employing the test in the study of schizophrenics, stated that impaired attention as measured by the CPT is "evident in schizophrenic patients regardless of clinical state; detectable before illness onset; apparently heritable; specific – in terms of distinct profile patterns – to schizophrenia, and predictive of later behavioral disturbance in susceptible individuals."

Because my earliest research at the U.S. Public Health Service Hospital in Lexington, Kentucky, in 1948-52, was directed towards problems of addiction, in addition to my schizophrenia research, I continued to carry out work with abused substances. In collaboration with Joseph Cochin, we demonstrated that in the rat there was tolerance to morphine after a single dose that could be expressed months later. Late in 1960 I began a series of experiments that have continued to today, directed towards elucidating the mechanisms involved in the rewarding effects of abused substances. This research is another story, but it has kept me busy for almost all of the last thirty years.

REFERENCES

1. Rosvold, H.E., Mirsky, A., Sarason, L., Bransome Jr, E.D., and Beck, L.H. (1956). A continuous performance test of brain damage. *Journal of Cons. Psychology* 20: 343-350.
2. Mirsky, A.F., and Kornetsky, C. (1964). On the dissimilar effects of drugs on the Digit Symbol Substitution and Continuous Performance Tests. *Psychopharmacologia* (Berlin), 5: 161-177.
3. Kornetsky, C., and Mirsky, A.F. (1966). On certain psychopharmacological and physiological differences between schizophrenic and normal persons. *Psychopharmacologia* (Berlin), 8: 309-318.
4. Vates, T., and Kornetsky, C. (1958). A comparison of some physiological changes in normal and schizophrenic subjects twelve hours after chlorpromazine administration. In *Abstracts of Fall Meeting: American Society for Pharmacology and Experimental Therapeutics* (p. 35).
5. Orzack, M.H., and Kornetsky, C. (1966). Attention dysfunction in chronic schizophrenia. *Archives of General Psychiatry* 14: 323-326.
6. Orzack, M., Kornetsky, C., and Freeman, H. (1967). The effects of daily administration of carphenazine on attention in the schizophrenic patients. *Psychopharmacologia* 11: 31-38.
7. Orzack, M.H., and Kornetsky, C. (1971). Environmental and familial predictors of attention behavior in chronic schizophrenics. *Journal of Psychiatric Research*, 9: 21-29.
8. Wohlberg, G.W., and Kornetsky, C. (1973). Sustained attention in remitted schizophrenics. *Archives of General Psychiatry*, 28: 533-537.
9. Kornetsky, C. (1976). Hyporesponsivity of chronic schizophrenic patients to dextroamphetamine. *Archives of General Psychiatry* 33: 1425-1428.
10. Angrist, B., and van Kammen, D.P. (1984). CNS stimulants as tools in the study of schizophrenia. *Trends in Neurosciences*, 7: 388-391.
11. van Kammen, D.P., Bunney Jr, W.E., Docherty, J.P., Marder, S.R., Ebert, M.H., Rosenblatt, J.E., and Rayner, J.N. (1982). D-amphetamine-induced heterogenous changes in psychotic behavior in schizophrenia. *American Journal of Psychiatry*, 139: 991-997.
12. Bradley, P.B. (1958). The central action of certain drugs in relation to the reticular formation of the brain. In H.H. Jasper, L.D. Proctor, R.S. Knighton, W.C. Noshay, and R.T. Costello (eds.), *Reticular Formation of the Brain* (pp. 123-149). Boston: Little, Brown.
13. Killam, K.F., and Killam, E.K. (1958). Drug action on pathways involving the reticular formation. In H.H. Jasper, L.D. Proctor, R.S. Knighton, W.C. Noshay, and R.T. Costello (eds.), *Reticular Formation of the Brain* (pp. 411-445). Boston: Little, Brown.
14. Kornetsky, C., and Eliasson, M. (1969). Reticular stimulation and chlorpromazine: an animal model for schizophrenic overarousal. *Science*, 165: 1273-1274.
15. Eliasson, M., and Kornetsky, C. (1972). Interaction effects of chlorpromazine and reticular stimulation on visual attention behavior in rats. *Psychonomic Science*, 26: 261-262.
16. Bain, G. (1980). The effects of norepinephrine perfusion of the mesencephalic reticular formation on behavior in the rat: Interaction with several neuroleptic drugs on a measure of sustained attention. Doctoral dissertation, Boston University.
17. Kornetsky, C., and Markowitz, R. (1975). Animal models and schizophrenia. In D. Ingle and H.M. Shein (eds.), *Model Systems in Biological Psychiatry* (pp. 26-50) Cambridge, MA: MIT Press.
18. Garcia-Rill, E., Biedermann, J.A., Chambers, T., Skinner, R.D., Mrak, R.E., Husain, M., and Karson, C.N. (1995). Mesopontine neurons in schizophrenia. *Neuroscience* 66: 321-335.
19. Cornblatt, B.A., and Keilp, J.G. (1994). Impaired attention, genetics, and the pathophysiology of schizophrenia. *Schizophrenic Bulletin* 20: 31-46.

RESEARCHING L-DOPA AND INDUCED PSYCHOSIS:
A Recollection

Sidney Merlis

Central Islip State Hospital in Central Islip, New York, was a typically large mental institution in a country-like setting on Long Island when I arrived there in 1951. It housed thousands of chronically ill patients, some of whom had been hospitalized for many years, forgotten, and essentially abandoned. The setting was overcrowded, noisy, and understaffed, with little or no privacy for patients. Large dormitory spaces were the rule, and individuals were more often segregated according to behaviour and convenience than need. Staff members tried heroically in many cases to ease the plight of the patients, despite a daily grind of repetitive and mostly unrewarding therapeutic routines. Central Islip State Hospital was duplicated across New York State, with the number of hospitalized patients numbering in the tens of thousands. In fact, within a thirty-mile radius of Central Islip on Long Island alone, there were more than twenty-five thousand in-patients. This type of facility was to be found in all states across the country.

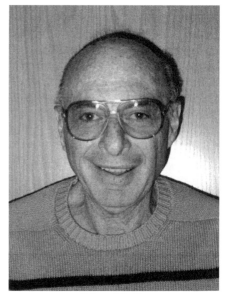

Sidney Merlis

At that time, the treatment choices were limited. There had been no significant innovations in therapy since the Second World War, except for penicillin for our "luetic" patients. Therapy was directed primarily towards controlling behaviour and the avoidance of injuries by patients to themselves or others. Traditional treatments then in use included chloral hydrate, paral-

Sidney Merlis received his medical degree in Nebraska in 1948. As Director of Research at Central Islip State Hospital in New York from the early 1950s through the 1970s, he led the studies of early clinical drug evaluation of psychopharmacological agents He was actively involved in clinical practice, focusing on psychoactive drug therapy in a variety of clinical disorders. He is a Life Fellow of the APA, ACP, and ACNP. His current interests include psychopharmacology and the delivery of health care for psychiatric patients.

Merlis was elected a fellow of the CINP in 1962. He presented a paper on "Polypharmacy: comparative residual symptom profiles" (Merlis, Sheppard and Francchia) at the 7th Congress, and coauthored papers on "The use of biological materials in the treatment of schizophrenia" (O'Neill, Turner and Merlis) and on "Hypnosis and psychotropic drugs, their interaction in mental patients" (Halpern and Merlis), presented at the 1st and 2nd Congresses, respectively.

dehyde (intravenously, intramuscularly, rectally, and orally), insulin coma therapy, cold wet towel packs, electro-shock therapy, and tub baths. The use of physical restraint was routine and frequent.

Remarkable changes began in the early fifties when I obtained chlorpromazine for clinical trials. After initial scepticism, I became enthusiastically involved in its use. The response of patients was remarkable: we saw rapid, meaningful, positive change in a significant number of our hitherto treatment-refractory patients, and improvement persisted as long as the medication was administered. As other phenothiazines became available, further salutary effects were observed.

It was decided at that time that research units would be established at several sites in the state hospitals of New York. Under the direction of Paul Hoch, then commissioner of the Department of Mental Hygiene, and the encouragement of the legendary Henry Brill, assistant commissioner and director of the Division of Research and Medical Services, who was an early exponent of this new chemical treatment, the research plans were put in place. Frank O'Neill, our hospital director, whose background included training in pathology as well as psychiatry, immediately saw the potential benefits. He was instrumental in arranging for the selection of Central Islip as the site of a research unit, and I became director of the new facility. Satisfactory clinical, laboratory, and neurosurgical spaces and all the required equipment were quickly made available on a high-priority basis.

Our mandate was to use a multidisciplinary approach, following those leads we felt to be most promising in order to obtain new knowledge that might benefit our patients. Our focus was to be on phase 2 investigations, including all areas of basic, as well as clinical, studies. Collaboration with academic institutions, the National Institute of Mental Health, and other research units was encouraged and obtained.

Two significant events shaped our course at that time and led to a series of studies on L-dopa and psychosis. The first was a serendipitous finding in our neurosurgical unit. During the course of a procedure on a patient with a psychotic disorder and concomitant severe parkinsonism, the anterior choroidal artery was accidentally severed. This produced an immediate and dramatic cessation of the very pronounced tremor of the patient, and the change persisted after the completion of surgery. Irving Cooper, our chief neurosurgeon, and his surgical team, which was affiliated with New York University and Bellevue Hospital, quickly grasped the significance of this finding and began a series of studies refining and expanding the procedure. With a stereotactic approach and pneumoencephalography as a guide, he was able to demonstrate that chemical ablation of the globus pallidus produced the same effects. These findings met with worldwide interest in the medical community and were used extensively as the treatment of choice in medically unresponsive patients with Parkinson's syndrome. The results were published in great detail in 1956.

The second event was less pleasant. We, along with others, observed that psychotic patients treated with phenothiazines were developing tremor and other symptoms of parkinsonism in varying degrees. In a survey of our population, we found that more than 5 percent of those treated with phenothiazines were affected, despite good clinical response. The question arose whether the neurosurgical findings of Cooper and his associates could in any way help to understand the underlying mechanism of the side effects seen in our phenothiazine treated patients. An alternative possibility was that a biochemical or metabolic anomaly in patients could explain the underlying mechanism of both the psychosis and the side effects of antipsychotic phenothiazine drugs. Our biochemical laboratories were already involved in a variety of research relevant to monoamines and especially to noradrenaline at the time that I decided, in the light of then-current hypotheses of Brodie and Schildkraut, that L-dopa might be useful in providing some of the answers.

By the mid-fifties our research division was involved in a variety of clinical psychophar-macological investigations on the behavioural effects of psychotomimetic agents. We were receiving funding from New York State and pharmaceutical companies, as well as significant seed money from the NIMH, where Jonathan Cole developed a network of early clinical evaluation units (ECDEU), involving multiple sites nationwide, as a means of validating clinical findings in the rapidly growing field of psychopharmacology. The Central Islip Research Division was one of the groups originally selected to participate. I was able to recruit a staff that included many creative investigators, among whom were the innovative Bill Turner, the solid Willie Krumholz, the inquisitive Art Wolpert, Charlie Sheppard, our chief psychol-ogist, Jose Yaryura-Tobias, an enthusiastic, irrepressible personality, and his colleague Bruce Diamond, as well as a host of others.

As we extended our clinical drug evaluations from phase 2 studies into clinical investiga-tions with antidepressant agents, Turner became interested in the long-acting monoamine oxidase inhibitors (MAOIs). His findings in laboratory studies with transmethylation, nicotin-amide, and serotonin in animal models were indicating behavioural changes when L-dopa was used. He hypothesized that L-dopa, being a norepinephrine precursor that enters the central nervous system, could perhaps enhance monoamine oxidase inhibition with possible favour-able clinical effects by protecting the available norepinephrine from intracellular desamin-ation. Turner was able to use pargyline, a long-acting MAOI available from Abbott Labora-tories. He studied a small sample of our patients with pargyline in conjunction with L-dopa. While some improvement was noted, the positive changes were overshadowed by side effects, including delirium, euphoria, and a cluster of amphetamine-like symptoms. He concluded that administering L-dopa together with a long acting MAOI was a potential avenue for further studies, but since the side effects of the combination were hazardous, studies with the combination should be restricted to hospitalized patients, using lower doses. Turner published his results in 1964.

In the years which followed, L-dopa became widely adopted as a therapy for parkinsonism in non-psychiatric patients. It has become obvious that the substance was a suitable tool for provoking psychopathology and for studying some of the biochemical correlates of the induced psychosis. Aware that further studies with L-dopa might increase our understanding of the psychotic process, our group continued its work. Yaryura-Tobias undertook studies using L-dopa as a tool of psychiatric research. He conducted a preliminary investigation of the effects of L-dopa on schizophrenic patients who were maintained on their pre-existing antipsychotic medication. His findings indicated an increase of auditory and visual hallucinations with worsening of paranoid thinking. Yaryura-Tobias therefore urged caution in further studies and postulated that L-dopa might not only worsen symptomatology, but also in some way serve as a precursor of some mental disease.

Animal studies using L-dopa seemed to reinforce some of the clinical observations. High-dose L-dopa administration produced catatonia, biting behaviour, irritability, increased sexual activity, aggressiveness, rage, and stupor. These findings were in keeping with reports in the literature which indicated that high doses of L-dopa used in the treatment parkinsonism in patients with a normal mental status induced mood and thought disorders in a considerable proportion of the patients. The incidence of psychopathologic symptoms was reported to be between 2.5 and 55 percent. The symptoms included delirium, perceptual changes, confusion, lack of judgment, impaired memory, acute anxiety, depression, and insomnia. While psychopathological symptoms were induced, patients neurological status improved.

In a letter to the editor of the *Journal of the American Medical Association* in 1970, Yaryura-Tobias reported that levodopa produced an increase in psychiatric symptoms, including an exacerbation of existing depression and auditory and visual hallucinations. He warned against the loosely supervised use of L-dopa, even in the non-psychotic population, because patients with a seemingly normal mental status had a tendency not to report the drug's psychiatric side effects spontaneously.

Yaryura-Tobias went further with his investigations, and based on findings in a study with a small sample size, he reported on the beneficial effects of L-dopa treatment on the verbal and communication skills of some patients. He postulated that dopamine and noradrenaline, for which L-dopa is a precursor, resembled stimulant drugs in their action. He further stated that L-dopa might be useful in enhancing psychotherapy in non-communicative patients. A reference was made to the possibility that it might also be helpful in autistic children.

We were able to follow up on these observations. The results of our work at Central Islip and the corroboration of our findings by other research teams led to the following conclusions:

1. L-dopa improves the neurological manifestations of parkinsonism, but can cause psychotic disorders similar to those seen in schizophrenia;
2. L-dopa worsens the symptoms of schizophrenic patients who do not display extrapyramidal signs;

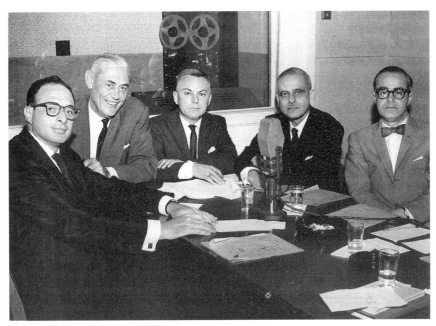

From left: Sidney Merlis, unidentified, Frank J. Ayd, Heinz E. Lehmann
and Fritz Freyhan

3. L-dopa aggravates the neuropsychiatric symptoms of schizophrenic patients with drug-induced Parkinsonism;

4. the effects of L-dopa are in line with the catecholamine hypothesis of schizophrenia;

5. there is some resemblance between the effects of L-dopa and certain psychotomimetic agents, such as mescaline and its derivatives in schizophrenia;

6. continued investigation of L-dopa might lead to further understanding of the genesis of psychotic disorders.

By the end of the sixties, a new picture was emerging in the large psychiatric hospitals. Treatment was becoming more effective; a greater choice of drugs were available; clinical improvement was more frequent; and deinstitutionalization was becoming the mantra of the psychiatric community. The remarkable advances in physiology, chemistry, and metabolism began to create opportunities for understanding the basic science of mental disorder. The early work of the fifties and sixties provided a base for the progress we have witnessed. L-dopa has earned its place in medical history as a research tool and as a treatment. Its use provided a link in a chain of events that was among the most exciting and productive episodes in psychiatric history. As I reviewed the material used in preparing this account, I felt that we were part of a revolutionary change in psychiatry and psychopharmacology – part of the thread of medical history.

OF MAGIC AND MEDICINE
George A. Ulett

When I was fourteen years old, a travelling magician came to our small town in southern Oregon. My friend, the son of the local theatre owner, and I were amazed by the miracles we saw. Later that day we climbed into the rafters above the stage and discovered how the tricks were done. Since then I have searched for the string or mirror behind every medical mystery. Now, sixty-four years later, I am learning the wisdom of such an approach.

I originally planned to become a psychologist (BA, Stanford, 1940). But then, at the University of Oregon School of Medicine (MS, 1942; PhD, 1944), I became interested in the neurosciences, and with my mentor, Professor Robert Dow, I set up the first EEG laboratory in the state of Oregon. After getting my MD (1944), I decided to become a neurosurgeon and took a residency at the Harvard Neurological Unit in the Boston City Hospital. The war was over (1946), and the army received me, along with other medical replacements. Colonel Corliss lined up his green recruits

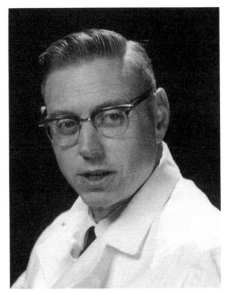

George A. Ulett

and said to the man next to me, "What training have you had?" The answer: "Nine months in surgery." "Fine," said the colonel, "You're head of surgery." I shuddered, was asked the same question, and answered, "Nine months of neurology." Said the colonel, "You are now chief of psychiatry!" And with that statement he changed my career. After a psychiatric residency with Professor Edwin Gildea at Washington University in St. Louis, I became director of psychiatry for the city of St. Louis, including the directorship of the acute psychiatric admitting centre, Malcolm Bliss Hospital. Together with John Stern (who later became chairman of the Department of Psychology at Washington University) and others, we established research

George A. Ulett was director of psychiatry for the city of St. Louis. There, with John Stern and others, he established research laboratories and from 1951 to 1961 published over seventy-five papers. In 1962 he became director of the State Department of Mental Health and created the Missouri Institute of Psychiatry, which became the Department of Psychiatry at the University of Missouri School of Medicine.

George A. Ulett was a fellow of the CINP in the 1960s. He presented papers on "Objective measures in psychopharmacology (methodology)" (Ulett, Heusler, and Callahan) and on "A clinical and EEG study of withdrawal syndromes in schizophrenic patients" (Ulett, Holden, Itil, and Keskiner) at the 2nd and 6th Congresses, respectively.

313

laboratories and from 1951 to 1961 published over seventy-five papers, including comparative evaluations of the new psychopharmacological agents which were just becoming available. Early studies with chlorpromazine gained me an invitation to present our work at a congress held in Nuremberg, Germany. I was to be the only speaker from the United States. The others were all German. My knowledge of the language was sparse, but a good friend, Austrian psychiatrist Leopold Hofstatter (who incidently did prefrontal lobotomies at the State Hospital), taught me to deliver my paper in perfect German with an Austrian accent. Afterwards I was asked questions in German. Not understanding a word that was said, I stood there with my mouth open like a *Dummkopf.*

In the Malcolm Bliss Hospital laboratories we did studies using electroencephalography with photic stimulation to study anxiety-proneness. We also introduced "photo-shock" in which, after sensitizing the patients with Azozol, we could produce either generalized or partial seizures at will by varying the parameters of flickering light. We compared this procedure with standard ECT and found the therapeutic effect to be the same, thus demonstrating that it was the generalized convulsion that healed depression. As our interest in the phenothiazines progressed, I developed a pocket drug dial showing the chemical structure of the newer phenothiazines that were being developed. In my job as director of psychiatry for St. Louis, I was proud that I had been able to accomplish the racial integration of psychiatric patients in the St. Louis City and State Hospitals.

In 1962 I became director of the State Department of Mental Health and created the Missouri Institute of Psychiatry. This was housed in a new multi-million-dollar building with lecture rooms, laboratories, and two hundred beds for psychiatric investigative studies. With the help of Dean Vernon Wilson of the University of Missouri (Columbia) School of Medicine, we became a separate Department of Psychiatry. I was chairman, Max Fink was our first medical and research director, and Amadeo Marazzi and Turan Itil joined us as research professors. Between 1962 and 1972 we published a total of 392 papers, with clinical emphasis on use of the new pharmacological agents.

Studies with Anton Heusler and others involved a comparison of clinical observations of EEG activity during the administration of various psycholeptic agents. These observations were made on long-term psychotic patients who had been refractory to any treatment. Our goal was to select the best agent for long-term therapy. We installed a photoelectric grid on the ward to measure changes in total activity of the group, sound-level meters to record changes in their verbal ability and special devices to measure sleep interruptions at night. We reported that EEG changes after withdrawal of each drug were long-lasting and that initial resting EEGs could be predictive of responsiveness to treatment by different drugs.

Turan Itil developed his method of using the computerized EEG for predicting the clinical actions of newly developed psychoactive drugs. He established a laboratory in Istanbul, Turkey, where many patients had never had any drug treatment. He invited us all to Istanbul for a conference on psychopharmacology. Our host was Necmetin Polvan, professor of neuropsychiatry at the local medical school. He invited us for a yachting trip on the Sea of Marmora, and I still have a vivid memory of Jonathan Cole diving from the top deck into the blue waters of the Bosporus. Our group had been doing work on hypnosis, a long-time interest of mine. From our EEG findings we suggested a neurobiological basis for the hypnotic state. While lecturing on the subject in Turkey, I was presented with a patient who had a hysterical hemiplegia. I was about to ameliorate her symptom with hypnosis when I found that she could not understand English and I could speak no Turkish. It was a first for me when I hypnotized her with the help of an interpreter.

As an early member of the US National Institutes of Health (NIH) study section on psychopharmacology, I recall active discussions between Leo Hollister, Henry Brill, Jonathan Cole, Heinz Lehmann, Burt Schiele, Gerald Klerman, and others. These were exciting days for the new science of neuropsychopharmacology. Psychopharmacology was a feature at all national meetings, and there I enjoyed the company of good friends such as Charlie Shagass and Doug Goldman. Doug told me about his "purple people," who had developed photosensitivity after long use of chlorpromazine. With Gerald Sarwer-Foner, he founded a new society, but they could not agree upon a name, and so it became known as GWAN, the "Group-Without-A-Name."

In the late 1960s I had been invited to Japan by a fine Japanese physician, Kodo Senshu, who was involved in translating textbooks from English into Japanese. He translated into Japanese my small psychiatric textbook, *A Synopsis of Contemporary Psychiatry*, and also my *Rorschach Introductory Manual*. These became the only two books I have written that I cannot read.

Senshu introduced me to acupuncture, which was not then known in the United States. He presented me with a book on the subject and a handful of needles. This got me started on what he said was a useful technique to employ when Western medicine failed. I had just begun the private practice of psychiatry and psychosomatic medicine, and I tried acupuncture on a few patients with some success. In 1972, after President Richard Nixon returned from China, "acupuncture" became a household word in the United States. Although I found that it was a helpful treatment, I was very sceptical of the metaphysical explanations and magical rituals that accompanied the practice. Again I searched for the "strings and mirrors," the physiological explanation of how acupuncture worked. After several trips to the East and to Scandinavia, I finally found physiological answers for this centuries-old Chinese folk medicine.

In 1972 our group at the University of Missouri received the first NIH grant to compare acupuncture and hypnosis for the relief of experimental pain. We demonstrated that acupuncture was not a psychological or hypnotic phenomenon and that, when electricity was added to needles placed in motor points, the modulation of pain was greatly improved. The ritual placement of needles in the ear was being promoted in the United States as a treatment for addiction. In Hong Kong I visited Dr. Wen, the neurosurgeon who first described the use of ear acupuncture for treating heroin addicts. I then found out that it was electrical stimulation, not the needle, that was the key to success. Apparently electricity stimulated the vagus innervation in the concha of the ear, thus ameliorating the sympathetic arousal produced by withdrawal from addicting drugs. It became clear to me that electrical stimulation was the crucial factor in acupuncture, and in 1982 I published *The Principles and Practice of Physiologic Acupuncture*.

In China I met Professor Ji Sheng Han, of Beijing Medical University, who had spent twenty-five years studying acupuncture. His findings were described in detail in his 1987 book, *The Neurochemical Basis of Pain Control by Acupuncture*. From my visits to his lab it became clear that what acupuncture is all about is getting electrical stimulation into the central nervous system. By serial studies of spinal fluid in humans after the administration of specific frequencies by his HANS stimulator, it was shown that different frequencies evoked the gene expression of different neurohormones. Han also showed that needles were no longer necessary: electrical stimulation through polymer conducting pads was sufficient. With this information and observations from my own experience, in 1992 I published *Beyond Yin and Yang: How Acupuncture Really Works.* In my practice I found the procedure useful for pain and a variety of psychosomatic and psychiatric problems. Combining acupuncture with my long-time interest in Pavlovian conditioning – while using imagery as the conditioning stimulus – I developed the technique of "conditioned healing with electroacupuncture," which I use daily in my practice.

I was unable to get NIH support to demonstrate my belief that electrical stimulation of body motor points for addiction was more effective than the ritual placement of unstimulated ear needles. So I collaborated with John Nichols, a friend in Australia, who ran a methadone clinic. His success rate was great, and in Australia we published *The Endorphin Connection,* a manual that is now used by the Australian VA for instruction in the use of the HANS stimulator, not only for the treatment of addiction but also for patients with post-traumatic stress disorder (PTSD).

As hypnosis and acupuncture come under the heading of "alternative medicine," my interest turned in that direction. Here I found there was much belief in magical methods that lacked scientific validity. Acupuncture was a major treatment used by holistic healers; however, the kind practised was often the mystical "meridian-theory acupuncture," which I had abandoned. The New Age cultic healers promoted many types of "mind/body medicine," touting them as imports from the East. I found better explanations in the Western concepts of "psycho/somatic medicine," as taught in our psychiatric residency training. Cannon's *Wisdom of the Body* and Jacobsen's *You Can Relax* gave better answers. The knowledge that most illnesses are self-healing, and that the placebo response adds immeasurably to the success rate of all therapies explains the "cures" of many holistic healers. When surveys showed that over one-third of all patients were turning to alternative medicine for "miracle healings," I decided that it was time to again look for the "strings and mirrors." I began to teach medical students to distinguish between the wheat and the chaff of alternative practices. From my course notes I wrote the book *Alternative Medicine or Magical Healing.* This has become the basis for my current teaching of physicians and allied health-care personnel. I am still practising psycho-somatic medicine and psychiatry in my private office using such basic treatments of alternative medicine as the new scientific no-needle acupuncture, hypnosis, and herbalism.

Thus the wheel has turned, and instead of studying FDA-approved psychoactive medications, my focus has turned towards unregulated herbal preparations and the ancient practices of medieval herbalists and turn-of-the-century travelling patent-medicine-show magicians. The search for "strings and mirrors" involves so-called natural, but potentially toxic, food alternatives that are not regularly monitored by the Food and Drug Administration.

WATCHING FOUR DECADES OF PSYCHOPHARMACOLOGY

Seymour Fisher

Some people believe that they control their own destiny. They are wrong! If we think about it, we will probably realize that most of the critical events in our lives have been strongly determined by chance. In my case, I simply happened to be in the right place at the right time.

My college education was interrupted in 1944 when I served two years in the U.S. armed forces. After I completed my bachelor's degree at New York University in May 1948, I was about to start looking for a job – *any* job – when by chance a friend mentioned that the U.S. Veterans Administration had just initiated a university-associated training program in clinical psychology leading to an advanced degree which provided a stipend during the training period. Having never taken a psychology course during my undergraduate years, I was not surprised when I was summarily rejected by three of the four programs to which I applied. However, James W. Layman, director of the program at the University of North Carolina,

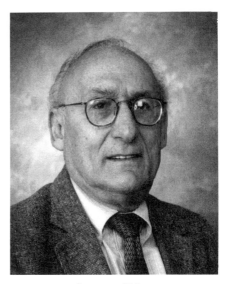

Seymour Fisher

took a huge chance on me and offered me a conditional acceptance if I received good grades in three psychology courses to be taken that summer. In September I moved to Chapel Hill,

Seymour Fisher completed studies at the Washington School of Psychiatry in 1955, then held a post as clinical psychologist at Walter Reed Army Institute of Research until 1958. Between 1958 and 1960 he was at the National Institute of Mental Health in Bethesda, Maryland. He went on to the Psychopharmacology Research Branch until 1963. Next, he served as professor of psychiatry (psychology) at the Boston University School of Medicine, from 1963 to 1978. There he was also director of research training and director of the Psychopharmacology Laboratory, Division of Psychiatry. From 1978 until the present, he has been professor and director of the Center for Medication Monitoring, Department of Psychiatry and Behavioral Sciences, University of Texas Medical Branch in Galveston, Texas.

Fisher was elected a fellow of the CINP in 1966. He presented papers on "Drug-set interaction: the effect of expectations on drug response in outpatients" (Fisher, Cole, Rickels and Uhlenhuth), on "The placebo reaction: thesis, antithesis, synthesis and hypothesis," and on "Hard-core anxiety in dental patients: implications for drug screening" (Fisher, Pillard and Yamada) at the 3rd, 5th and 6th Congresses, respectively; and coauthored a paper on "Comparability, acquiescence, and drug effects" (McNair, Kahn, Droppleman and Fisher), presented at the 5th Congress.

and four years later, in August 1952, I received my PhD after completing a dissertation on posthypnotic suggestion (1, 2). It was at Chapel Hill that Irvin S. Wolf taught me to think critically (as Ernest Hemingway phrased it: "The most essential gift [for a thinking person] is a built-in, shock-proof shit detector").

My first job was as a research psychologist at the Walter Reed Army Institute of Research in Washington, DC, where I extended my work on hypnosis, social influence, and psycho-therapy. (I had also been considered for an instructor's position at the University of Indiana, which would certainly have taken me in a different direction; by chance, however, I was not offered that position.) By the mid-1950s, reports were emerging about a number of new drugs that appeared to have dramatic therapeutic effects upon psychiatric patients who, for the most part, had previously been intractable to available treatments. Alas, my initial skepticism (paraphrasing William Osler, "use them fast, while they still work") was supported by all the research psychiatrists at Walter Reed – mainly psychoanalytically oriented – who dismissed the reports as "placebo effects."

I was most happy in that setting until, by chance, I received a letter in 1957 from Jonathan O. Cole of the National Institute of Mental Health (NIMH) informing me about a position (and a higher salary) in the newly-formed Psychopharmacology Service Center (PSC). Although I told Cole that I knew absolutely nothing about any drugs whatsoever, he offered me the position anyway. Working at the PSC I witnessed a revolution in psychiatric treatment as psychopharmacology became part of psychiatry and some psychiatrists came to be known as "psychopharmacologists." Best of all, I met – by chance – my future wife, Carmen. At the NIMH, Cole taught me many things about research administration.

Between 1958 and 1963 the PSC team at the NIMH attempted to advance knowledge in psychopharmacology primarily in three ways: by helping to improve the methodology of clinical trials, by stimulating and supporting research by U.S. and foreign academicians, and by conducting collaborative projects involving PSC staff. During my tenure the PSC was renamed the Psychopharmacology Research Branch. In 1958, when it became clear that child and adolescent disorders were being ignored, I organized the first national conference on psychopharmacology in children (3). As chief of the special studies unit, I also participated in various research projects on the influence of set, expectations, and milieu on the effects of drugs. By 1961 clinical studies of pharmacological intervention were being supplemented by neurobiological probes into questions of mechanism, and that led to the expanded label "neuro-psychopharmacologist."

In 1963, again by chance, I was offered a professorship at Boston University School of Medicine. Over the next fifteen years I headed a two-year research training program for advanced psychiatric residents and also served as director of the Psychopharmacology Labo-ratory, where Douglas McNair, Richard Kahn, Richard Pillard, James E. Barrett, and I conducted basic and clinical research on diagnosis and the effects of the new drugs of those years, including marijuana. In 1972, as program committee chairman of the American Psychopathological Association (APPA), I edited an issue of *Seminars in Psychiatry* entitled "Scientific Models and Psychopathology." It comprised papers presented by a group of distinguished speakers ranging from A (Nobel laureate Julius Axelrod) to Z (Joseph Zubin). The following year I also published papers from the program of the APPA's annual meeting (4).

Leadership in the Department of Psychiatry at Boston University was in upheaval in 1978, and I decided that it was time to leave. Robert Rose asked me to join him in developing the

Department of Psychiatry and Behavioral Sciences at the University of Texas Medical Branch in Galveston (UTMB), where he was to assume the chairmanship. Working with Bob Rose during his years at UTMB was a great pleasure which I shall always fondly remember. And at UTMB where I have remained, I currently serve as professor and director of the Center for Medication Monitoring. Over the years my research interests moved from investigating placebo effects, conducting clinical trials, and evaluating methods for the dissemination of drug information, into the area of pharmacoepidemiology and adverse drug effects. My additional academic responsibilities have involved sitting on various committees, leading resident seminars in research methodology, and writing papers whenever I think that I have a story worth telling. (It is not generally recognized that the reason academic politics are often so dirty is that the stakes are so low.)

In 1984 I was elected president of the American College of Neuropsychopharmacology, where I set up the first on-line access to all the abstracts of the college's meetings prior to the annual meeting. Although this toll-free service was used nationally that year, it was an idea before its time and could not be continued. The program from the meeting under my presidency was subsequently published (5). In 1988 I spent a sabbatical as visiting professor at both the Harvard Medical School (McLean Hospital) with Jon Cole and Boston University with Doug McNair. In 1995 I published a summary of an innovative method of using patient self-monitoring in postmarketing drug surveillance, developed over a ten-year period in collaboration with Stephen G. Bryant and Thomas A. Kent (6).

As I review these events, I can only conclude that the past four decades of psychopharmacology will probably best be remembered for their impact on the treatment of psychiatric patients. But I would like to suggest that, more importantly, psychopharmacology was the quintessential force which finally gave psychiatry a modicum of respectability in the halls of academic medicine. That came about in three major ways: along with their medical colleagues, psychiatrists now had developed their own empirically based pharmacopeia; psychologists and statisticians helped psychiatrists to realize that valid experimental designs and relatively well-defined behavioural assessment scales were necessary to evaluate the efficacy of new psychotropic compounds; and perhaps of greatest consequence, psychiatry was finally positioned to achieve the status of a clinical science, that is, to test a wide variety of clinical hypotheses and reject those opinions, beliefs, and hopes that could not be empirically supported. Whereas psychiatry had previously been infamous for clinging to the untested assertions of renowned authority figures, psychopharmacology soon brought about changes in clinical practice that reflected the outcome of rigorously controlled clinical trials; poor drugs were discarded for better ones. (Does anyone remember captodiame, or Suvren, from the late 1950s? – try spelling it backwards.) The evolution of this new academic attitude across much of contemporary psychiatry has been an auspicious development over the past forty years. But unfortunately, in some quarters there still exists the specious argument, "Since no one has been able to prove satisfactorily that what I am doing is *not* the best treatment for my patients, I will continue doing what I am doing." Psychiatry has a way to go before it completely replaces the image of the medicine man with that of the medical specialist.

The Collegium Internationale Neuro-Psychopharmacologicum should take great pride in its substantial contribution to the dramatic worldwide growth of the neurosciences and the incredible recent increase in new knowledge about brain-behaviour relationships made possible by experimental pharmacologic manipulations in vitro, in animals, and in man. Now, in 1998, research in neuropsychopharmacology and mind-brain-drug relationships intensifies, and new psychotropic agents appear on the market almost every year. "Psychopharmacology" has become so intrinsic to psychiatry that virtually all psychiatrists feel a need to be knowledgeable in psychopharmacology – so much, in fact, that one can safely and happily say that "psychopharmacology" as a distinctive clinical label is fast becoming obsolete.

After World War II most major medical schools in the United States had a single Department of Neuropsychiatry or Psychiatry & Neurology, later replaced by separate departments for each specialty. Don't be surprised if by the year 2013, turf wars notwithstanding, we see a trend for the return of combined departments (perhaps something like a "Department of Clinical and Basic Neuropsychiatry"?), reflecting the strong interdependence between brain and behaviour.

As we learn more about normal behaviour and its dependence upon neurobiologic functioning, we'll surely arrive at a better understanding of one of our great public health problems: the treatment of psychiatric disorders. On the darker side, there will also be forces operating to develop new drugs that can modify a wide range of behaviours only remotely related to genuine psychiatric disorders – with enormous potential for misuse. I can only hope that in the coming years the major emphasis on drug development will continue to be therapeutically oriented.

REFERENCES
1. Fisher, S. (1954). The role of expectancy in the performance of posthypnotic behavior. *Journal of Abnormal and Social Psychology,* 49: 503-507.
2. Fisher, S. (1955). An investigation of alleged conditioning phenomena under hypnosis. *Journal of Clinical and Experimental Hypnosis,* 3: 71-103.
3. Fisher, S. (ed.) (1959). *Child Research in Psychopharmacology.* Springfield, Ill.: Charles C. Thomas.
4. Fisher, S., and Freedman, A.M. (eds.) (1973). *Opiate Addiction: Origins and Treatment.* New York: Halsted Press.
5. Fisher, S., Raskin, A., and Uhlenhuth, E.H. (eds.) (1987). *Cocaine: Clinical and Biobehavioral Aspects.* New York: Oxford University Press.
6. Fisher, S. (1995). Patient self-monitoring: a challenging approach to pharmacoepidemiology. *Pharmacoepidemiology and Drug Safety,* 4: 359-378.

Memoirs from the Union of Soviet Socialist Republics

THE THREE FOUNDATION STONES OF THE LABORATORY OF PSYCHOPHARMACOLOGY

Izyaslav (Slava) Lapin

In October 1960 the city radio in Leningrad announced that the Bekhterev Psychoneurological Institute was opening a new laboratory – a psychopharmacology laboratory – and inviting applications for the position of scientific chief. I missed that announcement, but parents of a friend of mine brought it to my attention and encouraged me to apply. I was thirty years old at the time and a part-time assistant professor in the Department of Pharmacology at the Institute of Pediatrics, without any real prospect for a better position. Still, my first inclination was not to follow up the announcement. I felt that "psycho"-pharmacology, streamlined for political considerations to promulgate Pavlovian classical conditioning, was not something I would like to do. In the early 1950s, Pavlovian theory was proclaimed to be "the only progressive and appropriate approach for Soviet science" and subsequently the teaching of any alternative approaches was discouraged with the Freudian psychoanalytic and other psychodynamic approaches even prohibited. In 1960 every discipline in the Soviet Union which

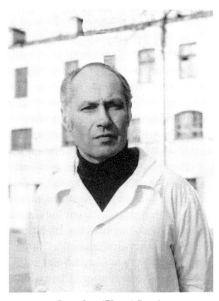

Izyaslav (Slava) Lapin

dealt with the "psyche" or was qualified by the prefix of "psycho," even clinical psychiatry, was squeezed into a Pavlovian politically motivated framework.

In spite of my feelings about the "position," I was persuaded by my friends to make a rational decision. So the next day I called the office of Dr. Boris Lebedev, the scientific director of the Institute, and got an appointment to meet him for the following week.

I went to see Lebedev without sending him in advance any information on my background or references. Although we virtually knew nothing of each other, he greeted me with a bright smile in an informal way. He seemed to be a nice person, just a few years my senior, about thirty-five to forty years old. It was easy talking to him and by the time we parted it was not

Izyaslav Petrovich Lapin has been chief of the Laboratory of Psychopharmacology at Bekhterev Psychoneurological Research Institute, St. Petersburg, since 1960. He has been Invited Consultant at hospitals in Leningrad, Moscow and Riga, and has lectured at the Pediatric Medical Institute, Leningrad, and the Medical Faculty of the University of Tartu in Estonia (1964-1988).

Lapin was elected a fellow of the CINP in 1994.

only he who knew that I was a specialist in internal medicine and pharmacology, but also I learnt that he was a psychiatrist.

During the interview I had the opportunity to clarify all the different issues I was concerned about, and from his answer to my first question I understood that the reason for deciding to open a psychopharmacology laboratory at the Institute was simply the feeling that, in 1960, a psychoneurological research institute like the Bekhterev was incomplete without such a laboratory. Similarly, from his answers to my other questions I felt relieved that it was certainly not his intention to set up a laboratory for the promulgation of Pavlovian theory and that I would be free to decide about the program of the laboratory. What he actually said was: "Everything will be up to you. Feel absolutely free. I do hope that you will soon orient yourself and find out which are the most promising areas of research in psychopharmacology."

"Feel absolutely free" sounded unbelievable for anyone in the Soviet Union in those years and especially for a young researcher. It was certainly sufficient for me to apply for the position.

At the end of the interview, I mentioned to him the names of some of my fellow pharmacologists as possible candidates for the "research staff" of the laboratory and Lebedev had no objection to any of my suggestions. I feel that I should add here that Lebedev remained supportive of our laboratory even after he became the director of the Bekhterev Institute in 1961, and even later on while an officer between 1964 and 1970 in the Mental Health Unit of the World Health Organization in Geneva. After his return from Geneva, Lebedev was appointed head of the department of psychiatry at the First Medical Institute of St. Petersburg. He stayed in that position until his untimely death in 1992.

Our psychopharmacology laboratory was opened on the 15th of November in 1960 with three researchers (including me), three laboratory assistants, and two technicians. It was the first psychopharmacology laboratory in the Soviet Union, as far as I know. My first research collaborators were Rebecca Khaunina and Eugene Schelkunov. (The three of us, later on, were referred to as the "old guard.)" Within a couple of years, Yuri Nuller, a psychiatrist, Irina Prakhie, a veterinarian, Maya Samsonova, a neurophysiologist, and Gregory Oxenkrug, an endocrinologist, joined our research team.

Initially, we had two large rooms on the third floor of the building with our animal quarters on the first. Within two years however, we practically took over the building with eight rooms on the second floor designated for pharmacological screening and behavioural pharmacology, and four rooms on the third floor for biochemistry. The budget of the Ministry of Health from the Russian Federation, to which our institute belonged, was extremely small. There was just no hope of funds for ordering supplies from abroad. Medicine and especially experimental medicine had a very low, if not the lowest priority in the Soviet Union. We were truly "self-made researchers."

From the very beginning and for about three decades, members of our team were *personae non gratae* in so far as the authorities were concerned. The reasons: we had no communist member in our laboratory, most of us were Jews (defying the antisemitic policy of the Soviet State by inviting suitable candidates to join the laboratory on "merit" exclusively), and we were young (with the mean age of the group below thirty). But we were a highly creative and hard-working group: familiar with the most recent developments in the field, fluent in English and some other foreign languages, and in regular correspondance about scientific matters with colleagues in other countries. This would have been "normal" for most countries, but not for Russia at the time. In the era of the Cold War and the Iron Curtain, our Western-oriented team provoked suspicion and envy, and as a result all of our foreign travel requests, regardless whether business or pleasure, were blocked by the "party bosses."

In this situation, any support we could get from colleagues and friends in other countries was of great importance. Fortunately we had many generous friends. Included among them were Bernard Brodie of the National Institutes of Health (NIH) in Bethesda, Maryland, who supplied us with chemicals, books, and reprints, and Daniel Bovet of the Istituto Superiore di Sanità in Rome, a Nobel laureate in medicine, who had updated us regularly about scientific meetings on psychopharmacology. He spent several days during his visit in our laboratory getting a grasp of not only what we were doing, but also how we were doing it. He also encouraged us to record our experiments on tapes and send the tapes to him for feedback. I learned from his feedback that he was especially impressed with our experiments in amphetamine-group toxicity and apomorphine aggression, pharmacological tests developed in our laboratory.

Both Brodie and Bovet invited us to spend some time in their laboratories. Brodie's formal invitation to become a visiting scientist at the NIH for a year was sent to me in 1964. It was one of the many invitations which had to be set aside for about twenty-five years. It was in 1990, almost two decades after Brodie passed away, that during the time of the "perestroika" I was finally allowed to visit and work at the NIH, invited by Irwin Kopin.

All through the years, from the very beginning, I operated the laboratory as a closely-knit team with a high spirit and an atmosphere which encouraged discussion. In our frequently held "round table laboratory conferences" we reviewed our findings, entertained possibilities for our prospective research and, as much as we could, decided about matters relevant to our work.

THE GABA STORY

Shortly after opening our laboratory we came to the conclusion that we needed to concentrate our research efforts on endogenous neuroactive metabolites which might be of interest in terms of developing new psychotropic drugs. At the time this decison was reached, our research group was greatly impressed by the inhibitory function of gamma-aminobutyric acid (GABA) in the central nervous system (CNS). In view of this, GABA seemed to be a rational choice for our research focus. An attractive feature of GABA was that it had only a little prior exposure to neuropharmacological research. In fact, there were only a few publications by Japanese and Italian authors on the mild anticonvulsant effects of two GABA-related drugs, i.e.,Gammalon (GABA) and Gamibetal (beta-hydroxy-GABA or GABA-OH).

When everything was ready to begin, however, an unexpected obstacle emerged. Reviewing the available information we learned that neither GABA, nor GABA-OH passed the blood-brain barrier. It seemed implausible, but not impossible that their therapeutic action (which we could not replicate) was due to some peripheral effects.

To be able to proceed with our plans we had to find a way to improve the penetration of GABA into the brain. One simple way that occurred to me was to increase the lipid solubility of the molecule, but for increasing lipid solubility phenyl derivatives of GABA were necessary, which we did not have and did know how to get. By a rather fortunate coincidence, just about that time Theodore Khvilivitsky, one of the professors of psychiatry at our institute, called me to ask a favour for one of his friends, a chemist, who was interested "in synthesizing something with psychotropic properties." So I met with Vsevolod Perekalin, the chemist, who was head of the Department of Organic Chemistry at the Institute of Pedagogics and whose department, by another miraculous coincidence, was engaged in the synthesis of GABA derivatives. Perekalin asked me which position of the phenyl ring is of primary interest to me, and by mobilizing all my modest knowledge about structure-activity relationships, I chose ß-phenyl-GABA as the substance with the phenyl ring "in the most suitable position" for our research. The substance I chose was called Phenigama, but was to become known as Phenibut after the Federal Commission of Nomenclature changed its name.

After the completion of the initial preclinical animal pharmacological studies (carried out by Rebecca Khaunina, Irina Prakhie, and myself) on mice, rats, rabbits, and cats, Phenibut was shown to pass the blood-brain barrier by Khaunina and Maslova. But findings in further pharmacological studies revealed that Phenibut did not alter either the concentration of GABA in the various brain regions or the activity of the enzymes involved in GABA metabolism, so it was suggested that it is a GABA-mimetic substance.

The pharmacological profile of Phenibut was found to be similar to that of meprobamate and diazepam; and its acute and chronic toxicity, as expected from a close relative of a natural amino acid, very low (LD50 in mice at 900 mg/kg), many times lower than for other psychotropic drugs. Contrary to expectations, however, Phenibut had no anticonvulsant properties, indicating that its activity could not be fully explained by the activities of GABA. It was only about twenty years later with the availability of receptor-binding technology that it was revealed that unlike GABA, which affects both the GABA-A and the GABA-B receptors, Phenibut and its p-chloro-phenyl derivative, baclophen, affect only the GABA-B receptor.

In clinical trials conducted under the direction of Professor Khvilivitsky, Phenibut was found to be an anxiolytic drug with hypnotic and antimanic effects. By 1964 the first publication on Phenibut was in print and in the same year our review (Lapin and Khaunina) of the drug was included in a monograph entitled *The Role of GABA in the Nervous System*, published by the Leningrad University Press.

Between 1964 and 1974 there were twenty-two articles published on Phenibut (including the reports of R. Khaunina and his associates on drug interactions and on the effects on endocrine functions), and by the end of the 1980s there were about three hundred articles on the drug in print. Since almost all of them were published in Russian, Phenibut remained unknown abroad.

To publish scientific papers in international journals was a highly complicated and time-consuming affair. The manuscript had to pass numerous commissions, and to submit the paper required approval by the Ministry of Health. This was particularly true for new drugs with a marketing potential. Without patent protection the use of Phenibut remained restricted to the USSR. Since the end of the 1960s it has been manufactured at the Chemical Factory in Olaine, Latvia, at the time one of the republics of the Soviet Union.

There are several true stories of Phenibut. One of them involves the visit of A. Keberle, the Swiss chemist, who synthesized baclophen (Cl-Phenibut) in the early 1970s. The visit took place at a time when he had already seen the pharmacological profile of his drug at home. Keberle was indeed surprised when Rebecca Khaunina showed him the protocols of her experiments from the early sixties with the pharmacological profile of CI-Phenibut (Baclofen) the substance he synthesized about ten years later.

Another true story of Phenibut involves the Apollo-Sojuz space flight in 1975. Apparently, as we learned from the Russian magazine *Ogoniek* (Spark), something went wrong with the

Sojuz capsule shortly before it was to join Apollo. Two days of repairs were in vain and the astronauts, completely exhausted after sleepless nights from the emotional and physical strain, were sending desperate messages to earth that it would not be possible to accomplish the link. Instead of approval for cancelling the mission, however, the astronauts were instructed by the flight center to take Phenibut, the drug they had been using in the course of their training. Complying with the command, waking refreshed after a restful sleep, the astronouts found and corrected the defect. Sojuz was ready to meet Apollo, as in a fairy tale with a happy end.

After the late 1960s, several research groups in the USSR collaborated with us on the further development of Phenibut. Included among them was the Department of Pharmacology at the Volgograd Medical Institute under the direction of Professor G. Kovalev. They studied the vascular effects of Phenibut and other GABA derivatives and gave an account of their findings in a monograph published in Volgograd in 1974.

In terms of psychopharmacology and pharmacopsychiatry however, the most valuable contributions to the knowledge base of Phenibut were made in the Department of Pharmacology at Tartu University in Estonia under the direction of Professor L. Allikments. Their intensive highly original research ranged from studies of Phenibut's receptor profile (GABA-A, GABA-B, benzodiazepine and dopamine receptors), through clinical trials conducted on Phenibut's nootropic (cognition-enhancing) effects, to studies designed for the delineation of its clinical profile (in neurotic and psychotic patients). The clinical profile of Phenibut was delineated in placebo-controlled studies and its nootropic effects were established in a placebo- and standard-controlled clinical trial with piracetam (Nootropil). The Tartu group published a monograph on their findings in 1990, in Russian (L. Allikmets, L. Mehilane, L. Rago, V. Vasar and A. Zarkovsky). They also published several papers on Phenibut between 1982 and 1990 in international journals in English.

Today, Phenibut is still widely used in Russia, for relieving chronic emotional stress and for the treatment of asthenic depression. It is also prescribed for post-traumatic patients, in children with stuttering, and for the control of the alcohol-withdrawal syndrome.

THE SEROTONIN STORY

Chronologically, serotonin was our second "hero" – not the substance in general, but serotonin in relation to the mechanism of action of antidepressants, tricyclics and monoamine oxidase inhibitors (MAOIs). It was just about the time our laboratory was opened that the Bekhterev Institute received a supply of imipramine (Tofranil) for clinical trials from the Geigy company in Basel. The psychiatrists of the Institute and our group alike were eager to get information about the mechanism of its antidepressant effect, but at the time there were only two or three publications about the pharmacology of imipramine. Moreover, the pharmacology of antidepressants generally was unknown territory on the map of psychopharmacology. This completely new area of research looked extremely tempting for us newcomers in psychopharmacology. We had an absolutely free hand in designing our research. There were no authorities in the field. There were no traditions.

We started from scratch and as a first step Schelkunov, Khaunina, Samsonova, and myself developed a battery for the screening of potential antidepressants. It included new pharmacological tests, such as apomorphine hypothermia in mice and pecking in pigeons, apomorphine agression and amphetamine stereotypy in rats; and biochemical assays for measuring brain monoamine oxidase levels and activity. Since two powerful groups of organic chemists agreed to supply us with bi-and tricyclic acyclic derivatives of iminodibenzyl and pheno-thiazine, we were ready to embark on screening to search for new drugs, using imipramine as the standard. We published our first review on the pharmacology of imipramine in 1964 in *Therapie,* a French journal, in appreciation of Professor Pierre Simon and his wife, Olga, who were the first to introduce our work in Western Europe. Four years later, in 1968, we also published the results of seven years of systematic research in screening for antidepressants in the *Proceedings of the Bekhterev Institute* (Leningrad) under the title Experimental Studies on Antidepressants, but this time in Russian. The most striking feature of our report was that, instead of opening up new avenues, as is customary in such reports, we were closing down some of the old ones. We focused attention on the fact that many screening tests, considered to be predictive, such as reserpine antagonism and amphetamine potentiation, are non-specific: by confounding sympathomimetic action with antidepressant properties they show only the "adrenopositive" component of the pharmacological activity of antidepressants. The component in the action of antidepressants we referred to as "adrenopositive" was not a determinant of the drugs' mood-elevating effect, but of the "motor-stimulating" action of antidepressants and related drugs. Amphetamine, cocaine, anticholinergics, and quaternary derivatives of antidepressants (which do not pass the blood-brain barrier) are all active on these tests without mood elevating effect in depressed patients. Our findings led to the nagging question that, if not the catecholamines, which of the other cerebral monoamines could be of importance in the mood-elevating effect of antidepressants.

On the basis of our own findings and information in the literature, we assumed that the cerebral monoamine responsible for the mood-elevating effect of antidepressants was seroto-nin (5-HT). Hence, we decided to set up a biochemical laboratory under the direction of Gregory Oxenkrug with the capability of measuring the following: 5-HT in human blood platelets and brain tissue; the uptake of 5-HT in the blood platelets of depressed, manic, and alcoholic patients; and the inhibition of the uptake of 5-HT by antidepressants and hormones. We decided to use the frog in our preclinical pharmacologic research, because in the frog 5-HT is the dominant monoamine in the brain with catecholamines present only in traces. The frog allowed us to observe the effect of drugs on 5-HT-ergic processes exclusively and to screen for "pure" 5-HT selective drugs. In the frog (in contrast to all other species) antidepressants potentiate the sedative effect of reserpine and 5-hydroxytryptophane (5-HTP) (with a linear relationship between the increase in sedation and the increase in the 5-HT concentration in the frog brain). Therefore, the frog provides a means for comparing selective serotonin reuptake inhibitors (SSRIs). Our systematic studies, in collaboration with Gregory Oxenkrug, led to the formulation of the hypothesis on the role of 5-HT in the antidepressant effect of drugs that we published in 1969 in *The Lancet* under the title "Intensification of the central serotoninergic processes as a possible determinant of the thymoleptic effect." Our findings in this area of research were presented in 1970 in the *Proceedings of the Bekhterev Institute* under the title "Serotonergic processes in the action of psychotropic drugs." For us, the 1960s were the years of serotonin. And with the sixties gone, the "Decade of Serotonin and Antidepressants" in our laboratory was over.

THE KYNURENINE STORY

Serotonin is one of the metabolic end-products of tryptophan. Simultaneously with our research on 5-HT, M. Sansonova was studying in our laboratory the pharmacology of the antidepressant effects of tryptophan. While meditating one day at the end of the 1960s about our research with tryptophan, I suddenly became keenly aware that, while there was an abundance of information on 5-HT (numerous volumes dealing with its role in sleep, aggression, aging, inflammation, etc), we were completely in the dark about the neuroactivity of other major metabolites of tryptophan, as for example the kynurenines. We apparently know that kynurenines are normal constituents of tissues in animals and humans, whereas we do not really know whether they are present in brain tissue. While we know the names and the chemical structures of the kynurenines, i. e., kynurenine (KYN), 3-hydroxykynurenine (3-OH-KYN), 3-hydroxyanthranilic acid, anthranilic acid, quinolinic acid (QUIN), kynurenine acid (KYNA), xanthurenic acid, and nicotinamide, we don't know whether any of these substances are neuroactive and if they are, what kind of activity they have.

To generate some information on these substances we started with the kynurenines (those which are listed in Mendeleyev's table) compound by compound, applying our physiological and pharmacological methods. Thanks to our foreign colleagues, who supplied us with the necessary "biochemicals" in the early 1970s, we were able to begin, first with an analysis of injected kynurenine preparations on the behaviour of animals, and subsequently with a study of interactions between the kynurenines and standard psychotropic drugs. During the 1970s and 1980s we were unable to measure the concentrations of kynurenines in the brain because of technical problems; the concentrations of KYN and 3-OH-KYN in the blood of psychiatric patients were measured in our laboratory by Ivan Ryzov.

The administration of kynurenines into the brain directly yielded findings which clearly indicated that kynurenines are neuroactive. By now it is recognized that KYNA, an indole-3-pyruvate, has anticonvulsant activity, with anxiolytic properties in animal models; on the other hand, KYN, 3-OH-KYN, and QUIN cause excitement and seizures. By now publications on the neuroactivity of kynurenines in the world literature exceed four hundred. There are at least three keywords for the kynurenines, i.e., "kynurenine," "kynurenic acid," and "quinolinic acid" in the *Current Contents.*

In closing I would like to add that in 1992 the name, "Psychopharmacology Laboratory," was changed. It was intended to be a punishment! Between 1989 and 1991 three researchers of the laboratory had emigrated to England or the United States, and the administration doubted that its "scientific chief," working at the National Institutes of Health in Bethesda at the time, would return, given the long history of discrimination and other troubles he had. Considering that setting up a "factory for immigrants" sets a bad example, the structure of the institute was reorganized; after the laboratory was combined with a small unit for clinical trials, the "psychopharmacology laboratory" became the "division of clinical and experimental psychopharmacology" of the Bekhterev Psychoneurological Institute. Although the name was changed, the activities and the facilities remained the same.

PSYCHOPHARMACOLOGY BEHIND THE IRON CURTAIN – THE UNFORGETTABLE SIXTIES

Gregory F. Oxenkrug

The Laboratory of Psychopharmacology at the Bekhterev Psychoneurological Research Institute in Leningrad (now St. Petersburg) was very young in the 1960s, both because it had only recently been established and because of the age of those working in it. I.P. Lapin, head of the laboratory (and my PhD adviser) was in his late thirties and only eleven years older than I. This was, by and large, the age range of our staff. Since for many years it was the only psychopharmacological laboratory in the Soviet Union, it received many visitors from the West, who were allowed in because of the relative liberalization of Soviet society in the early 1960s. It took the political courage of Professor Lapin and his remarkable knowledge of foreign languages to establish and maintain active contacts (including a vast correspondence) with our Western colleagues.

S. Gershon, E. Costa, I. Kopin, J. Knoll, M. Sandler, the late G. Klerman, and many others were among the welcome guests. We actively corresponded with W. Bunney, B. Carroll, A. Carlsson, A. Pletscher, the late B.B. Brodie, and others, who kindly provided us with information and reagents. Even H. Selye once asked us for reprints of our articles after a fire in his library. My personal acquaintance with Sandler and Kopin left an indelible mark on my life. It was so exciting to feel that one is part of the international scientific community and to be able to learn of new developments in the field at

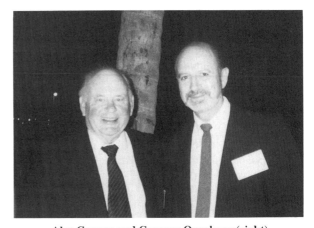

Alec Coppen and Gregory Oxenkrug (right)

Gregory F. Oxenkrug obtained his MD in 1965 from the Pavlov Medical School, and his doctorate in 1970 from the Bekhterev Psychoneurological Research Institute, Department of Psychopharmacology (St. Petersburg, Russia) where he stayed until 1979. In the United States, he has been a postdoctoral associate in the Department of Brain and Cognitive Sciences, at the Massachusetts Institute of Technology (1980-1982), professor of psychiatry and pharmacology at Wayne State University in Detroit (1982-1988), and professor of psychiatry at Brown University, Providence (1988-1994). Since 1994 he has been a professor of psychiatry at Tufts University, director of the Pineal Research Laboratory and Chairman, Department of Psychiatry at St. Elizabeth's Medical Center in Boston, where he continues his studies of the psychopharmacology of serotonin, N-acetylserotonin and melatonin.

Oxenkrug was elected a fellow of the CINP in 1996.

first hand. The field was very new, and the government had not (yet) required researchers "to develop psychopharmacology in accordance with the Marxist-Leninist philosophy," as was already the case in genetics and physiology. Initially, Lapin's huge library of reprints compensated for the general unavailability of scientific journals and monographs and for the restrictions imposed upon travel to scientific meetings.

However, this illusion of being in contact with the international scientific community soon started to fade away. (To be fair, travel was restricted for the rest of Soviet society as well.) In late 1960s Knoll, the professor of pharmacology in Budapest, invited me to spend a month in Hungary as a guest of the Hungarian Pharmacological Society. The administration at our institute refused even to call Moscow for permission: "We are not supposed to ask Moscow. We would send you if the initiative came from Moscow to do so." I decided to go as a private citizen during my annual leave. To do so, I needed a private invitation. Lapin called up the Department of Pharmacology in Budapest. It was August, and the only one there was a woman, Dr. A., who kindly agreed to send me the private invitation (although we had never heard of each other until that day). The government official figured out that the invitation was from a female. "You are a married person, and she is a woman... How come she invited you? Is she married?" I did not know, but realized that a negative answer would kill my project at once. "Yes, she is." "So, obtain the invitation from her husband." Lapin again telephoned Budapest. No, she was not married. Well, could she ask her father to invite me? I then presented her father's invitation as if it came from her husband.

This was my first and last trip abroad during my thirteen years with the laboratory. (A more dramatic experience was my unsuccessful attempt to visit Sandler's lab in London that I described and published in *Biogenic Amines*, under the title "Citizen Sandler, MAO-A inhibitors and melatonin") (1). I enjoyed every minute of my stay in Budapest and was able to demonstrate in the lab of K. Magyar the comparable effect of secondary (demethylated) and tertiary (dimethyl) beta-aminopropionyl dibenzazepine derivatives on the H-3-noradrenaline uptake in rat brain synaptosomes (2). These findings, together with findings in my previous studies, suggested that demethylation of the propionylic derivatives of imipramine – in variance with the propylic derivatives – was not associated with a decreased ability to inhibit serotonin (and noradrenaline) uptake. The development of drugs based on these studies, however, turned out to be almost impossible.

In the late 1960s Lapin introduced me to the patriarch of Soviet pharmacology, Professor M., who seemed very old, wise, and omnipotent. We enthusiastically told him about our serotonin hypothesis and expressed the hope that a new antidepressant could be developed – on the basis of our theory – by the intensification of serotoninergic processes (3). Professor M. replied: "You are lucky and naive guys. You came up with a new hypothesis and think that that is a big deal. Don't you realize that nobody in the government is interested in psychotropic medications since our party bosses and functionaries are not supposed to be crazy. And above all, our pharmaceutical industry cannot keep up with the demands for gauze and penicillin for Vietnam!"

Instead of developing a new drug, we thought that at least we could help with a new screening test for antidepressants. But our proposal to use the "frog test" for screening of potential serotoninergic antidepressants was rejected by the Soviet equivalent of the FDA. (The late R. Fuller, however, did use this test, together with many other tests, while studying fluoxetine). The test was based on the recognition that in frogs, whose brains contain predominantly serotonin, the serotoninergic component of potential antidepressants could be revealed, whereas in rodents, whose brains contain predominantly norepinephrine, the sero-toninergic component of potential antidepressants would remain hidden. Based on the differ-ence in the serotoninergic and noradrenergic components, in rodent brains, it was L-dopa and not 5-hydroxytrytophan that antagonized the reserpine induced sedation, whereas in the frog, it was 5-hydroxytrytophan, and not L-dopa which potentiated the sedative effect of reserpine (4). When I asked Professor M. the reason for the rejection of our proposals, he gave a deep sigh and told me that I was too young to remember the famous meetings of the Academy of the Soviet Union and the Medical Academy of the Soviet Union in 1948 and 1950 respectively, which resulted in the destruction of Soviet geneticists and physiologists. "Do you know what the main accusation levelled against Academician Orbeli and his colleagues was?" M. asked me. And he continued: "They were accused of the development of *frog physiology* instead of human physiology." (The accusation was certainly ridiculous and could be treated as a bad joke if it had not resulted in the loss of jobs, and even imprisonment, for some of the researchers.) "So – M. continued – I do not want anybody in the future to accuse you or me of developing *frog psychopharmacology*." I tried unsuccessfully to argue that we were proposing to use the frog merely as the test for screening antidepressants and not as the model of depression (5).

Almost thirty years later, while I was working with Sam Gershon at the Lafayette Clinic in Detroit, I ran across the abstract of a PhD thesis referring to the evaluation of melatonin in the "frog model of depression." I was very intrigued and wanted to know about this model. I thought that old Professor M. had turned out to be right after all: somebody had used frogs to develop a model of depression. It took an unusually long time for me to get the thesis, since the author, after obtaining her doctorate, had moved from South Africa to the United Kingdom and then to France in search of a position. It turned out that M. was even more right than I had thought: it was our frog test that was called "the frog model of depression," and it did demonstrate the antidepressant-like activity of melatonin, while the rodent test did not (6).

One might assume that the normal life of a researcher would include unrestricted contact with colleagues in the field (publications, visits, etc). When Professor Lapin and I decided to write up the serotonin hypothesis, I suggested that we submit it not only to the *Korsakoff Journal of Neurology and Psychiatry* (which as it turned out did not publish it), but also to *The Lancet*. The postal service would not deliver our paper without government approval. So we sent it (in Russian, of course) to the Ministry of Health in Moscow. The paper went through two reviews, one arranged by the Ministry of Health and the other by the Academy of Medical Sciences. It took almost two years for us to satisfy our anonymous reviewers, despite our arguments that it would be up to the editor of *The Lancet* to decide the fate of our manuscript. Eventually, we got "official permission to send abroad the manuscript of fifteen pages." This condition was very important since, although no reviewer ever read the English version of our paper, the number of pages in it had to be exactly the same as in the Russian.

After this experience, we started to ask our visitors from the West to take our manuscripts with them and submit them to Western journals for publication. Since we could not put our names on the manuscripts, and since our field of research was very similar to that of our guests, they could, if necessary, state to the customs officials that the papers were their own. This technique worked in most cases, although I remember getting a letter from one of the Western editors that read: "Dear Dr. Oxenkrug, I have received the manuscript that you asked Dr. N. during his visit to Leningrad to submit to our journal!" It was my luck that this particular letter was not opened by the authorities during their random check of our correspondence.

In most cases, however, our Western colleagues were wise and made the necessary corrections in our manuscripts without corresponding with us. I eventually had the pleasure of thanking most of them after my immigration to the United States in 1979. However, our technique eventually ran into an obstacle. Most of the Western journals sent fifty reprints free of charge to the author. These, as well as any correspondence from the West addressed to our institute, were registered by the special officer before they were passed on to us. So one day I was "congratulated" for one more publication in a Western journal. But I was also reprimanded because I had not obtained permission to submit my manuscript in the West and warned that such behaviour would not be tolerated in the future. It was a bad start for the year, the year that ended with the invasion of Afghanistan by the Soviet army (I could not predict that things would change so dramatically only ten or fifteen years later).

We, after all, were very lucky: our manuscript was accepted by *The Lancet* and our paper was well received. It was widely recognized by our colleagues and ended up as a citation classic (7). The publication on the role of cholinergic structures in antidepressant action in *Neuropsychopharmacology* by E.L. Schelkunov (8) from our laboratory remained virtually unnoticed. Based on his hypothesis, Professor Schelkunov had designed a new antidepressant and tried to develop it clinically. In those years, the rule was that drugs had to be administered in tablet form (and not as a powder) exclusively. A friend of his, a chemist, synthesized about 1 kg of the compound on his own time, but the equipment needed to prepare tablets was available only at Pharmacon (a pharmaceutical factory in Leningrad).

Schelkunov spent about a year in unsuccessful attempts to get the government to include the preparation of tablets of his compound in the annual plan for Pharmacon. Eventually he was told by some governmental official that he should study the mechanisms of drug action instead of inventing new drugs, and if he was going to continue to bother the government about this new drug, he would lose his job. The invention of new drugs, according to this officer, was the task of an institute in Moscow. Several years later, Schelkunov was invited to head the laboratory there, but he could not obtain permission from the Moscow police to reside in that city. (The government tried to keep people from moving to the big cities and at that time would grant residency permits only to construction workers.) Several years after my immigration to the United States, I was shocked and saddened to learn that Schelkunov had committed suicide at the age of forty-two. I cannot help but think that his unsuccessful struggle with the government bureaucrats contributed significantly to his suicide.

I was very lucky to work in Professor Lapin's laboratory during the exciting years of the 1960s, during the birth and rise of modern psychopharmacology. What I learned and experienced during that decade enabled me to restart my research in the United States, to have the honour of becoming an ACNP fellow and CINP member, and to participate in the CINP symposium on "5-HT and Psychiatry" at the time of Alec Coppen's presidency (9).

REFERENCES

1. Oxenkrug, G.F. (1993). Citizen Sandler, MAO-A inhibitors and melatonin. *Biogenic Amines,* 9: 465-468.
2. Oxenkrug, G.F. (1979). The equal effect of secondary and tertiary beta-aminopropionyl dibenzazepine derivatives on the H-3-NA uptake by rat brain synaptosomes. *Biochem. Pharmac.,* 78: 938-939.
3. Lapin, I.P., and Oxenkrug, G.F. (1969). Intensification of the central serotoninergic processes as a possible determinant of the thymoleptic effect. *Lancet,* 1: 32-39.
4. Lapin, I.P., and Oxenkrug, G.F. (1970). The frog as a subject for screening thymoleptic drugs. *J. Pharm. Pharmacol.,* 22: 781-783.

5. Poursolt, R.D., McArtur, R.A., and A. Lenegre (1993). Psychotropic screening procedures. In F. van Haaren (ed.), *Models in Behavioral Pharmacology* (pp.23-50). Elsevier Science Publishers.

6. Skene, D., and B. Potgieter (1981). Investigation of two models of depression. *S. African J. Sci.,* 77: 180-182.

7. Oxenkrug, G.F. (1987). *Current Contents,* 15(2): 16.

8. Schelkunov, E.L. (1967). Integrated effect of psychotropic drugs on the balance of cholino-, adreno-, and serotoninergic processes in the brain as a basis of their gross behavioral and therapeutic actions. *Neuropharmacology,* 5: 910-911.

9. Oxenkrug, G.F. (1991). The acute effect of monoamine oxidase inhibitors on serotonin conversion to melatonin. In M. Sandler, A. Coppen, and S. Harnett (eds.), *5-Hydroxytryptamine in Psychiatry: A Spectrum of Ideas* (pp.99-108). Oxford Univ. Press.

ACKNOWLEDGEMENT
The author highly appreciates the invaluable help of Karen Tsatuorian, PhD, in the preparation of this paper.

Other Memoirs

THE ESTABLISHMENT OF LABORATORIES (UK–US)

Roger W. Russell

During a recent visit to London I read in the *Sunday Express* a "Warning" that "fruit and veg could poison your child." Organophosphates (OP) were pronounced to be "The Deadly Dangers." This incident made me recall my personal involvement in psychopharmacology during the past half century.

Ever since my undergraduate years I have found it impossible to think in any other way than in terms of what I consider "the integrated organism," that is, in terms of basic properties that interact with each other. My own research has focused on the neurochemical and the behavioural aspects of the organism, and in most of my research I was involved in exploring hypotheses in animals, hypotheses that could not initially be tested on humans. In my master's thesis I reported on the effects of sodium amytal on memory. Later on I was involved in research on the behavioural effects of nitrous oxide, vitamin A deficiency, and thiamine deprivation. During World War II,

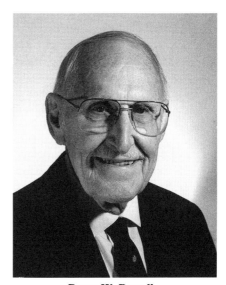

Roger W. Russell

I also studied the effects of mild hypoxia on psychomotor and mental skills in humans.

In 1949 I was appointed a Fulbright Advanced Research Scholar and given the responsibility of establishing an animal research laboratory at the Institute of Psychiatry in London. It was there that I made my first acquaintance with OPs. Questions had been raised in the British House of Commons about the hazards associated with the use of OP as an insecticide for the first time about forty years ago. For me, the research that was relevant to the "warning" printed in the *Sunday Express* in 1997 had begun almost half a century earlier!

Roger Wolcott Russell was born in Worcester, Massachusetts (USA), in 1914. After receiving his BA and MA from Clark University, he earned a PhD at the University of Virginia in 1939. He also holds a DSc from the University of London and honorary degrees from the University of Newcastle and Flinders University, both in Australia, where he taught for a number of years. Although his professional interests have strayed occasionally, the central core of his work has been in neurosciences, most specifically in psychopharmacology. He is currently a Lifetime Distinguished Fellow of the Center for the Neurobiology of Learning and Memory at the University of California, Irvine.

Russell was elected a fellow of the CINP in 1962.

In 1950 I was appointed to the chair in psychology at the University College of London (UCL). It was during those years that I became fully aware of the remarkable developments in the neurosciences in general and psychopharmacology in particular. No longer was it acceptable to limit knowledge to relationships between stimulus and response. We became interested in learning about the events intervening between these two variables, to "fill the empty organism."

It would be difficult to imagine a more stimulating environment than I found at UCL. Three members of the faculty were or were to become Nobel laureates in biophysics and physiology. Others of international reputation included F.R. Winton (Pharmacology) who, I believe, created one of the first university posts in psychopharmacology (the first appointee was one of my PhD students, H. Steinberg); E.H.F. Baldwin (Biochemistry); G.L. Brown (Physiology); J.Z. Young (Anatomy); and J.B.S. Haldane (Genetics, Biometrics). This environment allowed me not only to clarify my own ideas but also to evaluate concepts in a broad perspective.

Scientific societies provided opportunities for an interaction between researchers from different disciplines, which in turn contributed greatly to the development of psychopharmacology as a discipline that could stand on its own. A prime example of this was the meeting in which I participated in 1949, sponsored by the Society for Experimental Biology. In the course of a single meeting, E.D. Adrian (Cambridge, UK), who had received his Nobel prize in 1932, described his observations of the electrical activity of nerve cells; N. Tinbergen (Leiden, The Netherlands) called attention to biochemical events in the brain, and with K.Z. Lorenz (Altenberg, Germany) – both to receive the Nobel Prize in 1973 –, made a strong case for the inclusion of innate, instinctive behaviours as end points in the neurosciences. J. Konorski (Lodz, Poland) and J.Z.Young (London, UK) reported on their explorations into the mechanisms of learning; and K. Lashley (Harvard, USA) concluded on the basis of his many years of searching for specific sites of behavioural functions in the CNS that, "I sometimes feel, in reviewing the evidence on the localization of the memory trace, that the necessary conclusion is that learning is not possible." Later, on a train to London, he told me that, although he had made this remark tongue-in-cheek, it was his intention to pay more attention to the biochemistry and electrophysiology of the CNS. These were encouraging words for me, since we, at UCL, had already begun experiments using pharmacological tools to study the behavioural effects of neurochemical events.

The development of the neurosciences, and hence of psychopharmacology, also benefited early on from the wisdom of such organizations as the CIBA Foundation for the Promotion of International Cooperation in Medical and Chemical Research. In 1964 CIBA published a volume summarizing the presentations and discussions of the first British symposium on "Animal Behaviour and Drug Action." The symposium, which brought together some of the world's leading figures in psychopharmacology, emphasized the importance of interdisciplinary cooperation. W.S. Feldberg (London, UK) ended his introduction to one session with the comment: "When I think of how physiologists sometimes look on psychologists, and psychologists on biochemists, I cannot resist concluding ... that to speak ill of others is a dishonest way of praising ourselves. Thus, physiologists studying behaviours should beware of neglecting the methods of psychologists." The challenging questions I was asked during the discussion of my own contributions led me to conclude that my methods were not neglected!

In 1962 I was elected a fellow of the CINP, just five years after its formal inauguration. The 1991-92 directory of members lists eighty-four fellows whose association with the organization go back to those first five years. All of us are proud to have been able to contribute to the Collegium's development during that early period.

Psychopharmacology, as a coordinated discipline, was not born overnight and its birth was dependent on the appreciation of the contributions that the field could make to human mental and physical health, as well as to knowledge about the structures and functions of living organisms. This recognition could have been brought about only by those who chose to engage in clinical and or basic research. Such research was in turn dependent upon financial support. Recognition of the potential benefits of research in psychopharmacology finally led to the establishment of an advisory committee in psychopharmacology within the United States Public Health Service. I had just returned to the United States from London, and I was appointed a member of the first committee. Undoubtedly, the creation of this body did not mean that all the problems were solved. There remained the issue of how funds were to be allocated, for example. There were very competent psychologists and pharmacologists, but no psychopharmacologists at the time.

I remember an embarrassing episode that occurred, as I recall, during the second or third year of the committee's existence. We were called before the Finance Committee of the U.S. House of Representatives to explain why we had not spent all of the funds made available to us. Our answer was straightforward: we had not received a sufficient number of *worthy* proposals in *psychopharmacology*. Submissions from psychologists were naive in terms of which drugs were to be used and how, and those from pharmacologists fell short of knowledge on how to measure behaviour. (Such an observation seems incredible in the world of psychopharmacology today.) It was clear that the number of professionals qualified in the new discipline had to be increased.

My personal contribution to psychopharmacology, as well as that of my colleagues from the advisory committee, was the establishment of laboratories designed to investigate basic issues. My first laboratory was at Indiana University. It was a suitable site for the selection of postgraduate, doctoral students on the basis of their ability and sincere interest in the new discipline. I was able to attract two of the few highly recognized psychopharmacologists of the time to join me. One of them had prior research experience in the laboratories of an international pharmaceutical firm and the other in the laboratories of the federal government. Our research personnel also included a biochemist with a background in research at a major university. We greatly benefited from establishing a close relationship with pharmacologists and clinical researchers in the school of medicine of the university.

In 1967 I joined the faculty of the University of California, Irvine. My appointments in three departments – Psychobiology, Psychology, and Medical Pharmacology and Therapeutics – reflected my personal interests and perhaps also the uncertainty as to where psychopharmacology really belonged! By the time I arrived at Irvine, psychopharmacology had gained a firm standing in the biomedical sciences, and students of excellent promise were attracted to the field. In addition to providing courses for those at the graduate level, UCI developed a program for undergraduates called "Go for Honors." Students selected for this program were required to undertake original research projects under faculty supervision – projects that often led to publication in scientific journals. A major advantage for the participants of the program was that it made it possible for them to have an early start in the field.

For me personally, the rise of psychopharmacology had begun during my undergraduate years. It had grown in scope as knowledge in the biomedical sciences developed. By the close of the 1960s I could to assist another generation of students in experiencing some of the same satisfactions that I had felt a half-century earlier, but through interaction with a much more firmly established discipline. The CINP and its individual members have reason to be proud of the contributions that they have made to the development of psychopharmacology. It is to be hoped that the organization's role will continue as the discipline passes through its next half-century.

DRUGS AS TOOLS FOR UNDERSTANDING BRAIN AND BEHAVIOUR
(Italy–US)

Alberto Oliverio

When in 1964 I moved from the Istituto di Sanità (NIH) in Rome to the Physiology Department of the Karolinska Institute in Stockholm, my neuroscientific background did not directly involve psychopharmacology. My work experience in Rome with Daniel Bovet, who was awarded the 1957 Nobel Prize in Medicine for his work on a number of drugs – sulfonamides, sympathomimetic agents, curare-like and antihistaminic agents – was mostly limited to the role of the sympathetic system on cardiovascular regulation and on other adaptive mechanisms, such as catecholamine turnover in those immunosympathectomized mice that had just been produced by Rita Levi Montalcini in St. Louis and Rome, in her experiments on Nerve Growth Factor.

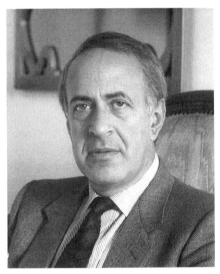

Alberto Oliverio

WHAT DO WE LEARN ABOUT THE BRAIN FROM THE PERIPHERY?

In Stockholm I spent one year with Ulf von Euler, a distinguished physiologist who had just discovered that noradrenaline was one of the main neurotransmitters and that its role was not confined to the sympathetic system. There were many foreign visiting scientists in von Euler's laboratory, and much excitement surrounded the batteries of "Sephadex" chromatographic columns, which, by means of a painstaking procedure, allowed for the extraction of noradrenaline from animal tissues and for its measurement by photofluorometric methods. It was in

Alberto Oliverio is professor of psychobiology at the Faculty of Biological Sciences, University of Rome, Italy, and director of the National Research Council Institute of Psychobiology and Psychopharmacology. He has worked at the Karolinska Institute in Stockholm, at the University of California in Los Angeles, at the Jackson Laboratory in Bar Harbor, Maine, and in various Italian and other research institutes. At present he is engaged in studying neurochemical and neurophysiological correlates of memory and the genetic approaches to stress.

Oliverio was elected a fellow of the CINP in 1968. He presented a paper on "Effects of cholinergic drugs on avoidance conditioning and maze learning of mice" (Oliverio, Bovet-Nitti and Bovet) at the 5th Congress.

1965 that Stockholm hosted the first international meeting on catecholamines at the Wenner Gren Centre. In a very crowded room and a smoky atmosphere – at that time, people smoked cigarettes without any feelings of guilt or social restrictions – I had a chance to discuss with experienced colleagues my first experiments on the effects of noradrenergic agents on different nervous functions, including the action of stressors such as cold on brain and behaviour.

A number of new drugs were screened in von Euler's laboratory, among them a rather odd one, decaborane, a rocket propellant that was very toxic but had the property of causing powerful noradrenaline – and other catecholamines – depletion in many tissues, including the brain. At that time, noradrenaline appeared to be the master key for opening all the secrets of the brain, and its role in relation to centrally acting drugs seemed as pivotal as that of dopamine a few years later. However, dopamine had yet to be discovered and the known neurotransmitters were just a lonely patrol of three or four neurochemicals, including acetylcholine, 5-hydroxytryptamine (Erspamer's enteramine), and of course, adrenaline. Like many other classical physiologists of his time, von Euler, who was to receive the 1970 Nobel Prize for his studies on catecholamines, had no doubt that it was possible to draw inferences concerning the central role of neurotransmitters and psychotropic agents in the brain by studying their role and effects at the periphery. Hence, my first projects in psychopharmacology were studies on the effects of catecholamine-depleting agents such as reserpine and decaborane on cardiac function and on cardiac noradrenaline turnover in animals exposed to cold and pretreated with noradrenergic, or anti-noradrenergic agents; I took on as well such classical subjects as the inhibition by phenoxybenzamine of the noradrenaline-releasing effect of tyramine. We could have interpreted our findings in a broader perspective if there had been more interaction with our "next door neighbors." But Professor Bjorn Uvnäs, director of the Department of Pharmacology, and Professor von Euler did not "network" to any great extent and this meant that also their co-workers had to stick to this "academic" rule. Because of the lack of interaction between the different departments, I could not take full advantage of my stay at the famous Farmakologiska Institutionen. It was just not possible for me, for example, to interact with Enzio Giacobini, who at the time was developing an interesting experimental model – the stretch receptor of the crayfish – for neuropharmacology and studying cholinergic functions.

FROM NICOTINE TO PSYCHOPHARMACOGENETICS

I was not really involved in much brain or behavioural research during my Swedish experience. Fortunately this "non-specific" background turned out to be very useful for me when I joined the Department of Pharmacology at the University of California at Los Angeles in 1965 as assistant research pharmacologist on a grant from the American Medical Association to study the effects of nicotine on behaviour and the central effects of nicotine and nicotinic agents.

While in Los Angeles I again joined Daniel Bovet, who was there, because of the availability of a number of different inbred strains of mice produced at the Jackson Laboratory in Bar Harbor, Maine. Though Los Angeles is on the opposite side of the United States from Bar Harbor, it was much easier for him to get inbred strains of Bar Harbor mice in L.A. than in Rome. Research on the effects of drugs on learning and memory was just taking off during those days in the United States and it was also much easier to interact from L.A. than from Rome with the team of James L. McGaugh, who had just been appointed professor at the

University of Irvine, and the team of Murray Jarvik at Yeshiva University in New York, who were working in this new area of research.

My first results on the effects of nicotine on behaviour indicated that, the effects were either stimulating or depressant depending on the genetic background of the animals, a fact that indicates how important individual differences are in terms of drug reactivity. I had similar findings with several nicotinic compounds in my research conducted in collaboration with R.B. Barlow and C.M. Thompson of the University of Edinburgh, and ever since that time my interest in psychopharmacology has been filtered through a genetic approach.

Although the term "psychopharmacogenetics" had still to be invented, several different research groups were already interested in the problem of individual reactivity to drugs from both a quantitative and qualitative point of view. A first screening of the behavioural effects of nicotine and nicotinic agents revealed clear-cut differences in different mouse strains. This offered a suitable model for studying the neurochemical and neurophysiological correlates of the genetically determined differences.

THE 1966 CINP SYMPOSIUM ON MEMORY AND LEARNING

I had the opportunity to report the preliminary results of our group (1) at the fifth CINP Congress on "Drug effects on memory and learning" in Washington, DC, in 1966. It was my first "big" symposium. Murray Jarvik, then professor of pharmacology at the Yeshiva University in New York City, played a significant "political" role by bringing together in our symposium American and both western and eastern European pharmacologists and physiologists. One of the latter was Jan Bure from Prague, well-known for his experiments on cortical spreading depression. There were not thousands of participants in the CINP symposium in Washington, just a few hundred, but I still remember it as an important occasion because it was one of the first meetings devoted to the problem of drugs and memory. Another historic meeting which brought together researchers working in the different areas of neuroscience (though the term had not yet come into use) was held in Puerto Rico in 1967 and organized by D.H. Efron. Both occasions, the CINP congress in Washington and the ACNP meeting in Puerto Rico, proved very useful in setting up collaborative projects with a number of colleagues. It was in Washington that I met Paul Mandel, the neurochemist from Strasbourg with whom I began a long-lasting collaboration.

THE GENETICS OF BEHAVIOUR

As a genetically-oriented pharmacologist, since 1965 I have tried to evaluate the effects of cholinergic, noradrenergic, and later dopaminergic agents in genetically distinct strains, i.e., in neuronal systems, with qualitatively and quantitatively distinct receptor patterns (2, 3, 4). For me, drugs were interesting mainly as tools for studying the brain and behaviour rather than for their possible therapeutic effects. As years passed, in experiment after experiment, I moved closer and closer towards the conclusion that the brains of different species, strains, or individuals are characterized by a huge diversification of expression of both nervous structures and behaviours.

In collaboration with Donald W. Bailey, Dietmar Biesold, Elaine Kempf, Paul Mandel, Giorgio Racagni, Pier Francesco Spano, Marco Trabucchi, and Jerzy Vetulani – to name just a few of the principal investigators – we found and described a large variability in the levels, turnover, and cerebral distribution of neurotransmitters responsible for different patterns of arousal and energy-deployment mechanisms. Furthermore, we described in the mouse during development and adult age intraspecies variations in brain chemistry, neurotransmitter turnover and in a number of morphological measures involving brain size, hippocampal volume, and hypothalamic or limbic organization. When considered in terms of learning and memory, these neurochemical, neurophysiological, and neuroanatomical variations result in both quantitative and qualitative memory differences, a fact that does not necessarily imply different "basic" memory mechanisms. Numerous findings indicate that the neurobiological mechanisms involved in memory consolidation are essentially similar within and across species, since they are based on almost identical functional or structural changes at the neuronal level. However, a number of sensory, arousal, attention, or emotional processes may impair or improve the different "basic" mechanisms of memory, i.e.,modulate mnestic processes. It is this modulation that is affected by different brain chemicals and by a number of drugs. It is much more difficult for drugs to affect "basic" or primary memory mechanisms – that is, to improve or depress memory consolidation processes – unless these agents, such as protein synthesis inhibitors, are injected in high doses into the brains of experimental animals.

NEUROPSYCHOPHARMACOLOGY AND THEORIES OF THE MIND

Our genetic or pharmacogenetic studies of brain and behaviour, including memory, were carried out mainly in the 1960s and early 1970s, when molecular neurobiology had not yet spread its wings. From time to time the genetic studies encountered opposition from radical political groups. They feared that it would legitimate social or class differences by implying that "all was in the genes," rather than in the culture. In Italy, where political life was quite radicalized, many psychiatrists, psychologists, and even neuropharmacologists tagged the genetic approach as conservative and likened it to a kind of rough reductionism and oversimplification of the brain's complexity. Despite these radical positions, the use of drugs as tools for studying brain functions and for understanding behaviour has proved one of the most important approaches to modern neuroscience. If today's theories of the mind reflect empirical evidence rather than abstract positions, it is due primarily to psychopharmacology but also to psychopharmacogenetics and behavioural genetics. Today my younger students do not fully appreciate the fact that, less than four decades ago, our knowledge of the brain was limited to a small number of neurochemical, neurophysiological, pharmacological, and clinical data. Thanks to several approaches based on healthy reductionism, such as those of the physiologist who hypothesized that what we know at the peripheral (nervous) level may be useful at the central level, we now know much more about cognition and emotion, and about some drugs that affect these processes.

REFERENCES
1. Oliverio, A., Bovet-Nitti, F., and Bovet, D. (1966). Effects of cholinergic drugs on avoidance conditioning and maze learning of mice. In Brill, H., Cole J.O., Deniker, P., Hippius, H., and Bradley, P.B. (eds.), Neuro-Psycho-pharmacology. Proceedings of the Fifth International Congress of the Collegium Internationale Neuro-Psycho-Pharmacologicum (Washington, D.C. 28th-31st March, 1966) (3rd Symposium on Drug Effects on Memory and Learning), Washington, DC. *Excerpta Medica International Congress Series,* 129 (213-219) Amsterdam: Excerpta Medica Foundation.
2. Oliverio, A., Castellano, C., and Puglisi-Allegra, S. (1983). Psychopharmacogenetics of opioids. *Trends in Pharmacological Sciences,* 4: 350-352.
3. Puglisi-Allegra, S., Cabib, S., Kempf, E., and Oliverio, A. (1990). Genotype-dependent adaptation of brain dopamine system to stress. In Puglisi-Allegra, S., and Oliverio, A. (eds.), *Psychobiology of Stress,* NATO ASI Series, vol.54 (pp. 171-182). Dordrecht: Kluwer Academic Publishers.
4. Cabib, S., Oliverio, A., Ventura, R., Lucchese, F., and Puglisi-Allegra, S. Brain dopamine receptor plasticity: testing a diathesis-stress hypothesis in an animal model. *Psychopharmacology* 132, 153-160.

SEROTONIN AND OBSESSIVE-COMPULSIVE DISORDER
(Argentina–US)

Jose A. Yaryura-Tobias

My first experience with psychopharmacology was as an intern in the emergency room of the Fernandez Hospital in Buenos Aires in the 1950s, when we used the French surgeon Henri Laborit's lytic cocktail to prevent shock in serious head-trauma by "artificial hibernation." It was about the same time, or just a little bit later that chlorpromazine, endorsed by Professor Jean Delay, was introduced in the treatment of psychotic patients. I witnessed the removal of the shackles and of the straitjacket, from patients in state psychiatric institutions; a new era in the history of psychiatry emerged in front of our eyes. By then I was on my way to becoming an internist, ready to leave for Saskatchewan (Canada) to do cancer research there. Although I was quite well acquainted with the work of Freud and his disciples, a career in psychiatry at that time was certainly not my first choice.

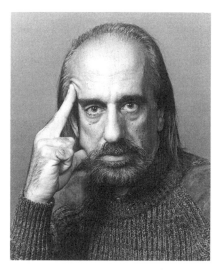

Jose A. Yaryura-Tobias

Saskatchewan was an exciting place in those years. The introduction of socialized medicine combined with a psychiatric revolution attracted attention to the Canadian province. It was in Saskatchewan in the mid-1950s that Drs. Abram Hoffer, John Smythies and Humphrey Osmond postulated their adrenochrome theory of schizophrenia, which led to the use of niacin in the treatment of schizophrenic patients. And it was in Saskatchewan in the early 1960s that the first buildings to house mental patients, in consideration of patients' psychotic experiences, were designed and erected. It was also in Saskatchewan that Humphrey Osmond, originally from England, coined the terms "hallucinogenic" and "psychedelic" drugs. Osmond offered me a "trip" on LSD (as a subject in one of his research protocols), but I was afraid of receiving a one-way ticket and declined the invitation.

Jose A. Yaryura-Tobias is a clinical research psychiatrist, a poet, and a fiction writer. He is the Medical Director of the Institute for BioBehavioral Treatment and Research. He is a Professor of Psychiatry at the Medical School of the New York University, N.Y., Visiting Professor of Psychiatry at the National University of Cuyo, Mendoza, Argentina, and Professor of Psychiatry at the University of El Salvador, Buenos Aires, Argentina. He has published over 200 scientific papers, and authored seven books in the specialty.

Yaryura-Tobias was elected a fellow of the CINP in 1972.

During my years in Saskatchewan I became very much interested in psychiatry and, after completing my residency training in internal medicine, I decided to start with a residency training in it. Early in my training I came across some patients who had symptoms resembling Parkinson's disease, and some other patients with tongue protrusion, a manifestation that was to become known as "bucco-oral dyskinesia." I was fascinated by what I saw and began to experiment with calcium gluconate in view of the possibility that some sort of hypocalcemia was the culprit. Actually, the use of calcium in Parkinson's disease had first been considered in the 1930s. It was around that time that I became interested in schizophrenia and in the extrapyramidal symptoms encountered in schizophrenic patients. For the next fifteen years I remained dedicated to the study of schizophrenia. Because I lived in a state hospital, I was able to interact continuously with both acute and chronic schizophrenic patients. My experience with them during those years had a major impact on my professional career. I can say today that what I learned by observing and interacting with patients provided the ideas for my research. It also gave a meaning to my professional life.

In 1967 I saw a patient suffering from Parkinson's disease who was jealous of his wife and would beat her up every time he went home for a visit. The patient was referred to me by Dr. Cotzias, who was at the time conducting a clinical trial with levodopa, a substance which on the basis of findings in the brains of patients with Parkinson's disease was expected to have therapeutic effects. In the course of my interview with the patient I learned that it was not every weekend, but only every other weekend that he became jealous of his wife. Puzzled by the episodic pattern of a patient's mental pathology, I decided to ask Cotzias for information on how the patient was being treated with levodopa in the research protocol. What I learned was that, "He is on levodopa for a week, followed by a week of placebo." I had got the answer I needed to postulate that levodopa can precipitate, aggravate, or even cause psychosis, notably schizophrenia. I published a series of papers, with S. Merlis and B. Diamond as co-authors, on findings which led to the levodopa theory of schizophrenia at Central Islip State Hospital in New York. The rest of the story is well known: the levodopa theory of schizophrenia emerged, then was replaced by the dopamine theory of schizophrenia with its ramifications.

I was back in Argentina, working in Buenos Aires in the early 1970s, when pimozide, an antipsychotic produced by Janssen Pharmaceuticals, was marketed there as a new drug. I decided to try it in some patients in group therapy with the diagnosis of paranoid-type schizophrenia. Since it was noted during the group therapy sessions that patients treated with the new drug were able to discuss their feelings of persecution, without giving up their false beliefs, I suggested that pimozide has a resocializing effect.

During my stay in Argentina, Professor Edmondo Fischer was active in Buenos Aires studying the properties of bufotenine, which he isolated from the urine of patients with schizophrenia. He believed that bufotenine is the psychotoxic substance responsible for the manifestations seen in schizophrenia. By now the bufotenine theory of schizophrenia has faded away, although the fact remains that shamans in North Africa use tobacco, prepared from the skin of *Bufo arenarum,* a toad with a high concentration of bufotenine in its skin, in tehir rituals to reach a high level of visual and auditory experiences.

I also helped Fischer to carry out his work on the therapeutic effect of phenylethylamine in depression. His contention that phenylethylamine has therapeutic effect in depression was based on reports which indicated a depletion of phenylethylamine in depressed patients. I used to bring his patients samples from the United States of d-phenylalanine, which they took to increase their phenylethylamine levels. Later on, similar work was carried out in Europe and

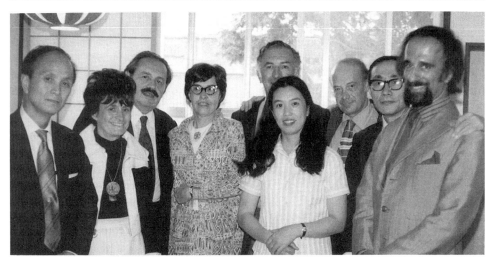

From left: Tetsuyo Fukuda, Mrs. Ch. Shagass, Edmondo Fischer, unidentified,
Charles Shagass, unidentified, George Winokur, unidentified and Jose A. Yaryura-Tobias

in the United States, with findings supportive of the therapeutic effect of phenylethylamine in depressed patients.

Since the late 1960s I have become increasingly involved in studying obsessive-compulsive disorder (OCD) and its pathophysiology and treatment. It was first in 1967 that Lopez Ibor Sr. from Spain, treated anorexia nervosa patients with clomipramine, obtaining favourable therapeutic effects. Later on I administered the drug in a severe case of OCD, and to my amazement the patient responded favourably to treatment. Subsequently we conducted a pilot study in the United States with clomipramine in OCD, which indicated therapeutic effects with the drug. We were able to verify our findings in the pilot study in a double-blind placebo-controlled study in OCD patients. Since I thought that serotonin was partially the culprit, with my wife, Dr. Neziroglu we put forward a serotonergic hypothesis for OCD which would explain that a serotonin reuptake inhibitor would have a therapeutic effect in obsessive compulsive disorder. Furthermore, we identified clomipramine as a specific anti-obsessive-compulsive drug. Our theory was supported by the "hyposerotoninemia" found in patients with OCD and by the favourable response of OCD patients to L-tryptophan. Today there is no longer any doubt that serotonin plays a role in the pathology of OCD. Our efforts to stimulate interest in OCD among our fellow researchers were successful. We have a substantial knowledge base about OCD today with clinical awareness of the part played by serotonin in the disorder. Moreover, there are several selective serotonin reuptake inhibitors available for treatment which are not only antidepressants but also anti-obsessive-compulsive drugs.

Today, we can see the development of a new generation of compounds with the promise of having a better therapeutic ratio than the old ones. They provide all but complete recovery. This, of course, is understandable, because the human being is a labyrinth, an open-ended system that continues to reveal a myriad of unexplored paths. What about all of those who preceded us in the challenging moments of research and discovery? They live in our memories and, we hope, in the memory of the younger generation of researchers, who must continue to break new ground in order to ease the pain of humankind.

FROM TRANSMETHYLATION TO OXIDATIVE MECHANISMS (UK–US)

John Smythies

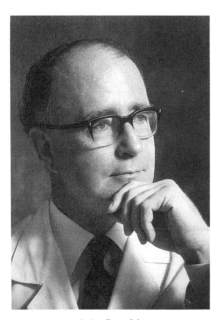

John Smythies

My own work during the last forty years has not been so much in the field of drug development as in developing biochemical theories that underlie certain areas of neuropsychopharmacology.

In 1951, six weeks into my first residency in psychiatry at St. George's Hospital, London, I became interested in mescaline after reading the accounts by Weir Mitchell and Havelock Ellis of the hallucinations it produces. As a minor poet I was impressed by the poetic beauty of the visions, and I decided to learn more about the subject. I soon came across Beringer's book *Der Meskalinrausch,* in which the chemical formula of mescaline was shown. The formula looked familiar to me, and I showed it to one of our medical students, Julian Redmill. "Ah, he said, adrenaline." Since mescaline produces a model psychosis, it seemed to me that schizophrenia might be associated with the production of a mescaline-like substance in the brain as a result of a disorder of adrenaline metabolism. My colleague at St. George's, Humphrey Osmond, took a keen interest in this new theory.

A few weeks later I happened to be in Cambridge and met John Harley-Mason, the organic chemist who had worked on the oxidative pathway of adrenaline metabolism. I told him about my ideas, and he worked out a possible biochemical mechanism by which a mescaline-like compound could be produced by O-methylation of adrenaline. This led in 1952 to the

John Smythies received his medical degree at Cambridge University and then did research with Bill Gibson, Harold Himwich, Hudson Hoagland, and Jack Eccles. He was reader in psychiatry at the University of Edinburgh for twelve years and C.B. Ireland Professor of Psychiatric Research at the University of Alabama Medical Center for sixteen years. His current academic affiliations are with the Institute of Neurology at the University of London and the Brain and Perception Laboratory at the University of California, San Diego.

Smythies became a fellow of the CINP during the 1960s. He presented a paper on "Structure-activity relationship studies on the effect of mescaline on the conditioned avoidance response in rats" (Smythies and Sykes) at the 4th Congress and was a formal discussant in Working Group 3 (Psychology and Experimental Psychopathology) at the same Congress.

publication of our paper, "Schizophrenia: a new approach" (Osmond and Smythies) in the *Journal of Mental Science* (now *British Journal of Psychiatry*), in which the first specific biochemical hypothesis of schizophrenia – the "transmethylation hypothesis" – was presented. Also in this paper the formula of metanephrine was shown for the first time. Five years later metanephrine was discovered by Julius Axelrod and others to be a normal metabolite of adrenaline. However, no evidence has ever been found to suggest that 0-methylated psychotomimetic derivatives of catecholamines play any role in schizophrenia itself. The importance of the transmethylation hypothesis was that, in an era when most psychiatrists believed in a psychogenic causation of schizophrenia (remember the "schizophrenogenic mother"?), it demonstrated for the first time that there might be a biochemical explanation for the causation of the disease. It therefore helped to direct the attention of researchers towards biochemical, rather than psychological, research strategies.

In later years my interest turned to the biochemical mechanism of transmethylation itself and I developed the second transmethylation hypothesis which implicated the mechanism of transmethylation – the one-carbon cycle – rather than abnormal endogenous O-methylated products. Since then much evidence has been obtained that there are disorders in this system. However, the abnormality is not specific for schizophrenia; it occurs in depression and other conditions as well (1).

In the early 1950s we turned our attention to the oxidative pathway of adrenaline metabolism, following a case – studied by my colleagues Abram Hoffer and Humphrey Osmond – of an asthmatic who had injected himself with oxidized pink adrenaline and had developed an acute psychotic reaction. So we tested the responsible agent, adrenochrome, in normal volunteers and showed that it produced subtle disorders of perception, ideation, and behaviour (without vivid visual hallucinations) not unlike those seen in certain cases of schizophrenia. This work was confirmed by groups in the United States, Czechoslovakia, and Germany. Therefore we suggested that schizophrenia might be associated with a disorder in the oxidative pathway rather than the transmethylation pathway of catecholamine metabolism. But all attempts to detect adrenochrome in vivo failed, and oxidative metabolites of catecholamines were dismissed as merely in vitro products of no clinical interest. Recently, however, it has become apparent that this conclusion was mistaken. Evidence has been obtained from various sources that aminochromes derived from catecholamines (i.e., dopamine and norepinephrine) are present in the brain (2). I have recently published three papers on the possible role of aminochromes in normal brain functions and in disease, i.e., Parkinson's disease and schizophrenia (3, 4, 5). However these publications appeared in the 1990s. After forty years in the wilderness, aminochromes, and the auto-oxidative pathway of catecholamine metabolism, are becoming the focus of increased interest and experimentation.

My work on the role of oxidative reactions in the brain led me to take a look at a wider field: the role of oxidative reactions and antioxidants in medicine in general. It is now becoming clear that oxidative stress plays a role in many illnesses, including atherosclerosis, cancer, diabetes, cataracts, and cystic fibrosis, as well as the brain disorders Alzheimer's and Parkinson's diseases. This evidence brings into focus the use of antioxidants as therapeutic agents in these diseases. There is now no doubt that a diet with a high intake of fruits and vegetables – and thus high in beneficial phytochemicals such as antioxidant vitamins and flavonoids – plays an essential role in preventative medicine. The only debate now is between those who believe that antioxidant supplementation to the diet is desirable and those who think it is not.

In the realm of public service, I spent some time during the 1960s as a consultant to the World Health Organization, coordinating research activities in different countries. This work provided me with an opportunity to meet psychopharmacologists from around the world, including my good friends the late Boris Lebedev, the late Marat Vartanian and Felix Vartanian from the former Soviet Union. I remember particularly feasting on the large tubs of caviar they brought with them from Russia.

Between 1955 and 1989 I continued my researches with various collaborators on halluci-nogenic drugs, in particular on structure-activity relationships of mescaline. We also studied endogenous hallucinogens such as dimethyltryptamine and O-methyl bufotenin, which we showed to be present in small amounts in the normal human CSF. However, the amounts are not increased in schizophrenia.

In addition, I have utilized my formal training as a neuroanatomist to make contributions to the field of functional neuroanatomy. These have included a book I wrote in 1968, when I was a fellow at the Neurosciences Research Program at the Massachusetts Institute of Technology with Frank Schmidt, which was called *Brain Mechanisms and Behaviour.*

My research strategy for forty years has been based on the idea that, in an era of ever-increasing specialization and the accumulation of enormous quantities of information, some generalists are needed to try to make sense of the whole picture. So I trained as a generalist and now concentrate on particular projects that integrate widely disparate disciplines within neuroscience: for example, my recent work on the biochemical mechanisms that operate at the glutamate synapse; the concepts of oxidative stress and antioxidant protection and their role in synaptic plasticity; and the role of the antioxidant properties of dopamine, together with the neurotoxic properties of its quinone metabolites, in the modulation by reinforcement of synaptic microanatomy. All these themes unite to provide a new theory of one aspect of the biochemical basis of learning and neurocomputation. I am now working on a textbook on the biochemical basis of schizophrenia. My particular mentors during this odyssey have been Heinrich Klüver, Lord Brain, Sir Francis Walshe, Sir Aubrey Lewis, Sir John Eccles, Oliver Zangwill, C.D. Broad, H.H. Price, Vilanayur Ramachandran, and Francis Crick.

REFERENCES

1. Smythies, J.R., Gottfries, C.-G., and Regland, B. (1996). Disturbances of one-carbon metabolism in neuropsychi-atric disorders: a review. *Biol. Psychiatr.,* 41: 230-233.
2. Smythies, J.R., and Galzigna, L. (in press). The oxidative metabolism of catecholamines in the brain: a review. *Biochim. Biophys. Acta.*
3. Smythies, J.R. (1996). On the function of neuromelanin. *Proc. R. Soc. (London) B*, 263: 487-489.
4. Smythies, J.R. (1997). The biochemical basis of synaptic plasticity and neural computation: a new theory. *Proc. R. Soc. (London) B,* 264: 575-579.
5. Smythies, J.R. (1997). Oxidative reactions and schizophrenia. *Schiz. Res.,* 24: 357-364.

CINP STORY

The Collegium Internationale Neuro-Psychopharmacologicum was founded in September 1957 during the Second World Congress of Psychiatry in Zurich. It was just about this time the Founders met, that the first effective antidepressants were discovered. The first antipsychotics, anxiolytics and mood stabilizers were already available for clinical use. There was excitement with great expectations. On the evening of September 3 (some claim; others argue for the 2nd or 9th), the founders of CINP held the inaugural meeting at the "buffet" of the Zurich railway station. It came at the end of one of the afternoon sessions of the psychopharmacology symposium, and some members might perhaps have been surprised at receiving the invitation to this genteel station restaurant.

The success of the first international symposium on psychotropic drugs, held in Milan in the spring of 1957, had made apparent the need for such a professional association in psychopharmacology. It was Silvio Garattini, then associate professor of pharmacology at the Milan University, who did the work of organizing the symposium and Emilio Trabucchi, the professor of pharmacology, who chaired it.

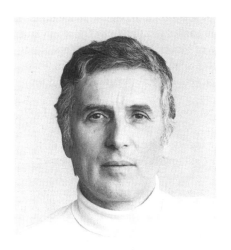
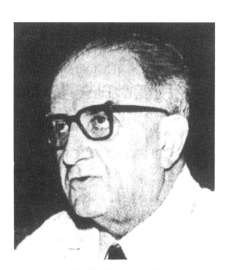

Silvio Garattini   **Emilio Trabucchi**

The spirit in Milan was high and stimulating. During the symposium it had been Corneille Radouco-Thomas, a Roumanian-born pharmacologist then in Geneva, and Wolfgang de Boor, a Heidelberg psychiatrist and member of Kurt Schneider's historic department, who formally proposed establishing an association dedicated to psychopharmacology. Among the Milan participants there was a small but enthusiastic group who wanted to found the new society without delay, even before leaving Milan. But Ernst Rothlin decided to slow the pace. Rothlin, the scientific director of Sandoz for well over a decade, was a powerful man. He was at the time of the Milan symposium president of the International Pharmacological Society, and perhaps he wanted them to clear it. The exact story is lost. What is known is that Rothlin had been aware that the four major Swiss companies had observers in Milan. He apparently was also sure that he could count on their support.

In any event, a few months later in Zurich, during the meeting of the 2nd World Congress of Psychiatry, Rothlin seemed to have succeeded in enlisting the support of these four companies and was ready to preside over CINP at its first meeting. While seeming to collaborate with the people who had been present at the Milan meeting, between the two meetings, Rothlin in fact handpicked the 33 individuals who were invited that evening to the buffet of the Zurich station.

The Constitution of the new association said that its members "shall meet from time to time to consider and discuss matters related to neuropsychopharmacology," promote the discipline all around the world, consult on the development of drugs, and advise official bodies.

Rothlin remained President through two terms, but internal squabbles led to the resignation of both secretaries, Herman Denber and Corneille Radouco-Thomas, at the time of the second congress in Basel two years later. Rothlin had an authoritarian personality, but in addition he had demanded central control over the finances. This did not sit well with some of the American members, who wanted money raised in the States to support the American delegation. At that meeting Paul Hoch became president, having been earlier president-elect. Born in Hungary, Hoch was at the time Commissioner of the Division of Mental Health in New York State. Hoch was followed as president by Hans Hoff (Austria), Jean Delay (France), F.G. Valdecasas (Spain), and Heinz Lehmann (Canada). Lehmann was the last president during the period covered in this volume.

In spite of the growing tension within the executive, the membership of the Collegium steadily increased during the 1960s (see Appendix: Membership). By 1979, the CINP had become a truly international organization with the ability to make a substantial difference in the development of the field. The proceedings of the congresses over these years provide a record of what happend.

In the following sections we present information on the growth and structure of the organization. Readers curious about how the balance of membership among the countries changed, or the composition of the executive body altered, will find much of interest. Readers can also follow the appearance and disappearance of the drugs talked about at CINP meetings, follow the shifts in the topics selected, and identify the chief players in drug development.

Memoirs of Fellows

RECOLLECTIONS OF THE FOUNDING OF CINP

Frank J. Ayd, Jr

When I received an invitation to participate in a meeting on psychotropic drugs that was to be held in Milan in May 1957, I was excited and challenged. I was excited by the prospect of exchanging ideas with colleagues from various parts of the world with whom I shared an engrossing interest in the newly developing fields of psychopharmacology and psycho-pharmacotherapy. I had the privilege of meeting some of these colleagues in 1956 when I toured psychiatric centres in England, Scotland, Belgium, Germany, Switzerland, France, and Italy, and I looked forward to another opportunity to exchange ideas and data with them.

I was challenged by the invitation because the meeting was to be held at the same time that one of my daughters would be making her first Holy Communion. I had vowed that I would never miss anything that was important to my children. Since, on the other hand, I did not want to miss the Milan meeting, I decided that I would take my wife, who was then pregnant

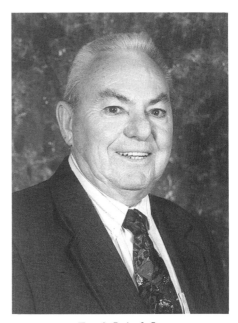

Frank J. Ayd, Jr.

with our eleventh child, and our daughter to Rome, where our daughter would receive her first Communion. Arrangements were made for the sacrament, and she received her first Communion in St. Peter's Basilica. My wife, my daughter, and I then had a private audience with His Holiness, Pope Pius XII. In addition, Mrs. Ayd and I were guests at a special celebration of the Pope's birthday. Hence, we went to Milan saturated with very happy memories.

Of all the Popes who have reigned in the Catholic Church, Pope Pius XII had the greatest interest in medicine. During his papacy, he addressed more medical groups and wrote more

Frank J. Ayd, Jr. is a pioneer in psychopharmacology, and one of the twelve founders of the American College of Neuropsychopharmacology. He is an internationally known psychiatrist, lecturer, and author of many publications including *Ayd's Lexicon of Psychiatry, Neurology, and the Neurosciences.* He is the recipient of numerous awards including the ACNP Paul Hoch Award (1988), the ACNP Distinguished Service Award (1993), and the Open Mind Award in Psychiatry presented by the Janssen Research Council.

Ayd was elected a fellow of the CINP in 1974. He presented papers on "A clinical analysis of the differential effects of phenothiazine derivatives" and on "Chlorpromazine: ten years' experience" at the 1st and 3rd Congresses, respectively.

on medicine, human research, and the ethics of medical practice than any of his predecessors. His addresses to medical gatherings and his writings on various aspects of the subject are published in a large tome. I was aware of this fact before the private audience that my wife, my daughter, and I had with him. Hence, I was not surprised when he asked me about the Milan meeting, which I told him that I was to attend. I shared with him the information I had, and at the conclusion of our private audience, I promised to let him know what transpired at the Milan symposium, a promise that I kept. For many reasons, I was very pleased that His Holiness accepted the invitation to address the First International Congress of the CINP, held in Rome in the next year from September 8 to 13, 1958.

The Milan meeting was as exciting and as educational as I had anticipated. Because of my readings and what I had learned in my tour of psychiatric centres in Europe a year earlier, I arrived in Milan cognizant of the fact that the years between 1951 and 1957 could best be characterized as probably the most chaotic in the annals of psychiatry and perhaps also of pharmacology. In those few years a plethora of neuroleptics had been synthesized, and many were being clinically evaluated. Also during that period, meprobamate, imipramine, iproniazid and other psychotropic drugs were being tested.

This cascade of psychoactive drugs resulted in prescriptions for millions of patients by physicians and psychiatrists, many of whom knew little or nothing about the nature of the illnesses they were treating, or of the pharmacology of the drugs they were prescribing. One must bear in mind that the first edition of the American Psychiatric Association's *Diagnostic and Statistical Manual* was published only two years before chlorpromazine and reserpine were approved for marketing by the Food and Drug Administration in the United States and five years before the discussion at Milan of the need for a collegium in neuropsychopharmacology.

In the early 1950s the number of residents in psychiatry was really quite small everywhere in the world. Furthermore, very few, if any, of these residents in training were being exposed to the principles and practice of biological psychiatry in more than an elementary way. At that time there was no generally accepted International Classification of Diseases, and diagnostic tests were limited to the Rorschach, the Minnesota Multiphasic Personality Inventory, the Wechsler, and a few other tests for organicity.

In the early days of psychopharmacology I was dismayed by the lack of communication between psychiatrists and pharmacologists and other scientists, despite an urgent need for such contact. Few psychiatrists knew pharmacologists interested in psychotropic drugs, and the latter therefore received scant feedback from the clinicians doing the preliminary research on the new psychopharmaceuticals. Precious little was known in the early years of psychopharmacotherapy about how to measure blood levels of these new drugs or about their pharmacokinetics and pharmacodynamics. Nor was there much known about the biological basis of psychiatric disorders. Ralph Gerard's sage aphorism that "Behind every twisted thought is a twisted molecule," was prescient of the advent of molecular psychiatry, which at the time of the founding of the CINP was dependent on concepts not yet verified.

Every pioneer in psychopharmacotherapy can attest that in the early years of psychopharmacology there was a marked resistance to such therapy by many leaders in psychiatry. In fact, many of the pioneers were ridiculed and denigrated by colleagues faithful to psychodynamic concepts about the etiology of psychiatric disorders and to the unproven efficacy of psychoanalytic psychotherapy.

When I journeyed to Milan for the spring 1957 meeting, I was very aware that what was diagnosed as schizophrenia in one part of the world would not be so diagnosed in another. I also was cognizant of the lack of skills in the emerging art and science of psychopharmacotherapy. In 1957, with little more than anecdotal case reports based on uncontrolled observational data, the pioneers in psychopharmacotherapy nevertheless became convinced of the potential benefits of its use, and persisted in their efforts to master the art and science of rational, safe, and effective prescribing.

During the few days of the Milan meeting, as I listened to colleagues primarily from Europe and North America, I was favourably impressed with their awareness of what needed to be done if psychiatric patients were to be the beneficiaries of psychopharmacotherapy. I was inspired by their determination to improve the care of those afflicted with psychiatric disorders, for whom, until the advent of the first psychotropics, little could be done. I was proud to have as mentors men of such stature, who, prior to the advent of chlorpromazine and reserpine, had devoted their energies and time to patients with very poor prognoses.

It is important to stress that the first patients treated with neuroleptics were chronically ill persons who had proved refractory to all prior therapies, psychological and physical. Not only had many spent a significant part of their lives as prisoners of psychoses for which there were no effective therapies, but they also were victims of the deteriorating effects of decades of institutionalization. When psychopharmacotherapy was in its nascence, the portals of the wards in many psychiatric hospitals could have had inscribed on them: "Abandon hope all ye who enter here." Happily for the hundreds of thousands of chronic psychotics and the many victims of other psychiatric disorders, most of the pioneers in psychopharmacology were astute clinicians. Their observations of the responses of these early patients formed the clinical and scientific basis of the advances of the next forty years.

By 1955 I had become convinced of the need for communication between psychiatrists and other scientists, a conviction that I expressed to as many colleagues as possible, especially during my 1956 tour through Europe. I soon realized that this need for communication was also recognized by many colleagues and by the pharmaceutical industry and governmental regulatory agencies. The growing acknowledgment that clinical researchers and basic scientists must be in better contact with one another was evident at the Milan meeting. Hence, I was pleasantly surprised when, during the gathering, it was announced that a special meeting would be held for those interested in exploring the founding of a society of psychopharmacologists, to be composed of psychiatrists, pharmacologists, psychologists, and others interested in psychopharmacology.

Most of those present at this special meeting favoured the formation of an organization open to all professionals interested in psychopharmacotherapy and psychopharmacology. However, Ernst Rothlin, a very influential man who at that time was president of the International Pharmacological Society, opposed the idea. He suggested that the establishment of a new college be postponed to September 1957, when the Second World Congress of Psychiatry would be held in Zurich. I was one of those who were disappointed that Rothlin's suggestion prevailed.

At the Milan meeting it was agreed that the founding session would be held in Zurich. But Professor Emilio Trabucchi declined an invitation to become president of the new organization. Rothlin then agreed to be its founding president. In the four months between the end of the Milan meeting in May 1957 and the opening of the Second World Congress of Psychiatry, a handful of men met regularly to formulate plans for the CINP. They made the decision to restrict membership in the organization to psychiatrists and pharmacologists involved in research with the new psychopharmaceuticals, a decision that was quite controversial; but again Rothlin prevailed.

I attended the Second World Congress of Psychiatry in Zurich. During this meeting a selected number of psychopharmacologists and other scientists received an invitation from Rothlin to a buffet dinner at the Zurich railway station. Among the invitees to this dinner were some who had attended and others who had not attended the Milan meeting. I did not receive an invitation to the dinner, but the next day I learned from friends who had been there that during the meal Rothlin had presented the attendees with a slate of officers which included himself as president and Professor Trabucchi as vice-president. The CINP was formed that night by a show of hands, and the decision was made that the first meeting would be held in Rome in September 1958.

There are those who think that politics played a major role in the founding of the CINP. There is some evidence to support this view. Nevertheless, those who were prominent in its establishment deserve our gratitude. The history of the organization also documents that Emilio Trabucchi, Silvio Garattini, and Corneille Radouco-Thomas warrant recognition as major contributors to its founding. In fact, the Milan meeting should be considered the point of origin of the CINP, and Radouco-Thomas should be given special credit for proposing that the new organization be named the Collegium Internationale Neuro-Psychopharmacologicum.

I also attended the first meeting of the CINP, held in Rome in September 1958, which was known as the First International Congress of Neuropsychopharmacology. It was a splendidly organized and executed scientific meeting that attracted several hundred psychiatrists, pharmacologists, psychologists, and other professionals from all parts of the world. It was impressive not only because of its organization, its elegant receptions at historic sites, and the special audience with Pope Pius XII at his summer residence, Castel Gandolfo, but also because of the quality of the diverse scientific presentations. The address delivered by the Pope at Castel Gandolfo was a remarkable demonstration of his knowledge of the new psychopharmaceuticals, the emergence of psychopharmacology, and the importance of these new developments in medicine and pharmacology for humankind (see Appendix: 1.1 Extract from Pope Pius XIIth's Address).

I left Rome convinced that I had participated in an historic conference at which, for the first time, large numbers of psychiatrists, pharmacologists, and other professionals had openly exchanged ideas that augured well for the future of biological theories about the etiology and treatment of psychiatric illnesses. I was proud to be a part of the CINP.

At the time, it was impossible for me to envision the impact these events would have on my personal and professional life. Since 1958 I have attended the majority of CINP meetings, and my life has been enriched by the hundreds of fine men and women whom I have come to count among my true friends.

RECOLLECTIONS OF THE FIRST CINP MEETING

Gerald J. Sarwer-Foner

There was a good rapport and friendship among the relatively small number of individuals working in psychopharmacology during the early days of the field. A considerable proportion of them met and presented papers at the Second World Congress of Psychiatry in Zurich in 1957, where Nathan Kline had organized, with the help of Jean Delay and Heinz Lehmann, a very comprehensive Psychopharmacology Symposium (1).

Henry Ey, Ewen Cameron, and Lopez-Ibor, Sr., were central to the planning and implementation of the World Psychiatric Association in the time that the new field of psychopharmacology emerged internationally. Since the spirit of worldwide scientific collaboration was alive and well, it did not seem strange to see the relatively small group of workers in psychopharmacology wanting to organize an international college for this rapidly developing discipline.

The Collegium Internationale Neuro-Psychopharmacologicum was founded on September 3, 1957 during the Second World Congress of Psychiatry in Zurich. A distinguished slate of officers were elected at the inaugural meeting; the decision was also reached that the Collegium would have its first international congress in Rome in 1958.

Thus, prospective members of the Collegium, including the North Americans, largely from the United States but with a good representation from Canada, went to Rome for this auspicious occasion. Some of us North Americans, including the late Hassan Azima, H.C.B. Denber, the late Nathan S. Kline, Sidney Malitz, and myself, had agreed prior to the meeting about where we would be staying in Rome.

I arrived several days before the meeting to check into a small room in the Hotel Grand Flora; Nathan Kline, next door at the Excelsior Hotel, had, with his usual panache, booked a suite. Many of us met, talked, and promenaded with friends and colleagues in front of the hotels for several days before the meeting opened on September 9th. European and British friends were seen, including Brian Ackner, the affable, courteous, and ever helpful Professor Frederick Mielke of Heidelberg, then working in Zurich, and other European colleagues.

Frederick Mielke was a particular friend, a man of great integrity and personal courage, who had dared, just after the Second World War, to raise the issue of medical war crimes in Germany. He had met most of us before, or during the Second World Congress in Zurich in 1957. Living there, he had been extremely

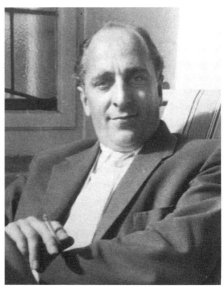

Frederick Mielke

helpful to all of the North Americans, including the late Leo Alexander.

The North Americans intermingled well with the British, European, and other participants. Mielke introduced me to German and Swiss colleagues with familiar names whom I had not previously met. It was a severe blow, several months after the meeting, to receive unexpectedly a letter from his family, informing me of his death from leukemia. But it was good to see him and be with him at this meeting, when Rome was beautiful, hospitable, and full of life.

On September 8th, through an American starlet friend of Nathan Kline, Mielke and I were invited to dinner in the Borghesi Gardens attended by that year's Italian film greats (including Anna Magnani of *Bitter Rice* fame). As a result, I got to bed late, slept in, and missed the opening ceremonies, which, as you will see, was just as well.

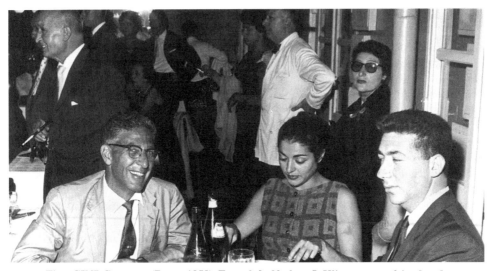

First CINP Congress (Rome 1958). From left: Nathan S. Kline, actress friend and Gerald J. Sarwer-Foner (right)

Several important professors were to give opening papers with profound commentary on the field. Professor Aubrey Lewis (he had not yet been knighted) of the Maudsley chaired the opening ceremonies. I had never had the opportunity to talk to him until then, though we had met in an off-hand way. Professor Lewis was an avid reader and a very erudite psychiatrist with a broad knowledge of the field. He was known for maintaining the highest standards of academic discussion, including its critical aspects. All of his colleagues, Professor D. Michael Shepherd, and their registrars bore testimony to this. Professor D. Ewen Cameron who was then chairman of the Department of Psychiatry, McGill University, was slated to give one of the main papers, a review of the current status of the field, for this opening ceremony.

The standard of scientific papers throughout the meeting was very high, as you would expect from these presenters. The meeting brought together clinicians, biochemists, geneticists, and basic scientists working in psychopharmacology, along with their older colleagues, who were well versed in psychiatry and who were incorporating the new data from neuro- and psycho-pharmacology. The interpersonal relationships were as important as the formal papers. Pharmacologists such as Alfred Pletscher and C. Radouco-Thomas rubbed shoulders with basic science researchers and research clinicians such as Turan Itil, Max Fink, Fritz Freyhan, Sidney Malitz, Seymour Kety, P. B. Bradley, and with European professors of note such as W. A. Stoll and J. Odegard. Henry Brill's importance was widely recognized for having put into place for the entire New York State Mental Hospitals System both the clinical (inpatient and outpatient) and the research structures of the new psychopharmacology. Professor Linford W. Rees was another British professor of note who knew many of us well.

The importance of the new Collegium was recognized by His Holiness, Pope Pius XII, who received the Collegium members in a special gathering at his summer palace, Castel Gandolfo. The Catholics occupied, by mutual consent of their colleagues, the first four rows from which they were greeted by the Pontiff along with the officers of the Collegium. This was a moving experience for everyone.

A condensed version of my own paper on "Some Psychodynamic and Neurological Aspects of Paradoxical Behavioral Reactions" was published as part of the "Proceedings" of this meeting in *Neuropsychopharmacology*, edited by Bradley, Deniker, and Radouco-Thomas (2).

The scope and extent of neuropsychopharmacology had already been very evident in Zurich but its rapid progression was even clearer at this meeting. We all knew that this new Collegium Internationale would quickly grow and prosper.

At the end of the meeting, I found myself at the Rome Airport with Professor Aubrey Lewis, flying to London, and we sat down and talked together. After a while he said "Tell me, how do you pronounce your name?" I told him, and he said, "Curious: that's how I pronounced it." He explained that he, as chairman of the opening session, after Professor D. Ewen Cameron's address, asked, "Would Dr. Sarwer-Foner care to discuss this paper?" and when there was silence Lewis asked Professor Cameron, "Did I say that right?" Cameron said, "What?" and he said, "You know, Sarwer-Foner, that man in your Department," to which the reply was "Oh, yes." Lewis looked at me expectantly.

This broke the ice. I felt completely at ease with him, sensing his underlying empathy and kindness. I then told him that after completion of my residency training I became a junior member of Cameron's department at McGill where I worked first as consultant in psychiatry and quickly became Director of Psychiatric Research at Queen Mary Veterans–Montreal's military hospital under Travis Dancey's direction. At the time, though possibly familiar with my scientific work, Cameron had little personal contact with me. Actually, Cameron may not have liked the idea of a junior member of his department discussing his review of the field paper. I consider it, therefore, a happy accident that I had missed the opening session.

Professor Lewis listened with sympathy, some laughter, understanding, and warmth. This was the beginning of a bond between us. He always received me cordially, and we remained friendly for the rest of his life.

I am happy to say that Cameron and I became friends as he got to know me personally and followed my progress. I left McGill, as an associate professor of psychiatry and director of psychiatry at one of the teaching hospitals (the Queen Elizabeth), to become professor of psychiatry and director of the Department of Psychiatry, Ottawa General Hospital, at the University of Ottawa, Faculty of Medicine, on January 1, 1971.

I was elected fellow of the Collegium in 1962, when Paul Hoch was President, Hans Hoff president elect and Pierre Deniker our first councillor. In the Collegium my most valuable contribution lay, perhaps, in liaison and consultation roles with the French, British and Irish in particular. I also worked with other Europeans (Italian, Scandinavian, German, Swiss, Greek, and Yugoslavian) members as well as with Australian, New Zealand, Indian, Japanese and Yugoslavian) members as well as with Australian, New Zealand, Indian, Japanese, and African colleagues. In this regard, I helped many who sought training in psychiatry to come to McGill. I played a significant role in relating their work to ours in North America, inviting them onto scientific programs, and to present papers, as well as facilitating friendly collaborations through meeting Canadian and American colleagues. Much of this related to scientific meetings of such groups as the American Psychiatric Association, the Canadian Psychiatric Association, the Quebec Psychiatric Association, and international gatherings as well as those of the Collegium.

At the World Congress of Psychiatry in Montreal in 1961, where I was a member of the organizing committee, I was delegated to greet the chartered aircraft bringing the French scientists to the Quebec meeting of the Collegium. These activities, undoubtedly, had some influence on my being named in 1974 to chair of the Scientific Program Committee of the 6th World Congress of Psychiatry, Honolulu, 1977.

I enjoyed acting as interpreter, friend, and guide to Professor Jean Delay when he presided at the Washington meeting of the CINP, and later I chaired the symposium at the American Psychiatric Association's meeting, with Pierre Deniker as vice chairman, on "Therapeutic Agents Available in France But Not yet Available in The United States." These are small examples of ongoing friendships and liaison activities with my fellow psychiatrists and researchers in the neurosciences, a significant number of whom I first met and worked with in the early days of the Collegium Internationale Neuro-Psychopharmacologicum.

REFERENCES

1. Kline, N.S. (ed.) (1959). Psychopharmacology Frontiers: Proceedings of the Psychopharmacology Symposium of the 2nd International Congress of Psychiatry, Zurich 1957 (533 pages). Boston: Little Brown & Co.

2. Sarwer-Foner, G.J., (1959). Some psychodynamic and neurological aspects of the "paradoxical behavioral reactions," presented at the 1st International Congress of the Collegium Internationale Neuropsychopharmacologicum, Rome, Italy, Sept. 9-13, 1958. In P.B. Bradley, P. Deniker, and C. Radoucco-Thomas (eds.). Neuropsychopharmacology (Vol. I. pp. 680-682), Amsterdam: North Holland Publishing Co.

THE BIRTH OF THE CINP: FROM MILAN TO ZURICH

Jean Thuillier

THE MILAN SYMPOSIUM

In May 1957, Professor Emilio Trabucchi organized an international symposium on psychotropic drugs. The meeting was held in Milan and attended by several hundred experts of the new field from all around the world.

It was on the morning of May 11, 1957, while Rothlin, Trabucchi, Deniker, Denber, and I were having breakfast together, that we began to contemplate the founding of a society that could facilitate communication between clinical psychiatrists and pharmacologists, as had been done so effectively at the Milan Symposium.

Ernst Rothlin was receptive to the idea and was confident that he could secure the necessary support from the four major Swiss pharmaceutical companies with headquarters in Basel, i.e., Sandoz, the company of which he was the scientific director, Hoffmann LaRoche, CIBA, and Geigy. These four companies,

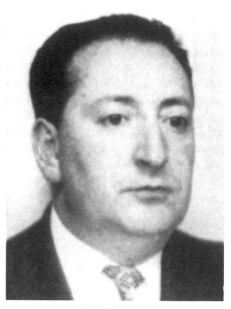

Jean Thuillier

Jean Thuillier is the former head of clinical psychiatry at Sainte-Anne's Hospital in Paris. With an interest in bridging psychiatry and pharmacology, he was first to set up an experimental psychiatry laboratory in 1950. He was director of INSERM's first neuropsychopharmacology laboratory and the founding president of the European Federation of Medicinal Chemistry.

Thuillier is one of the founders of the CINP and served as treasurer on the 3rd and 4th Executives. He presented papers on "Utilisation des rats gyrostatiques pour les essais de drogues psychotropes" (Thuillier et Nakajima), on "Antagonisme central et périphérique. Étude de l'ester dimethylaminoéthylique de l'acide p-chlorophenoxyacétique (Centrophenoxine)" (Thuillier et Nakajima), and on "Étude neuropharmacologique de la p-fluorophenylsulfone (Fluorésone)" (Thuillier, Rumpf, and G. Thuillier) at the 1st, 2nd, and 3rd Congresses respectively. He coauthored papers on "Inactivation de la serotonine par la ceruloplasmine. Influence des drogues psychotropes sur cette réaction" (Nakajima and Thuillier), and on "Inhibition in vivo du pouvoir oxydatif du sérum par des drogues agissant sur l'hypothalamus (reserpine, ascorbate de reserpine, Centrophenoxine)" (Nakajima et Thuillier) at the 1st and 2nd Congresses respectively. He was a formal discussant of the third Symposium (Comparison of abnormal behavioural states induced by psychotropic drugs in animals and man) at the 1st Congress, and of the 1st Symposium (The problem of antagonists to psychotropic drugs) at the 2nd Congress.

which together represented over 10 percent of the world's output of pharmaceutical products, were already involved in psychotropic research and had all sent observers to the Milan symposium.

We decided that the new society should be inaugurated during the Second World Congress of Psychiatry, which was to be held in Zurich from September 1 to September 6 in that year. Thus we had little more than three months to prepare the statutes of the prospective society and to convene the inaugural meeting which was to be attended by a selected group of psychiatrists and pharmacologists. The new society was to be called the Collegium Internationale Neuro-Psychopharmacologicum. We had already come to think of it, however, as the CINP.

THE ZURICH CONGRESS

The Zurich Congress had a large attendance, including many of the key figures of American psychiatry. Rothlin was president of the congress and C.C. Jung was chairman of the session on psychotropic drugs.

As the head of clinical and pharmacological research of Sandoz, Rothlin was primarily responsible for the company's significant growth in those years. His work on ergot alkaloids had helped to increase the revenues of the company considerably; about the time of the founding of the CINP, the revenues of Sandoz were still on the increase. As was the case with many of the researchers working with the international pharmaceutical industry in Basel, Rothlin had travelled around the world several times, visiting company affiliates, research centres, and universities. He spoke seven languages fluently, a skill that helped him in conducting international business.

In following up the decisions reached during the Milan symposium, Rothlin had prepared the statutes of the Collegium, and forwarded them to Denber, Deniker, Trabucchi, and me. As someone who was used to acting independently, he had already decided, based on the preliminary list of attendees, who would be invited to the founders' meeting. He had also asked each of us, as well as Kline, Rinkel, and Denber for input in general, but espcially regarding our respective countries.

We had decided to limit membership in the Collegium to those psychiatrists and pharmacologists who had demonstrated experience with the new drugs. The selection of psychiatrists was simple, but the choice of pharmacologists presented some difficulty. As expected, there were some highly animated discussions. Emilio Trabucchi, who came by train from Milan, had brought his own impressive list of names. He wanted to keep the doors wide open and admit everybody into the Collegium, maintaining that it was the only way to raise awareness of this new discipline.

Trabucchi always spoke French or Italian during our meetings, since he had virtually no knowledge of any other language. Whenever he was not satisfied with a suggestion, he would first smile and say that it was very good, and then follow with a long explanation of why he found it unacceptable. Things sorted themselves out in the end, however.

Following a preliminary meeting at which we reached a consensus, it was decided to hold the CINP's inaugural meeting in the buffet of the Zurich train station. Rothlin had told us that the food was good and inexpensive there. Meanwhile, everyone who was selected to be invited received their personal invitation for the dinner. The event took place on September 9, at 8:30 p.m., and the meal was followed by Rothlin's speech, in which he gave an account of events relevant to the dinner invitation and the prospective founding of the society which was to become the CINP. He expressed his thanks to Trabucchi, Deniker, Denber, and me. He repeated his speech in French, German, Italian, and Spanish. By the time he reached the end, a few people were yawning.

The attendees were called upon to indicate, by a show of hands, their acceptance of the invitation to become founding members of the Collegium. A second vote was held to confirm the adoption of the statutes and the election of the executive committee, on which I was to serve. The vote for both was unanimous.

Some attendees felt that the name Collegium Internationale Neuro-Psychopharmacologicum was too long, and the use of Latin obsolete. Finally, it was decided that the first congress of the Collegium would be held in the next year (1958).

Once again, Emilio Trabucchi proposed Italy as a venue, declaring that we would be welcomed in Rome with open arms. The exceptional organization of the Milan Symposium was sufficient reason for us to accept his proposal. As an expression of our appreciation and respect, as well as to facilitate the official procedures, he was unanimously elected chairman of the organizing committee of the first CINP congress.

In so far as I was concerned, I was quite happy. As both a psychiatrist and a pharmacologist, I could fully appreciate what was taking place. I was witnessing the founding of a society which was to serve the reuniting of psychiatry with traditional medicine. As one of the first researchers working in the field, I found it exciting to be surrounded by such a large number of my fellow psychopharmacologists.

NOTES FROM ANOTHER TIME AND PLACE

Herman C.B. Denber

I had been in family practice for about three years (1947 to 1950), when I realized that 80 percent of my patients really required the services of a psychiatrist. At that time, psychiatry was riding high in the medical world, and on February 1, 1950, I began a psychiatric residency at Manhattan State Hospital in New York. I had done research as a medical student some years before, and since I was interested in becoming engaged in research again, I was pleased to see that psychiatry opened up a vast horizon for original investigations.

Shortly after Heinz Lehmann's presentation on chlorpromazine, which created great excitement at the meeting of the American Psychiatric Association in 1953, I was visited by the late Bill Kirsch from Smith, Kline and French to discuss the implementation of a study with chlorpromazine at Manhattan State Hospital. Interestingly enough, he had just come from a visit to Cornell Medical School, where little interest was expressed in his new compound. (It should be noted here that academia in the United States at the time was strictly psycho-analytically-oriented with almost all the heads of departments psychoanalysts, and the training programs so oriented).

Subsequent to Bill Kirsch's visit, I conducted a study with chlorpromazine in 1500 patients with the help of two assistants. It was the largest sample of patients treated with chlorpromazine for investigational purposes in the United States and yielded "extraordinary changes" in the hospital environment. By the time it was completed, the "agitated wards" at Manhattan State Hospital were no longer "agitated." Our striking results became the subject of an article in *Life* magazine and a television program of the National Broadcasting Corporation (NBC).

Herman C.B. Denber was born, brought up, and educated in New York City, graduated from New York University (A.B., 1938), and earned his MD from the University of Geneva Faculty of Medicine in 1943. He also received an MS (1963) and PhD (1967) from New York University. After three years in family practice, he began a psychiatric residency at Manhattan State Hospital in 1950, where he was named Director of Psychiatric Research five years later. The major thrust of the research program was in psychopharmacology and molecular biology. In 1972 he completed psychoanalytic training with the American Institute of Psychoanalysis and was subsequently affiliated with medical schools at the universities of Lausanne, Florida, Louisville, and Ottawa. He retired in 1982.

Denber was a founding member of the CINP and served as secretary of the 1st and 2nd Executives. He presented papers on "Biochemical findings during the mescaline-induced state, with observations on the blocking action of different psychotropic drugs"; on "Comparative analysis of drug trials in Europe and the United States"; on "Clinical response to pharmacotherapy in different settings"; on "Molecular biology and psychiatry" (Denber and Teller), and on "Studies on mescaline XX: comparative effects of phenothiazines, amphetamine and amobarbital sodium on C^{14}-mescaline content in the rat brain after intravenous or intraperitoneal injection" (Denber and Teller) at the 2nd, 3rd, 5th, and 6th Congresses, respectively. He co-authored a paper on "Binding of psychotropic drugs to soluble proteins" (Teller and Denber), presented at the 5th Congress.

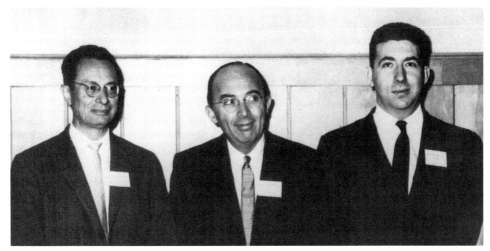

From left: Daniel Ginestet, Herman C. B. Denber and Gerald J. Sarwer-Foner

The price for the extraordinarily successful treatment was side effects, including extrapyramidal reactions, skin rash, and icterus, and we noted that they were encountered in a considerably higher proportion of patients than reported in the European literature. The dosage might have been an explanation. But even if the American dosages differed greatly from the English, they were rather close to the French. To pursue matters further, one day in 1954 Henry Brill, the associate commissioner of mental hygiene for research in New York, called me to suggest that I make a three-country tour of Europe (England, France, and Switzerland) to meet the various research groups who had worked with chlorpromazine and discuss the findings with them.

It was in 1957, about one year after the trip which followed Brill's call, that I attended the International Conference on Psychotropic Drugs in Milan, presided over by Emilio Trabucchi. The sessions were very exciting and the atmosphere charged as speaker after speaker described results with the new drugs that had never been seen before. Some of us, Corneille Raduoco-Thomas, Jean Thuillier, Philip Bradley, Ernst Rothlin, with two or three others, met to discuss the need for a group that would come together regularly to talk about current research, and decided to form a society devoted to the new drugs in psychiatry. We felt that it should be a fairly small group (the number originally chosen was two hundred) which would meet each year in a different city in Europe or the United States.

Final plans were drawn up later on in the year (1957) at the 2nd World Congress of Psychiatric in Zurich, Switzerland. An executive committee was formed, and at my insistence, Pierre Deniker was included. The presidency was offered to Professor Trabucchi, but he declined and eventually Ernst Rothlin assumed the chair. Raduoco-Thomas and I became the secretaries.

A word about the name: originally, we believed that the group should be called the International Collegium for Psychopharmacology. However, Professor Rothlin argued that eventually neurologists would become members, and he suggested the term "neuropsychopharmacology." He was unrelenting on the question, and finally the name Collegium Internationale Neuro-Psychopharmacologicum (CINP) was adopted.

There was some discussion about the possibility of creating a journal of psychopharmacology through the Collegium. While this was endorsed by the Executive, there were dissenting voices from some of the more senior members, each of whom also apparently nurtured the idea of a journal. This was made clear some years later when several journals of psychopharmacology were launched.

The first CINP meeting, which was held in Rome in 1958, was an outstanding success. The executive committee charged me with inviting American and Canadian participants, while Radouco-Thomas issued the invitations for Europe. The program decided by the executive encompassed a wide range of subjects pertaining to the new field of psychopharmacology. The various symposia and original papers generated a great deal of enthusiasm, and the demand for membership grew. At the same time, various problems began to develop. Since the American contingent was the largest and had the firmest financial support, there were demands that these monies be sent to the central office and placed under Rothlin's direction. Many members wanted their colleagues to be included and were hurt when they did not succeed with their request. Although the original aim was to restrict membership to two hundred, it was soon clear that this rule would have to be changed, and it eventually was.

The executive committee initially met between one and four times a year since there were innumerable issues to be discussed and acted upon. These meetings, led by Rothlin, were occasionally acrimonious, and some problems were really never solved to the satisfaction of the committee members. Eventually, at the Basel meeting in 1960, a new executive committee was formed. Lacking support from the more senior members of the Collegium, Raduoco-Thomas and I stepped down. In the years which followed, I have withdrawn more and more from the affairs of the Collegium, even from participation in its various Congresses, of which I was one of the founders.

It was a great privilege to have been part of the initial executive committee of the CINP. From this vantage point it was possible to observe the rapid advances in the new field of psychopharmacology. In retrospect, I think that the choice of subjects for the first several CINP meetings accurately reflected the state of the art at the time. The committee as a whole was very much aware of the research underway in various European and North American centres and the direction these studies were taking. The programs for the Congresses were structured to reflect this research.

It is interesting to observe current events in light of past history. I often wonder what would have happened if chlorpromazine had been introduced today and to what degree regulatory agencies would have interfered with the development of new psychotropic compounds. Psychopharmacological studies in the 1950s and 1960s do not resemble those of the 1990s. Clinical observations were primary, and double-blind trials as we know them today were neither required nor done. Informed consent was unknown. With legal staffs in all state hospitals today, I shudder at the thought of securing informed consent from a psychotic, or even a non-psychotic patient and the family. There were no institutional review boards to pass through, with their sometimes interminable waiting periods, and initiation of a study resulted from discussion between the investigator and the sponsor. Initially, there were no rating scales either, and reports were given in a narrative fashion (from which I believe one gets a much better idea of clinical drug action than from the "p" values, "chi square," and so on). Very little laboratory work accompanied drug trials, since it was not required. Various investigators had their own interests, such as psychological testing, EEG, and biochemistry (hepatic profiles).

It was only after some cases of agranulocytosis were observed that greater attention was paid to the leucocyte count.

In view of the newness of the field, its vast therapeutic potential, and general staff interest, initiation of a drug trial was not very difficult, although one must remember that psychoanalysis was still considered to be *the* treatment for mental illness. Since I was in psychoanalytic training at the time, I could look at both sides of the coin. There were always naysayers, but in the face of something new, such was to be expected. Presentation at meetings and the publication of results were no problem: there were no peer reviews, and the editor's decision was final. It was generally known that efforts were constantly being made to influence the content of reports. Frequently, sponsors offered to "write the paper for" the researcher. My reply was always, "If I sign it, I write it."

Everything changed in 1962 with the thalidomide episode. I still remember the meeting in Washington at which Frances Kelsey spoke, telling how she had not passed thalidomide. It was clear that this was not done for any specific reason; rather, bureaucratic inertia had carried the day. Since that time the FDA has become an integral partner in all new drug investigations, asking for more and more "supportive evidence." It also approves (or not) the study protocols. The question I always ask myself is, "Has all this improved therapeutic drug research?" The recent episode in which dexfenfluramine was ordered withdrawn from use in spite of multiple "safeguards" should give us much to think about. As I wrote in my *Textbook of Clinical Psychopharmacology*: "There are no safe drugs; only safe doctors."

I have lived through a stimulating time, a time whose excitement has now ended. I think that the next important period will begin when the membrane defects in mental illness are determined. The CINP will continue to move forward and upward as younger investigators and clinicians enter the field. I believe, however, that the final answers will come from the laboratory and will be tested on the wards.

A WOMAN PSYCHOPHARMACOLOGIST IN THE CINP: VICE-PRESIDENT OF THE SEVENTH EXECUTIVE

Hannah Steinberg

Although I had been closely involved in the CINP from the beginning and knew the main *dramatis personae,* I did not seek office or membership of committees and probably wouldn't have succeeded if I had, since I was, for some years, more or less the only woman scientist who was not regarded as an "assistant." To begin with, the CINP was very much a male kingdom, and I have a sneaking feeling that for a long time the most important decisions were made in the privacy of the men's loo. Interestingly, an affectionate obituary for Paul Hoch by Fritz Freyhan at the Birmingham Congress in 1964 about a proposed Hoch memorial review lecture ends with the recommendation, "let the lecturer be a *man* [my italics], who can keep alive this legacy..." Fortunately things have moved on a bit.

There was one ghastly general meeting at the 2nd Congress in Basel, where *inter alia* major differences of opinion were aired between a group of people at the front left and another at the top right of a steeply-raked lecture theatre. As far as I could gather, it was to do with who should be the next president. Professor Deniker (of chlorpromazine fame together with Delay) was proposed several times and each time responded with an emphatic, "Je ne suis pas candidat." A noisy shouting and desk-banging match took over the meeting for some time, all of which was probably just the sporadic airing of national and international competition. Apparently Deniker did not regard it as etiquette to become president until after Delay, who was senior to him, held this position. I was sitting next to Professor (later Sir) Jack Gaddum, who was quite distressed by so much shouting and squabbling. He was one of our special guest speakers, and I heard him ask repeatedly, "What am I doing here?" However, peace was eventually restored and Professor Paul Hoch was elected unopposed, with Professor Hans Hoff as president-elect. Professor Delay, he of chlorpromazine, poetry and the French Academy sword, did in fact become president in 1966.

Some years later I found myself a vice-president (unsure whether I was elected or appointed) and admitted to the inner councils of the Collegium. This was most interesting and gave me various splendid "working lunches." I soon learnt that, in most of the discussions – though officially they were about trends, finance, membership, meeting venues and programs – the most important underlying issues were prestige and status, i.e., who should hold office or be allowed to organize, chair, and edit symposia and other meetings. In an interdisciplinary and international organization it was obviously vital to achieve a fair balance, and my impression was that after a certain amount of horse-trading they got it more or less right; obviously members of the executive and committees had an inbuilt advantage, and lesser lights were often disappointed, especially as the membership grew larger and the meetings not much longer, with plenty of parallel sessions.

The politics of science have never had much appeal for me and I did not think that I was particularly good at them. I was therefore surprised and pleased to be asked to co-organize and chair a symposium at the ninth Congress in Paris in 1974. My French counterpart and I got on well. One preliminary committee meeting had to be held in an airport lounge in Germany, and on a Sunday. It got pretty argumentative, with some members reverting to their mother tongue (luckily I could manage French and German as well as English) and talking at cross purposes. Also it was getting dark and we all had planes to catch, and so in desperation I resorted to Latin "in nocte concilium" and we agreed and broke up soon after that.

Paris might have been my last CINP meeting. Four years earlier, in 1970, I had become Europe's first Professor of Psychopharmacology and continued research work with colleagues and students, especially on opiate dependence and lithium, for both of which we developed successful rodent models. But the climate in my home faculty had changed as a result of new appointments who

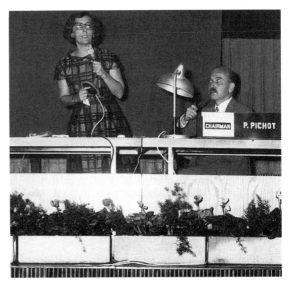

Hannah Steinberg (lecturing) and Pierre Pichot (chairing)

were most interested in classical pharmacology and not particularly sympathetic to psychopharmacology or me. As a result I could never invite a CINP meeting or even a distinguished guest lecturer to London and reciprocate the warm hospitality which I had received from so many others in many countries and which would have given us more prominence within the CINP.

Thus for our new work we turned to other outlets nearer home, which luckily were plentiful, even if our resources were not. One Friday 13th, Elizabeth Sykes, Christina Davies, Clare Stanford and I made an unexpected discovery. Since our interest in behavioural effects of drug combinations was now easier to satisfy because of the development of proper computers, we co-administered an antidepressant with a benzodiazepine. This may have seemed an odd combination at the time, (despite the existence of "Limbitrol," Roche), but we learnt later that it was common to conduct clinical trials of antidepressants with "drug-free" patients who were nevertheless allowed their nightly benzodiazepine to help them sleep! We were somewhat startled by this state of affairs, which was not usually mentioned in publications, but also of course pleased, since it gave a human dimension to our rodent work. Anyway, what happened to our mice with particular mixtures of the two kinds of drug was that they energetically and conspicuously walked backwards (1).

Elizabeth Sykes and I were invited back by Professor Netter of Giessen University to present this work to a symposium at the sixteenth CINP Congress in Munich. This was most successful and made us feel that we were back in the swing. A good deal of this work is still to be fully published (2,3). We hope that we are correct in thinking that it has widespread implications (4).

To return to the Executive, I have to admit that, partly because of being female and partly because of my lack of clout in London, I never regarded myself as particularly influential at meetings (as for example Philip Bradley was with ease), though I enjoyed discussions and sometimes won a point. My main concern was then, as it is now, that organizations should be open, especially to young people, and not become cabals of a few favoured colleagues who are "on the inside," as the song goes, with the hungry commoners being allowed glimpses from without. Because CINP quite rightly moved its meetings all over the world, travel to them was often costly and travel funds were and are increasingly scarce. So, unless one had an invitation, many young budding and existing members could not afford membership fees or meetings.

I have the impression that the CINP is still wrestling with these problems, especially since there are now several European and regional psychopharmacology societies of which the British Association for Psychopharmacology (BAP), the European College of Neuropsychopharmacology (ECNP) and the European Behavioural Pharmacology Society (EBPS) are successful examples. Nonetheless, and despite the international telecommunication revolution, with its Internet, video conferencing and such – like CINP retains the distinction of having been first in the field and is likely to remain the international forum from which much honey flows.

REFERENCES
1. Stanford, C. Steinberg, H., Sykes, E.A. and Davies, C.E. (1986). Backward walking unaccompanied by other components of the 5HT syndrome. *Brit. Assoc. Psychophamacol.* Abstract C24.
2. Davies, C.E., Stanford, C., Steinberg, H. and Sykes, E.A. (1986). Unusual behavioural and binding effects after coadministration of denbuterol and chlordiazepoxide in mice. *Brit. J. Pharmac.* 9:531-61.
3. Steinberg, H., Stanford, C., Sykes, E.A. and Davies, C.E. (1986). Antidepressants and chlordiazepoxide cause backward walking. *Psychopharmacology* 89:S35
4. Hughes, M., Sykes, E.A. and Steinberg, H. (1992). Drug interactions represented by high resolution computer graphics. *Neuroreport* 3:625-628.

COMMENTS FROM THE PRESIDENT OF THE
SEVENTH EXECUTIVE

Heinz E. Lehmann

I don't remember many details of my presidency of the CINP in 1970, but I do recall that, at the time, I was rather unwilling to accept this position. It was, of course, a great honour to be chosen for it from among the world's leading experts in psychopharmacology, but frankly, I do not even remember the procedure for the choice. Was there a vote? And if there were voters at that time, were they only the members of the council or the whole membership? Or was there just a gentlemanly discussion ending in a final consensus? Something like that must have taken place in order to agree on the candidates.

I was not an eager candidate. For one thing, I had a lot of work to do at home: my research and clinical work at the hospital, much travelling as a member of the Canadian Royal Commission on the Non-medical Use of Drugs, and taking over the chairmanship of the Department of Psychiatry at McGill University. (If I remember right, I had said to the dean, when he told me that I was the leading candidate for the post, that I needed to be chairman of the department "like a hole in the head" – but I had finally accepted it.)

The main reason for my reluctance to accept executive positions was that I never liked administrative work, that I knew little about it and was not good at it. What I did not know was that I would be under much political pressure to accept the presidency of the CINP in 1970, the first time that our meeting would take place in a city behind the Iron Curtain, in Prague. In the midst of the Cold War, that was a rather daring plan.

You see, I was a Canadian. And Canada had the reputation of being a quiet, civilized, but somewhat bland and dull country that did not threaten anyone – some thought it was perhaps a wimpy country – and it roused little hostility anywhere. Nor did it provoke much political jealousy in other countries. That was a rather unique position. On the other hand, candidates

Heinz E. Lehmann is emeritus professor of psychiatry of McGill University. Born and educated in Germany, he published the first paper on chlorpromazine in the English language. Recipient of the Lasker Award, the Order of Canada and numerous other distinctions, Lehmann was chairman of the Department of Psychiatry at McGill and served as president of both the International and American College of Neuropsychopharmacology.

Heinz E. Lehmann is an honorary fellow of the CINP; he was elected a fellow in 1958. Lehmann was President of the 7th Executive and delivered his presidential address on "Crises and conflicts in neuropsychopharmacology" at the Prague Congress in 1970. He presented papers on "Measurement of changes in human behaviour under the effects of psychotropic drugs" (Lehmann and Knight), on "Differences in behavioural effects in humans" and on "Tranquillizers: clinical insufficiencies and needs" at the 2nd, 5th, and 6th Congresses respectively. He coauthored a paper on "Predictors of therapeutic responsivity to thiothixene in schizophrenics" (Ban, Lehmann, Sterlin and Saxena) at the 6th Congress and was a formal discussant in Working Group 6 (Dynamics and significance of psychopharmacological intervention in psychiatry) at the 4th Congress.

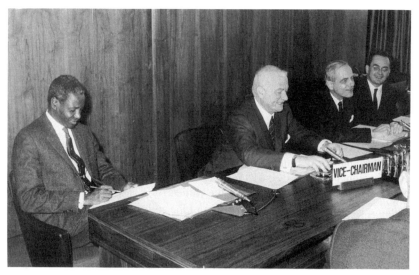

Working group at WHO.
From left: Thomas Lambo, Pierre Deniker, Heinz E. Lehmann and Boris Lebedev

for the presidency from the European countries and the United States had a lot of difficulties with each other. In fact they had much more than I ever dreamed of, although I was not entirely naive about the issue either. "For God's sake, not that person from ... – they are all so unbearably arrogant" ... "That country thinks they are the only ones who always know what's right" ... "Those people have been pushy all along. What do they want to prove?" ... "A president from ... at our first meeting behind the Iron Curtain? Impossible!" ... "That country has not got anyone who really knows anything" ... "That country again?!"

I don't remember who said what about which country – and I would not tell if I did remember – but that was what I heard when a representative of the maligned country was not in the room. Apparently, few people on the council bad-mouthed Canada. So, *faute de mieux,* I was elected. Nothing personal, just business. The Czechs gave us a fine reception. I remember two trumpeters, one standing on each side of me, at the opening ceremony. I remember Prague, the beautiful city – and the huge holes in the pavements, the magnificent buildings that needed sandblasting badly, and the people on the street with expressions of a mix of suspicion and sadness. Taking it all together, our meeting in Prague was more of an emotional experience than a scientific one. At least for me.

The   Collegium

THE FOUNDERS

Ernst Rothlin's thirty-three invited guests to the "buffet dinner" at the Zurich Railway station (September 3, 1957) became the Founders of CINP.

At the time of founding, CINP was a European-American organization with twenty-four of its thirty-three founders from Europe and nine from the Americas:

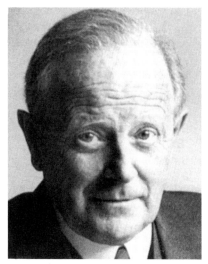

Ernst Rothlin

COUNTRY	NUMBER	WORK
France	5	Clinicians: 5
United Kingdom	4	Clinicians: 3
		Basic Scientist: 1
United States	4	Clinicians: 3
		Basic Scientist: 1
Canada	3	Clinicians: 3
Italy	3	Clinician: 1
		Basic Scientists: 2
The Netherlands	3	Clinicians: 3
Switzerland	3	Clinician: 1
		Basic Scientists: 2
Austria	2	Clinicians: 2
Germany	2	Clinicians: 2
Venezuela	1	Clinician: 1
Denmark	1	Clinician: 1
Norway	1	Clinician: 1
Peru	1	Clinician: 1

Although one of CINP's main objectives was the facilitation of communication among the disciplines involved, the founders' group consisted mainly of clinicians (27 of 33) with or without academic affiliation, and only a few pure basic scientists (6 of 33). And even from the very limited number of basic researchers, one was a drug company executive.

Information on founders' country representation, and work are given in Appendix 2.3.

THE MEMBERSHIP

During the period from 1957 to 1970 the membership of the CINP grew ten-fold. Because of missing records it was not possible to establish with any certainty when 139 of the members were elected. However, based on existing records, by 1970 CINP had 341 members.

COUNTRY	1957	1958	1960	1962	1964	1966	1968	1970	N/A
Australia				1	1	1	1	1	2
Austria	2	2	2	2	3	4	4	4	6
Belgium				1	2	2	2	3	6
Brazil									4
Bulgaria							1	1	2
Canada	3	4	4	6	6	6	8	9	12
Ceylon									1
Czechoslovakia				1	1	4	4	7	7
Denmark	1	2	2	3	3	4	4	4	14
Finland									1
France	5	10	10	16	19	22	24	25	37
Germany	2	2	2	12	15	18	18	19	34
Great Britain	4	5	5	6	10	11	13	17	31
Hong Kong						1	1	1	1
Hungary				1	1	1	1	1	2
India								1	1
Ireland					1	1	1	1	1
Israel							1	1	1
Italy	3	5	5	7	8	11	13	13	19
Japan				1	1	1	1	1	4
Mexico									1
Netherlands	3	3	3	3	3	4	5	5	5
Norway	1	1	1	1	1	1	1	1	2
Peru	1	1	1	2	2	2	2	2	2
Poland				1	1	1	1	1	1
Portugal									2
Romania									1
Spain									6
Sweden		2	2	5	5	6	6	6	10
Switzerland	3	6	6	6	8	11	13	15	26
Turkey									1
United States	4	21	23	34	35	43	51	60	95
Venezuela	1	1	1	1	1	1	1	1	1
Yugoslavia						1	1	2	2
TOTAL:	*33*	*65*	*67*	*110*	*127*	*157*	*178*	*202*	*341*

Thirty-four countries were represented, with the largest number from the United States (95 members), followed by France (37 members), Germany (34 members), Great Britain (31 members), Switzerland (26 members), Italy (19 members), Denmark (14 members), Canada (12 members) and Sweden (10 members).

Almost one-third of the total membership of CINP was from the United States, and well over two-thirds came from the United States, France, Germany and Great Britain together.

Further details regarding CINP membership, in terms of the country representation and year of election to membership, are given in Appendix 2.4.

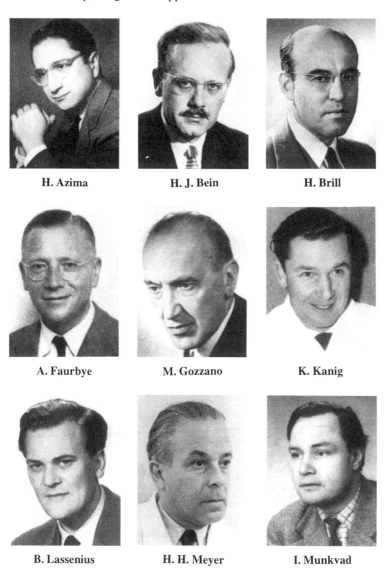

H. Azima   H. J. Bein   H. Brill

A. Faurbye   M. Gozzano   K. Kanig

B. Lassenius   H. H. Meyer   I. Munkvad

THE EXECUTIVES

Between 1957 and 1970 the Collegium had seven Executive Committees with forty-two members serving as Officers for a total of seventy-seven times.

In terms of the country representation of its Executives, the CINP was a European-North American organization from 1957 to 1970. During that period thirty-nine of the forty-two members serving as Officers and seventy-four of the seventy-seven Officers on the Executive came from Europe (30 and 54 respectively) and North America (9 and 20 respectively):

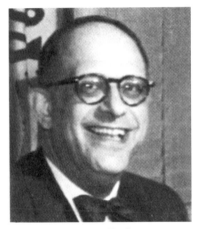

Paul H. Hoch

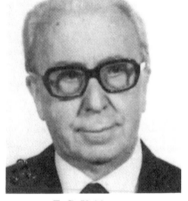

F. G. Valdecasas

COUNTRY	NUMBER	
	Members Serving as Officers	Officers Serving on Executive
United States	7	17
France	4	11
Switzerland	5	9
United Kingdom	4	9
Germany	4	7
Austria	2	5
Spain	2	4
Canada	2	3
Italy	3	3
Australia	2	2
Denmark	2	2
Belgium	1	1
Czechoslovakia	1	1
Norway	1	1
Peru	1	1
Poland	1	1
TOTAL	*42*	*77*

The Executive represents the leadership of the organization. Considering that well over 50 percent (24 of 42) of the members serving as Officers and that 53 of 77 of the Officers serving on the Executive were from one of the five most industrialized countries, i.e., United States (9 and 17 respectively), France (4 and 11 respectively), Switzerland (5 and 9 respectively), and Germany (4 and 7 respectively), the leadership of CINP during the 1960s represented a small segment even of Europe and the Americas (with a vested interest in perpetuating the status quo) and was dependent entirely on second-hand information on the state of psycho-pharmacology and the needs in the pharmacotherapy of mental illness outside the richest countries of the world.

The President of the 1st and 2nd Executives (the same person) was from Switzerland, and of the subsequent, five Executives numerous representatives were from the United States, Austria, France, Spain and Canada. The Treasurer of the 1st and 2nd Executives was from Switzerland, of the 3rd and 4th from France, and of the 5th, 6th and 7th from the United Kingdom. Five of the seven Presidents were clinicians, whereas one (serving two terms) was a basic scientist. All but one of the Presidents (who was affiliated with the pharmaceutical industry at the time of his presidency) were from the academy.

Information on the country representation of the 42 members serving as Officers and on the offices held by the officers in the seven Executives is given in Appendix 2.5. (see Executives). The same Appendix also includes the country profile of each of the seven Executives during the period from 1957 to 1970.

THE PROGRAMS

During the 1960s, CINP congresses alternated between open (Rome, Munich, Washington and Prague) and closed (Basel, Birmingham and Tarragona) meetings. The closed congresses were restricted to the membership and one invited guest of each member.

The programs of the seven congresses reflect the changes in the various interests in psychopharmacology during the 1960s. An outline of these programs is presented in Appendix 2.6. (see Programs).

A presidential address was delivered at six of the seven congresses. Extracts (in English) of the addresses by Hoff (delivered in German) and Delay (delivered in French) at the third and the fifth congresses are presented in relevant appendices. Pope Pius XII addressed the first congress (see Extract in Appendix 1.1).

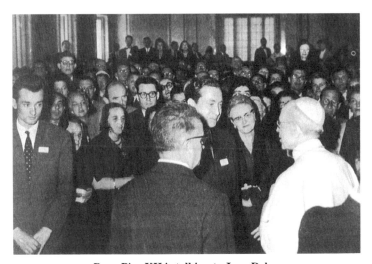

Pope Pius XII is talking to Jean Delay

The proceedings of each of the first seven congresses were published. A review of the proceedings of the fifth congress is presented in Appendix 1.4.

CINP congresses were directly and indirectly supported by the pharmaceutical industry. Direct support for the first four congresses was given by nine, four, twelve, and twenty-one companies respectively. There is no information available regarding direct support for the fifth, sixth and seventh congresses. Indirect support given to professionals for attending the congress by the drug companies is acknowledged in the proceedings of the first three meetings.

APPENDICES

1 Extracts and Reviews

1.1 EXTRACT FROM THE ADDRESS OF POPE PIUS XII TO THE FIRST CINP CONGRESS IN ROME
Delivered On September 9, 1958

Published in Acta Apostolicae Sedis – Commentarim Officiale
Translated from French by Jean-François Dreyfus.[*] Extracted from the English translation.

Gentlemen, you would not like to have the first congress of the Collegium Internationale Neuro-psychopharmacologicum at any other place but in Rome, the Eternal City. The goals of this first international psychopharmacology congress, in keeping with the goals of your organization, are the promotion of research and information exchanges, together with the promotion of co-operation between the clinical disciplines and basic sciences dealing with psychopharmacology. Particular attention is also to be paid, and we emphasize this with pleasure, to medico-social problems which arise from the use of psychotropic medication in psychiatric therapy.

RECENT PROGRESS IN NEUROPSYCHOPHARMACOLOGY

Time and again, mankind has shown interest in influencing psychic functions. Alcohol and opiates, for instance, are universally known for the transient euphoria and the relaxation they induce. The barbiturates exert a depressing actvity on the central nervous system. However, in recent years, new kinds of medication have attracted attention. One can characterize them by their ability to sedate without inducing sleepiness. Psychopharmacology, which studies these new drugs, distinguishes them from "psychotomimetics", which are used experimentally to induce changes that mimic those seen in mental illness, and from "tranquilizers", which exert a sedating effect. The new drugs are of interest not only to laboratories but also to clinicians, whom they help in treating psychoses, and especially severe psychoses with marked excitation.

The first among these new drugs was chlorpromazine. Its use led to therapeutic success and even cures in about 80 percent of patients with acute psychoses accompanied by psychomotor excitation. The most astonishing results with chlorpromazine have been in the treatment of the paranoid schizophrenias, acute confusional states and chronic hallucinatory delusions. The results are less clear-cut in endogenous depressive psychoses and are only modest in the psychoneuroses, unless anxiety symptoms are especially severe.

Chlorpromazine, used in 1952 as the first of these drugs, was the result of laboratory research, whereas reserpine, also introduced in 1952, was extracted from the *Rauwolfia serpentina* plant. The roots of this plant have been used in the Far East since ancient times to treat some mental disorders. In 1582, a physician and naturalist, Leonard Rauwolf, brought back some specimens of the plant from India, but it is only in our time, since 1931, that its properties have been systematically studied. Widely used to fight hypertension, due to its

---

[*] Jean-Francois Dreyfus was elected a Fellow of CINP in 1976.

relative safety and long duration of action, reserpine provides remarkable effects in the treatment of the mentally ill and particularly of schizophrenic patients. In addition to these two major drugs, let us note also meprobamate, initially used to treat muscular spasms and tensions, now primarily used in psychiatry for the relief of anxiety in outpatients.

The usefulness of these drugs, and of many others of a similar type, is dramatically evident in psychiatric clinics and hospitals, where patients are often admitted who are irrational and are a danger to their environment. Since the introduction of these drugs, the use of constraining means, electroshock and barbiturates has decreased. The entire atmosphere of the institution is transformed, providing patients a much more normalizing setting, allowing them to take part in therapeutic activities and to establish closer relationships with their relatives.

There are also new treatment methods – new tranquilizers – for neuroses. Even in normal life, it often happens that excessive tension, provoked by professional or familial problems or by impending danger, is relieved by psychotropic medications, which enable the person to face a situation with more strength and calm. There is however a danger to the public if these drugs, and especially the minor tranquilizers, are used without control, merely to avoid fears and tensions which are a part of an active life.

It is difficult to predict the future of psychotropic drugs. The initial results indicate that an important step has been taken in the treatment of mental illness and especially of schizophrenia. However there are also warnings against unguarded enthusiasm. Several questions, indeed fundamental ones, are waiting for an answer, in particular how psychotropic drugs act on the central nervous system. One can only admire the everlasting perseverance of researchers, in rooting out the secrets of delicate biochemical mechanisms in order to establish the precise site of action of drugs. In this infinitely complex domain, you seem determined to understand the mechanisms step by step. This will provide a solid pharmacological basis for practical applications, in order to benefit from all possible therapeutic advantages.

Even more difficult is the relationship between psychiatry and neuropsychopharmacology. Does the psychotherapeutic medication act on the cause of the disease, or does it only modify, more or less temporarily, the severity of some symptoms, leaving the roots, the causes untouched? Are central nervous system changes a cause or a result of emotional disorders? Some authors note that their experimental findings indicated still unidentified physical causes. On the other hand, there are psychiatrists who emphasize the psychogenic nature of mental disorders. They appreciate that tranquilizing medications facilitate the dialogue between a patient and his physician but remind us that an improvement in social behaviour brought about by drugs does not mean that the difficulties have been resolved. It is the personality in its totality that has to be treated. It would not be in the interest of patients to help them to cover up, or conceal, their personal difficulties by providing them with drugs that lead to a superficial adaptation to social reality.

MORAL REQUIREMENTS

We shall now address the moral principles relevant to your field. While you are dealing with man as the subject of science, and are trying to use all the means available to you to modify his behaviour and cure his physical and mental illnesses, we will look at man, here, as a person, a subject responsible for his actions, involved in a destiny that he has to accomplish while remaining faithful to his conscience and his God. For this we will have to examine the norms which determine the actions and responsibilities of a neuropsychopharmacologist and of anyone who uses the discoveries that psychopharmacology offers.

A conscientious physician instinctively needs to be guided by a medical deontology, rather than just referring to empirical rules. In our address to the 13th Congress of the International Society for Applied Psychology on April 10, 1958, we brought to attention the fact that in America, a Medical Deontology Code has been published that was based on the answers of 7500 members of the American Psychological Association. We are certain that this Code provides for norms which stem from an objective moral order. We are certain that you share this point of view. It may seem superfluous to speak again about the dignity of human life. But we are now looking not at your sincere, devoted and generous care for patients, but at something even deeper, your attitude towards other persons. What is the basis of human dignity as an existential value? What should be our position in relation to it?

Moral order requires us to have esteem for others, to be considerate towards them, to be respectful to them. A human being is indeed the noblest of all visible creatures; he has been made in the image and is similar to the Creator. Even if he is mentally ill, even if he is a slave of his instincts or has fallen lower even than animal life, he remains a person who has been created by God and destined to become his immediate possession. This fact should determine the attitude you will take towards him.

On many occasions already we have had the opportunity to remind you of our position, and in particular in our address to the First International Congress of Neurohistopathology on the 14th of September 1952. We discussed at the time the three circumstances that justify the research and treatment methods of modern medicine: scientific interest, individual concern, and caring for the community. We have emphasized that, even if the research is justified, one still has to examine, for each particular case, whether the acts posed do not violate superior moral norms. Scientific interest, concern for the individual, and preoccupation with the community are not absolute values and do not necessarily guarantee that every right will be upheld.

We have made the same points to the members of the Applied Psychology Congress on April 10th, 1958; there too one needed to judge whether certain research and treatment methods were compatible with the rights of the person when research is performed. We have stated that one had to ensure that the process in question conformed to the subject's rights and whether he was capable of giving his consent to it. If the answer is positive, one has to ask oneself if the consent has really been given and in conformity with natural rights, if there has not been a mistake, ignorance or deception, if the person has the competence to consent, and finally if it does not violate a third party's rights. We have thoroughly stressed that such consent does not always guarantee that the intervention is legitimate. We can only repeat ourselves, stressing again that the medical justification of a process does not necessarily mean that it is morally permissible.

To decide on technical questions, in which the theologian has no direct competence in individual cases and circumstances, you may remind yourself that man has a right to use his own body and his superior faculties, but cannot dispose of them since he has received them from God, on whom he is still dependent. It may be that while using his rights, he mutilates or destroys a part of himself, if it is necessary for the well-being of the whole organism. But in doing so he is not encroaching on divine rights, since he is only acting to safeguard a superior good, to save life, for instance. The good of the whole then justifies sacrificing a part.

But just as single organs are subordinate to the whole organism, the whole organism is subordinate to the spiritual finality of the whole person (him- or herself). Medical experiments, whether physical or psychic, may, on the one hand cause some damage to organs and functions, but on the other hand, they may be quite legitimate, because they are in agreement with the person's welfare and do not trespass against the limits set by the Creator to the right a human has to dispose of himself. These principles evidently apply to experiments in psychopharmacology. We had the opportunity to read in the documents that we received, a report on an experiment in artificially-induced delirium, in which thirty healthy persons and twenty-four psychiatric patients participated. Have the fifty-four persons assented to this experiment, and in a way that would be sufficient and acceptable with regards to natural law? Here, as in the other cases, the facts of the case must undergo a thorough examination.

It is the observance of moral order which confers value and dignity on human actions. Everyone has the duty to recognize and to respect this moral order both in himself and in others. This is the obligation that we now stress in the field of psychotropic medication use because it has become so common.

In our address to the Italian Society of Anesthesiology, on February 24, 1957, we already discarded one objection that could have been raised on the basis of the Catholic doctrine on suffering. Some invoke the example of Christ refusing the wine mixed with myrrh that was offered to him. We then answered at that time that, in principle, there was nothing against the use of treatments aiming at decreasing or suppressing pain. Renouncing their use could be and was often a sign of Christian heroism. But we also added that it would be a mistake to pretend that pain is an indispensable condition of this heroism. Similar principles may be applied to the soothing effect of the narcotics on pain; as to their suppression of consciousness, it depends on motivations and consequences. Since narcotics are not in opposition to a religious or moral obligation, if there are serious reasons for their use, one may even give them to dying persons, if they consent. Euthanasia, the will to provoke death, is obviously condemned by ethics. But if a dying person consents to it, it is permissible to use narcotics in moderation to soothe pain even if they hasten death. Truly in such a case, death is not desirable but is inescapable and proportionate motivations allow for measures which will hasten death.

One should not fear that respecting the laws of conscience or, if one prefers, of faith and ethics, would hamper or even prevent the exercise of your profession. In the above-mentioned address of April 10, 1958, we have already specified some norms which facilitate solving concrete questions of interest to psychologists. These may also be of concern to you, such as, for instance, using "lie-detectors", psychotropic drugs to conduct narcoanalysis, hypnosis, and so on. We divided intrinsically immoral actions into three groups: those which are characterized by direct opposition to moral order, those performed by persons who are not entitled to do so, and those leading to unjustifiable dangers. Psychologists, and those whose moral consciences are well-formed, must be able to decide easily if the measures they propose fall in one of these categories.

You are also aware that the careless use of psychotropic or other medications may lead to morally unacceptable situations. In several regions, many such drugs are available to the public with no medical control, though such controls may not be in themselves, as experience shows, sufficient to prevent indiscriminate use. Moreover, some countries show an alarming tolerance of some laboratory experiments and some clinical procedures. We do not wish to require here the help of authorities but rather to enlist that of the physicians themselves, and especially those with authority in the profession. We are convinced, indeed, that there exists a natural medical ethics, based on sound judgment and the responsible awareness of doctors themselves, and we wish its influence to be ever increasing.

We have, gentlemen, sincere esteem for your works, for the objectives to which you aspire, and for the results you have already obtained. Going through papers and books published in your field, it is easy to see that you are providing precious services to science and mankind. We have seen that you are able to help much suffering and distress that, only three or four years ago, was beyond the reach of medical science. You are now in a position to restore mental health to many patients, and we sincerely share the joy that this confers.

In the present state of scientific development, further progress can only be made through widespread international collaboration: the present Congress is vivid evidence of such collaboration. One wishes that this might expand not only to all the different disciplines of psychopharmacology, but also to all psychiatrists and psychotherapists, in a word to all those who take care of the mentally ill.

If you adopt a positive attitude towards those moral values we have evoked, you will perform your professional duties with the firmness and the quiet safety that is required by the seriousness of your responsibilities. You will then be for your patients, and for your colleagues, a guide, a counsellor, and a help, meriting both their confidence and their esteem.

Gentlemen, we hope that the first Congress of the "Collegium Internationale Neuro-psychopharmacologicum" might give a strong impetus to the magnificent efforts of researchers and clinicians and help them to new victories. May the Lord be with you in your work! We implore Him eagerly and we give as a pledge to you, your families and your collaborators, our apostolic blessing.

1.2 EXTRACT OF HANS HOFF'S PRESIDENTIAL ADDRESS
Delivered at the Fourth CINP Congress in Birmingham in 1964

Translated and extracted from the German original by Helmut Beckmann

In his presidential address delivered in 1964 at the fourth CINP congress in Birmingham, Hans Hoff talked about the close relationship between the CINP and the clinical practice of psychiatry. He pointed out that clinical psychiatrists were elected repeatedly to the presidency of CINP.

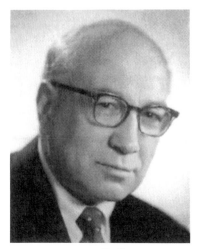

Hans Hoff

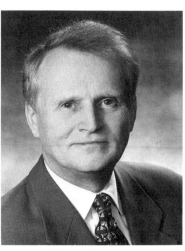

Helmut Beckmann

Hoff emphasized the important role neuroleptics have played in clinical psychiatry and enumerated some of the major benefits of the new drugs. Among them he referred first to the changed millieu of psychiatric hospitals in which treatment and patient care take place without physical restraints in a calm and tranquil environment. With conditions in psychiatric hospitals

---

* Helmut Beckmann completed his residency training in psychiatry at the universities of Heidelberg and Munich. Subsequently he was a Visiting Scientist at the National Institute of Mental Health in Bethseda, and later on a lecturer in the Department of Psychiatry at the University of Munich. Since 1985 he has been the Chairman and Head of the Department of Psychiatry at the University of Würzburg in Germany.

Beckmann was elected a fellow of the CINP in 1976. He was Vice President of the 17th, 18th and 19th and President-Elect of the 20th executive.

resembling those in general hospitals, the fear of psychiatry has decreased. By relieving patients from the pressure of their pathological emotions psychotropic drugs have helped to facilitate communication and opened up the possibility of understanding patients' experiences during the episodes of their illness.

Hoff also raised the question of whether neuroleptic medication should be regarded as specifically antipsychotic and argued that even if this is not the case, by reducing emotional pressure, neuroleptics rendered the pathological process of psychoses recognizable.

In an entirely different perspective he pointed out that LSD-25 seemed to provide a model for studying the pathogenesis of schizophrenia, anticholinergics were a model for studying the pathogenesis of exogenous psychoses. The recognition of the relationship between antidepressant effects and cerebral serotonin reuptake inhibition and interference of cerebral monoamine breakdown, facilitated the understanding of depression. Furthermore, findings of a dopamine-deficiency in the neostriatal areas of patients with Parkinson's disease provided a better understanding of the pathology of this disorder.

Hoff stressed the need to integrate neuropsychopharmacological findings with recent advances in neurophysiological knowledge. He also expressed his notion of a close link between motor functions, emotional functions, and the vegetative nervous system, with each system being inseparable from the other. By influencing one component of the system he maintained that the others would inevitably be modified too. Within his frame of reference, thymoleptics and neuroleptics are not separable in a strict sense, even if antidepressants were considered to be illness-specific to a greater extent than neuroleptics. The use of antidepressants has yielded a clear change in the attitude of depressed patients towards treatment. The frequent refusal of ECT was replaced by acceptance of treatment with an antidepressant.

Hoff also pointed out some of the problems which may arise from treatment with the new antidepressants. He considered the growing tendency towards outpatient care to be a danger, because the takeover of psychiatric care from psychiatrists by general practitioners can lead to an increased risk of suicide. He underlined the need for close contact with depressed patients.

Finally, Hoff made some comments about tranquilizers. He considered combined administration of an antidepressant with a tranquilizer a desirable practice in depression, and in the management of withdrawal symptoms in alcoholism and drugs. The danger of tranquilizer abuse in Hoff's opinion did not arise from the drugs, but rather from the thoughtless manner displayed by many physicians in administering them. Since doctors may prescribe a tranquilizer before understanding the nature of the disease, there is also a danger of a general deterioration of diagnostics.

In his concluding remarks, Hoff emphasized that administering drugs requires a great sense of responsibility in everyday clinical practice. He cited Wagner-Jauregg: "All a physician's work and research must be dedicated to one aim: helping the ill person."

1.3 EXTRACT FROM JEAN DELAY'S PRESIDENTIAL ADDRESS
Delivered at the Fifth CINP Congress in Washington

Translated from the French original by Jean-François Dreyfus
Extracted from the English translation

The meeting that opens today in Washington is the fifth Congress organized by the Collegium Internationale Neuro-Psychopharmacologicum (CINP), an organization founded in September 1957, in Zurich. The CINP is a body for international co-operation that provides a platform for representatives of different disciplines, united by a common interest in psychotropic drugs, to meet.

One of the pioneers of the field, our former president, Paul Hoch, professor of psychiatry at Columbia University, Director for Mental Health in New York State, has passed away since our last meeting. Everyone appreciated his organizational abilities, his dynamism, the wisdom of his advice, and his commitment to our collegium. Paul Hoch was in charge of establishing the scientific program of the present congress and of co-ordinating its implementation.

Psychopharmacology is an interdisciplinary field which is of interest to chemists and pharmacologists; physicians and physiologists; psychologists and sociologists. Modern psychopharmacology distinguishes itself from purely empirical knowledge (in fact quite different from it), by its striving to become a scientific discipline. The young science is an ancient art. One of the oldest dreams of mankind has been to cure mental disorders using herbs or philtres. The history of medicinal plants is evidence that psychopharmacology was known in ancient times. It is a captivating task to try to divide facts from legend, placebo effects from psychopharmacological effects, and magic from chemistry in studying the psychological powers ascribed to plants such as mandrake, hashish, passiflora and belladonna, *Rauwolfia serpentina*, and coca.

Homer, in the *Odyssey*, speaks of pharmakon, which he also calls nepenthes. Nepenthes, which means lack of sorrow, had the power to soothe psychic pain by producing a sort of emotional neutrality. What was nepenthes? Probably opium, the ancestor of all tranquilizing agents. True, the ataractic effects of opiates are widely different from those induced by neuroleptics, and the latter are far easier to use for therapeutic purposes, but all of them pose the same psychopharmacological problem: whether it is possible to change emotions through the use of a drug.

Another example, almost as far-reaching, is that of the medicinal plants with a psychological effect used by Aztec priests in the ancient civilization of Mexico. In initiation ceremonies, they employed these plants to help communicate with the divine, and give people access to the supernatural world. Even though the trance states and miraculous cures attained in these states of collective ecstasy have been long considered by psychiatrists as hysterical phenomena, it appears nowadays that they were at least partly related to psychopharmacology. Amongst these hallucinogenic plants, one could find peyotl, teonanacatl and ololiuqui. Peyotl contains mescaline, teonanacatl contains psilocybine and psilocyne, ololiuqui contains LSD derivatives and the amide of the d-isolysergic acid. The millenary cult of the Mexican mushroom,

Psylocibe mexicana, is explained today by its psychotropic principle. Conditions that we currently study under the name of artificially-induced psychoses were known to these ancient priests, and the cult around collective ingestion of hallucinogenic substances shows they understood, in their way, how environment and milieu influence the response to psychotropic substances.

For a number of years, and especially since 1952, the year of the discovery of a centrally-acting phenothiazine, chlorpromazine,we in psychiatry have witnessed an extraordinary growth in the number and diversity of psychotropic drugs available to physicians. One is somewhat embarrassed by this proliferation of drug families and would appreciate having an easy scheme for clinical orientation. For this purpose, it may be useful to have recourse to an elementary and purely clinical systematic classification.

The word psychotropic, since it is so general, is suitable for designating the whole set of chemical substances, natural or artificial, which have a psychological tropism, i.e., able to modify mental activity, with no prejudgement as to the type of this modification. Clinicians have a large variety of psychotropic drugs causing different kinds of behavioural change on demand. Depending on whether they generate a depressant (leptic), stimulating (analeptic), or deviating (dysleptic) effect on mental functions, it is convenient to divide them into three groups and to specify in each of these groups whether the predominant effect of a drug is on mood or alertness, on the affective or intellectual state, or in the thymic or noetic sphere.

In the psycholeptic group, we find all the substances that depress mental activity, whether this lowering in psychological tone is related to a decrease in alertness, to a reduction of intellectual energy or to a relaxation of emotional tension. This vast group can be divided into subgroups, the two principal being alertness-depressants (nooleptics) and mood-depressants (thymoleptics). Alertness-depressants, i.e., depressants of the vigilance function that regulates sleep-wake cycles, include all hypnotics whether barbiturates or not. Mood-depressants, i.e.,depressants of the thymic function, which regulates oscillations of the emotional tone between a pathetic and an apathetic pole, include all tranquilizing agents, the action of which is characterized by changing an apathetic status to a pathetic one. Tranquilizers are sometimes called ataractics, since ataraxia is by definition an absence of emotional disorder, the status of someone that cannot be roused (although it seems an exaggeration to speak of true ataraxia in relation with most tranquilizers). Let us also note that the distinction of hypnotics and tranquilizers is a relative one given that, at low doses, barbiturates are tranquilizers and at high doses, tranquilizers enhance sleep.

There is a type of major tranquilizer, the neuroleptics, which should be separated from the rest. They attract particular interest because of their remarkable effects in the chemotherapy of psychoses. The neuroleptics comprise phenothiazines, reserpine and butyrophenones. Neuroleptics owe their name to the psychomotor neurological syndrome, or more exactly the psycholeptic syndrome they produce. This neurological syndrome ranges from a simple decrease of mimic to severe extrapyramidal, Parkinson-like symptoms. Indeed, the extra-pyramidal system always has a role in the definition of neuroleptics. It is another question whether the severity of the extrapyramidal syndrome bears a relation to the intensity of therapeutic effects.

In the psychoanaleptic group, we have all the substances that stimulate mental activity by an increase in alertness which may reach the level of insomnia, an increase in intellectual energy, or an increase of emotional tone which may reach the level of anxiety or euphoria. This vast group may be divided into subgroups, with the two main groups being stimulants of vigilance (noo-analeptics) and stimulants of mood (thymoanaleptics). Stimulants of vigilance comprise all psychotonic amines which facilitate intellectual functioning. In contrast to the barbiturates, which produce sleep, phenamines produce insomnia. Mood stimulants comprise all drugs that can induce an increase in emotional tone; some of them have an antidepressant effect which makes them effective in depressive states. One thinks, for example, of the hydrazines and imipramine, which are so effective that their use led to a reduction in the use of electroconvulsive therapy. Nevertheless, the distinction between stimulants of vigilance and mood is schematic. A psychotonic effect may be accompanied by euphoria, and the antidepressant effect of iproniazide or imipramine may be associated with insomnia. In the antidepressants, there is a clinical interest in grouping under a particular heading the monoamine oxidase inhibitors, not because of a well-established correlation between monoamine oxidase inhibition and the antidepressant effect of these drugs, but because from a practical point of view, a clinician has to be able to distinguish those drugs from other antidepressants with which they may be incompatible.

In the psychodysleptic group, we include all substances which distort mental activity and can cause delusions. These drugs may cause hallucinations, oneroid states, confusion or depersonalization. Examples of such drugs are mescaline, the peyotl alkaloid, lysergamide or LSD-25, and psilocybine and anticholinergic substances such as Ditran. From a pharmacological point of view, one may distinguish among the hallucinogens, the indoles, such as LSD-25 or psilocybine, and the anticholinergic drugs such as Ditran. All psychodysleptics may induce psychoses and are, therefore, also called psychotomimetics.

This clinical classification of psychotropics will become more complicated and evolved as correlations between types of pharmacological structures and types of psychological reactions, and between the topographical distribution of psychotropics in the brain and biochemical and neurophysiological mechanisms become known.

One of the most striking aspects of the transformation in psychiatry by biological therapy in general, and by chemotherapy in particular, is the profound modification of clinical pictures and their evolution. With treatment, psychopathology is rapidly changing. Classical forms, as described in books and handbooks, are being replaced by atypical forms that require modifying descriptions and concepts. Our earlier descriptions were made at a time when psychiatry had no therapeutic means of modifying the clinical picture; one had to let the disease follow its natural course. The clinician's craft consisted mainly of predicting whether a disorder would lead to chronicity or would spontaneously remit. Today, our major task, as for any physician, is to decide which treatment is indicated, and to prescribe, in Klett's words, the right drug for the right patient.

At the beginning of psychopharmacology the changes achieved were so obvious that it was easy, for instance, to agree on the improvement by chlorpromazine of agitated states or acute attacks of unequivocal mania. But as psychotropic drugs increased in number and grew more diverse, some difficulty arose. The first difficulty is with nosography, which needs to be reorganized: treatment has yielded transitional entities, a sign that the standard morbid forms are nosologically heterogeneous. Another difficulty is related to the assessment of change in the course of treatment with drugs, i.e., the evaluation of results. Recently, major progress has been made towards a more homogeneous and more objective assessment through the use of psychometric methods. Experience has shown that clinicians agree most easily on elementary symptoms; on their mere presence or absence. As well, some psychiatrists object to rating scales, the use of which tends towards simplification and quantification. However, rating scales should not interfere with traditional clinical observation, which remains irreplaceable.

Clinical psychopharmacology forces psychiatrists to think in terms of physiology. It also directs research towards biological substrates for mental disorders, regardless whether neurological or humoral. Absence of anatomically-discernible lesions in endogenous psychoses does not mean that there are no such lesions detectable with the employment of neurophysiological or biochemical techniques. The possibility of inducing and controlling psychopathological symptoms by psychotropic drugs supports this notion.

Psychotropic drugs act on psychic functions insofar as they are cerebral functions. It is true that one cannot localize a specific centre for a particular psychic function, yet for the psychic function to operate, a specialized cerebral mechanism with multiple connections must be at work.

Neurophysiology has already identified the functions of some of the key parts of the brain. Accordingly, the role of the diencephalon and reticular formation lies in the regulation of wakefulness and sleep (in disturbances of vigilance and consciousness), the role of hypothalamic and limbic structures in the regulation of mood and emotional tone (in mood disturbances), the role of the mamillary bodies and connected structures in the memory circuit (disturbances of memory and perception), and the role of the cortex in psychomotor regulation (in disturbances in psychomotor activity and orientation).

Human psychopharmacology allows us to study the relationship between psychological functioning and the activity of these structures. In the field of emotions, for example, data from human experiments involving psychopharmacology enable us to assert that emotion is a cerebral phenomenon, not only in its expression but also as an affection. It is not only the outward behaviour of the manic or depressed patient which is corrected by neuroleptics or antidepressants but the fundamental mood disturbance which underlies these syndromes. In the field of consciousness, the findings in animal experiments indicate the cerebral origin of the sleep-wake cycle, its pharmacodynamic variations, and its electroencephalographic correlations with cortico-reticular activations and inhibitions. Human psychopharmacology adds information to the analysis of behavioural data by "experimental introspection," which allows us to study the correspondences between the changes in alertness and the level of consciousness.

Pharmacological production of syndromes commonly observed in human psychoses suggests the involvement of similar cerebral structures. But there is a prior question. Are artificial psychoses analogous or identical to human psychoses? Analogy or identity, these are the very words that were used by Moreau de Tours to set the stage for the debate, as early as 1845, in his book *Hashish and Lunacy*. His conclusions pointed toward identity as the answer, whereas others asserted analogy.

Artificially-induced psychoses with dysleptic drugs are acute exogenous psychoses, the symptomatology of which is dependent on the drug and the host. These acute exogenous experimental psychoses do not differ from acute exogenous psychoses observed in clinical work, and it is also often extremely difficult to distinguish them from endogenous psychoses.

In the search for a biochemical injury in psychoses, much work is focused on the metabolism of biogenic amines in order to detect metabolites which are not found in normal subjects. In this area of research, investigations of the metabolism of amino-acids and biogenic amines (such as catecholamines or indolamines) or of the role of cerebral enzymes, have been added to the classical studies of carbohydrate metabolism in cerebral functioning.

Recent discoveries in molecular biology allow us to envisage new directions, such as, for instance, analyzing relationships between ribonucleic acid and memory. One of the most fruitful perspectives in molecular biochemistry concerns the genetic control of the cerebral enzymes that govern active substances in the brain. This explains the importance of research on genetic coding. Psychiatry is directly involved with the development of genetic bio-chemistry, since heredity remains the principal factor in mental disorders.

As powerful as the biological movement may be, other methods and other treatments should not be neglected. It would be absurd for a psychiatrist to deprive his patient of such powerful resources as psychotherapy and social therapy, just because he is enthralled by psychophar-macology. Psychiatry should not be reduced to chemistry. In mental medicine, the doctor-pa-tient relationship is fundamental, and the quality of this relationship plays a major role in treatment, whatever the means used. While we may not agree on theories, in practice our first duty as therapists is to use every possible means to treat disease. This eclectic attitude is not shared by some psychoanalysts who continue to think that their method alone qualifies for therapy.

The resistance of the most orthodox psychoanalysts to psychopharmacology should itself be analyzed. A frequently-invoked argument is that psychotropic drugs would hinder, and may even prevent, transference for the patient in therapy. Another argument is that improvement brought about by psychotropic drugs may diminish the need for psychotherapy. In opposition to this contention, Paul Hoch wrote that the idea that a patient should be deeply uncomfortable for psychotherapy to be effective is an old shibboleth that has never been proven and that should be thoroughly re-examined in light of recent knowledge. Not only has chemotherapy not restricted the indication for psychotherapy but the new drugs have on the contrary widely increased the need for psychotherapy, since it is now applicable to illnesses that before would never have benefited from such therapy.

Drugs also allow pharmacodynamic explorations for psychotherapeutic purposes, as for instance narcoanalysis, weck analysis, and so on. Narcoanalysis, which uses barbiturates may appear to be the opposite to weck analysis performed with amphetamines, but there is often a major advantage to combining them, for example by using sodium amobarbitone and methylamphetamine, in a subnarcosis with amphetamines. This method is so useful for the clinician for diagnostic purposes, that for my own part, I prescribe it as routinely as I request psychometric assessment or electroencephalography. From a therapeutic point of view, subnarcosis with amphetamines provides spectacular results in some cases, as in the case of traumatic neuroses, but more often it only plays an adjuvant role and has to be used temporarily at some stages of psychotherapy for psychoses and neuroses alike. As to oneiroanalysis by oneirogenic drugs such as LSD-25 and psilocybine, it is both an exploration and a therapeutic method. Its results, and the various reservations about dysleptic use, will be the focus in one of our symposiums which is specifically centred on this front-page topic.

Social retraining and rehabilitation techniques through work have now become quite important in psychiatry. As Sir Aubrey Lewis wrote some years ago: If we had to choose between dropping all new psychotropic drugs or dropping all industrial rehabilitation units and the other social means we use, there should be no hesitation in our choice, drugs would have to go. Happily, we do not have to make such a decision since chemotherapy and social therapy are not opposed but complementary; they help each other. By reducing unrest, aggressiveness, negativism and more generally the dangerousness of mentally-ill patients, chemotherapy has greatly facilitated the use of social retraining and rehabilitation. Similarly, by changing living conditions in psychiatric hospitals, psychotropic drugs have rendered necessary the redesign of such institutions, entailing improvements in housing and in the patients' social framework. Patients previously treated in closed wards may be treated in outpatient facilities, without being committed to hospital. And patients who were previously treated in open wards may be treated in outpatient facilities without hospitalization. This leads to structural changes even if one does not yet envisage the disappearance of psychiatric hospitals. One has to stand firm against the present trend of avoiding at all costs committing psychiatric patients to hospital and pretending that mental patients can now be treated just as any other inpatients. This does not take into account that the psychiatric patient may be dangerous to others or to himself, and recent treatments have not suppressed this danger factor. Also, one has to stand firm against the trend towards drastically shortening the hospital stay of patients and towards discharging patients as soon as some improvement has been noted. These premature discharges are quite risky since in some cases symptoms are only transiently concealed by chemotherapy. If the latter is interrupted or if surveillance is insufficient, forensic accidents occur which could have been avoided by a longer-lasting hospital stay. Therapeutic progress allows a freer social regimen for mentally ill patients, but freeing should be conducted carefully and progressively.

As an introduction to our work sessions, I have tried to sketch the point of view of a clinician on psychopharmacological perspectives in psychiatry, at least those that can be envisaged currently. It is certain that they will be increased and transformed in the years to come. The psychotropic era, which has sometimes been called the tranquilizer era, is just at the beginning, and the results that have already been attained justify great expectations.

Considering the amount of ongoing work, it appears that tranquilizers do not have a similar effect on those taking them and those studying them. The former are pacified by them; the latter are stimulated as again and again the drugs raise new problems. More than giving answers, exploring the psychotropics raises questions which keep us in a productive state of tension, without which there would be neither search nor discovery. So much research, performed simultaneously in so many countries, is a good omen for the future of psychopharmacology. Through the diversity of their work, psychopharmacologists show a common will, and where there is a will, there will, one day or the other, be a way.

1.4 A REVIEW OF THE FIFTH CONGRESS

Leo E. Hollister

NEURO-PSYCHOPHARMACOLOGY: PROCEEDINGS OF THE FIFTH INTER-
NATIONAL CONGRESS OF THE COLLEGIUM INTERNATIONALE NEURO-
PSYCHOPHARMACOLOGICUM. H. Brill, J.O. Cole, P. Deniker, H. Hippius, and
P.B. Bradley, editors. International Congress Series no. 129. Amsterdam: Excerpta
Medica Foundation, 1967.

The fifth meeting of the Collegium Internationale Neuro-psychopharmacologicum (CINP)
was held in Washington, DC from March 28 to 31, 1966. This meeting was the first to be held
in the United States, appropriately in the nation's capital. It was the last to feature simultaneous
translation: English, French, or German, depending upon the speaker's preference. Soon after,
probably by virtue of the recalcitrance of the British and Americans, English – sometimes
impeccable and sometimes broken – became the international language of science.

The meeting was convened by the president, Jean Delay, one of the pioneers of the
psychiatric drug revolution. Most international meetings like to trot out some Nobel Prize
winners; at this meeting the honour fell to Daniel Bovet, who had developed the concept of
antihistamine drugs. A future Nobelist, Julius Axelrod, was also a participant. Several
individuals who ultimately became presidents of the CINP were on the program: Eric Jacobsen,
Pierre Deniker, Heinz Lehmann, Leo Hollister, and Paul Janssen (as well as Oakley Ray and
the late Al DiMascio, esteemed executive secretaries of the American College of Neuropsychopharmacology at different periods).

The meeting was organized around fourteen symposia and five paired concurrent sessions.
Even a partial record of the meeting, as reported in the book under review, came to 1275 pages.
As has been the case ever since, CINP meetings covered a number of disciplines and the topics
considered were diverse. No brief review can do justice to all the information presented. My
attempt here will be to summarize highlights, as seen from my own perspective, and to try,
when possible, to put them into historical context.

SYMPOSIUM 1: RESEARCH METHODOLOGIES

Clinical trial methodology was still of considerable interest. By then, the concept of the
parallel-group, controlled clinical trial was accepted. Difficulties still remained in establishing
consistent clinical diagnoses, a problem that continues today despite many earnest attempts
over the years to clarify the issues. Problems associated with multiclinic trials were also of
importance, as well as the difficulties in obtaining representative samples of patients, a result
of pretreatment by general physicians and the reluctance of prospects to be exposed to placebo
or ECT and to continue in a study for as long as four weeks. A Medical Research Council (UK)
multiclinic study reported results which might not be much different today: one-third of
depressed patients did well on placebo alone; one-sixth eventually required ECT regardless
of drug treatment; patients initially treated with imipramine or ECT did better than those who
received placebo or phenelzine.

SYMPOSIUM 2: DIFFERENCES BETWEEN SEDATIVE-HYPNOTIC, TRANQUILIZER, AND NEUROLEPTIC DRUGS

Concern still existed regarding differences between the neuroleptics, on the one hand, and sedative-hypnotics and tranquilizers (the latter referring to what we would now call antianxiety drugs), on the other. It seemed easy to note many differences between the neuroleptics and the other two classes of drugs, but it was still difficult to show convincing differences between classic sedative-hypnotics and the newer tranquilizers.

SYMPOSIUM 3: DRUG EFFECTS ON MEMORY AND LEARNING

The idea that memory could be encoded by RNA or polypeptides, a hypothesis originated by Holger Hyden in the 1940s, seemed strengthened by the observations from several laboratories that memory could be impaired by drugs which blocked synthesis of proteins or RNA. The idea that memories could be transferred from one animal to another by intracisternal infusions of RNA or, even more preposterous, by one animal eating the other, still had some credence, absurd though it now sounds.

SYMPOSIUM 4: DRUG ABUSE AND DEPENDENCE

Drug dependence studies had not yet become dominated by behavioural pharmacologists; the brief symposium on this subject had no such studies. Data from patients treated with neuroleptics indicated that these drugs would produce a withdrawal reaction if suddenly stopped. However, physical dependence does not equate with abuse, and abuse of neuroleptics, even today, is quite rare. On the other hand, such studies indicated that withdrawal from long-term treatment with any psychoactive drug is likely to produce a reaction as the brain compensates for the effects of the drug. Jaffe reported on the current modes of treatment of opiate dependence. In principle, the paper would not be much different today. He referred to the various non-pharmacological approaches, cited studies of cyclazocine, a mixed agonist-antagonist (substitute buprenorphine today), and early studies with methadone maintenance. Levo-methidyl (LAAM), a long-acting methadone, may now supplant methadone, but it is remarkable how little has been changed in principle over the years.

SYMPOSIUM 5: MECHANISMS OF DRUG ACTION

Mechanisms of action of various drugs were of interest, but could not be studied with the vast sophistication that current methods allow. Various neuroleptics were ranked on their ability to antagonize amphetamine effects as well as prevent "shock", both in rats. The ranking was almost identical with that achieved some years later by measuring dopamine D-2 receptor blockade in the brain. A chemical approach showed that the accumulation of homovanillic acid (a dopamine metabolite) was much greater in rat brainstem after neuroleptics than after other drugs, such as tricyclics and meprobamate. Similar findings emerged from the rat caudate nucleus. A number of data led to the hypothesis that neuroleptics act by blocking the action of dopamine in the brain. Thus, only a few years after Carlsson first proposed dopamine as a neurotransmitter of consequence in drug action, the dopamine hypothesis was well under way. Axelrod's group provided data which indicated that tricyclic antidepressants might act by inhibiting uptake of norepinephrine but not dopamine, a new mechanism for terminating synaptic transmission.

SYMPOSIUM 6: ANTICHOLINERGIC DRUGS

The symposium on anticholinergics was summarized by a number of short papers relating to the effects of these drugs on the electroencephalogram and their propensity to be hallucinogens. Cholinergic mechanisms were still of interest, and only twelve to fifteen years previously was acetylcholine known brain neurotransmitter.

SYMPOSIUM 7: PSYCHOTOMIMETICS

The mid-1960s were the heyday of psychotomimetic drugs. Many hoped that understanding their action might help reveal the biochemical basis of naturally occurring psychoses, which they were supposed to model. Many people thought that these drugs might be useful in improving psychotherapy, and studies of LSD for the treatment of alcoholics were just beginning. However, the disappointing results with these drugs led to a period of disillusionment, so that few studies were done after 1970. It would only be in the 1990s that some interest in them reappeared.

SYMPOSIUM 8: DRUG COMBINATIONS

Use of drug combinations began early in clinical psychopharmacology. Probably the first combination of antipsychotics was that of chlorpromazine and reserpine. Results were different in two studies, one of which showed some benefit, while the other did not. At this meeting, reports were made on studies of combinations of chlorpromazine with chlordiazexopide, none of which was more effective than chlorpromazine alone. A combination of trifluoperazine and tranylcypromine was thought to act more quickly than the former drug alone. This combination was ultimately marketed with little success. In animal studies, the combination of dextroamphetamine and amobarbital produced more initial increase in activity than either drug alone, suggesting a novel action of the combination. However, no difference in initial increase in activity was noted between either drug alone, a most surprising finding. Such combinations were marketed, primarily for treating anxiety, but rapidly followed the barbiturates into obsolescence following the introduction of the benzodiazepines.

SYMPOSIUM 9: FACTORS INFLUENCING DRUG RESPONSES

Many factors other than the pharmacodynamic actions of drugs may alter clinical responses. These factors might be called "metapharmacological." How does one explain differences in responses among various clinics participating in a multiclinic trial? Different milieux, observers, or physicians? Differences in response rates of schizophrenics to a phenothiazine were marked when patients in an American clinic were compared with those in a German one. This result led to the hypothesis that genetic influences might explain such differences. However, this experience has not been replicated. The interaction between the attitudes of treating physicians and the acquiescence of patients has been shown in studies comparing diazepam with placebo in anxious patients. Doctors with little interest in mechanical things obtained better outcomes from either the active drug or the placebo than those whose interest in mechanical vocations was highest. On the other hand, the patient factor of acquiescence showed a marked difference in outcome. Differences between drug and placebo were greater in patients with low acquiescence than those rated high. The concept of placebo reactors was explored, and it was concluded that some patients might be so considered.

SYMPOSIUM 10: SIDE EFFECTS OF DRUG TOXICITY

Side effects and complications of psychotherapeutic drugs were of considerable interest. The interaction of monoamine oxidase inhibitors (MAOIs) with cheese or other drugs was recognized. Fear of this interaction probably delayed any widespread use of MAOIs for some years thereafter. The syndrome of tardive dyskinesia had been described, but little was yet known about predisposing factors other than long-term use. The skin-eye syndrome from chlorpromazine attracted the interest of dermatologists and ophthalmologists. The skin pigmentation (so-called purple people) was thought to be due to binding of the drug to melanin. However, the mechanism of cataract formation was still controversial. No doubt the recognition of this unusual effect of chlorpromazine, as well as the advent of the piperazine phenothiazines and haloperidol, led to a marked decline in its use. Sudden death associated with antipsychotics has remained controversial. One proposed explanation was intimal thickening in small arteries and arterioles. However, work on this was never confirmed. Shortly after, it became evident that death was due to physiological, rather than anatomical, changes. To this day, the validity of this concept is argued. About 300,000 to 400,000 sudden deaths occur each year in the United States; it is difficult to separate from these large numbers the relatively few such instances that occur during drug therapy.

SYMPOSIUM 11: SPECIFIC INDICATIONS FOR DRUGS

A matter of interest at that time was trying to find the right drug for the right patient. By classifying depressed patients as anxious, hostile, or retarded, it was possible to show that tricyclics were most clearly beneficial in retarded (endogenous) depressions. Trying to find specific drugs for the various syndromes of schizophrenia was more difficult; investigators cautioned against expecting too much. Non-specific factors complicated evaluation of anti-anxiety and antidepressant drugs. The greater the amount of initial anxiety, the greater the response to meprobamate. The periodicity of depressions also complicated matters, as the natural history of the disorder led to a number of spontaneous remissions. The chronicity of depression was not then fully recognized. Nosological problems abounded. The French classification of psychoses was quite different from that in the United States, almost to the point of making translation impossible. Using the Inpatient Multidimensional Psychiatric Inventory, it was possible to delineate thirteen psychotic syndromes; none of these were prominent in negative symptoms, a concept which arose much later. The specific response of patients with phobic anxiety to imipramine, as compared with little response from placebo and worsening with chlorpromazine, led to the splitting of the newly named panic disorder from other anxiety disorders.

SYMPOSIUM 12: ANIMAL MODELS

Although in 1966 a number of animal models existed for anxiety and aggression, none had been developed for depression and schizophrenia. Considerable evidence had evolved concerning the role of catecholamines in drug actions. It was apparent that norepinephrine uptake was reduced by tricyclics, such as desipramine and protriptyline, and also that drugs which increased dopamine synthesis as well as blocking receptors had antipsychotic action. The reward pathway in the brain was considered to be noradrenergic; we now believe that it is dopaminergic. Quite probably the error might have been due to chemical methods not sensitive enough to measure differences between these two catecholamines. Taming of aggressive animals with various psychotherapeutic drugs, especially when this could be done without markedly impairing consciousness, was considered to be a reliable indicator of the effectiveness of neuroleptics.

SYMPOSIUM 13: CLASSICAL CONDITIONING

Classical Pavlovian conditioning was discussed by many contributors. Gantt put the matter most succinctly: "It is quite likely that in psychiatric diseases the action of the drug is determined more by the type or temperament of the individual than by the clinical diagnosis or the disease symptomatology." The concept of a conditioned abstinence syndrome affecting relapse to drug abuse was described by Wikler; this concept still has heuristic value. It is somewhat surprising that Len Cook was not on the program. His demonstration that the conditioned avoidance reaction could differentiate antipsychotic drugs from other types and help discover new compounds had a lasting effect on the search for new drugs.

SYMPOSIUM 14: DRUGS AS TOOLS

Drugs may be tools as well as treatments, allowing inferences to be drawn about some of the pathophysiologic mechanisms of psychiatric disorders. The sedation threshold, which measures the amount of a sedative required to produce a given degree of sedation, had been extended to a stimulation threshold. However, this concept has not been further broadened to include other drugs. These tests have suggested that schizophrenics, rather than being less aware of their surroundings, may be hyperaroused. The two most important hypotheses framed from the action of drugs have been the amine hypothesis of depression and the dopamine hypothesis of schizophrenia. Neither was clearly evident at the time of this meeting, however.

INDIVIDUAL COMMUNICATIONS

As might be expected, these covered a wide range of topics, many of which had also been discussed in the symposia. One paper, which might have portended the future, was a discussion of the antipsychotic effects of a number of compounds with a 6-7-6 ring structure, the dibenzoxapines. Clozapine, one of this class of drugs, was synthesized only a few years later. A combination of thioridazine and chlordiazepoxide was found to be as effective in half-doses (200 mg/day of thioridazine) as in full doses. Adding the benzodiazepine did not enhance the effectiveness. Had we been alert in considering this paper, we might have concluded that the usual doses of antipsychotics being used were too large, and the epoch of low-dose therapy might have started earlier.

The paper with the most engaging title was "Molecular biology and psychiatry." It was only two short paragraphs in length and was mainly concerned with the role of nucleic acids in memory formation, a topic that had been considered in more detail in symposium 12. The era of molecular medicine began in 1949 with the discovery that an aberrant structure of hemoglobin caused sickle-cell anemia. Who could have guessed that, thirty years after this meeting, we would have a journal called *Molecular Psychiatry?*

SUMMARY

We are always the prisoners of our preconceptions and the methods available to us. In 1966 we were only twelve to fourteen years into the revolution in thinking created by the new psychotropic drugs. The methods available then were primitive compared to our current repertoire. Yet the participants in the fifth CINP meeting came up with enough new insights to demand respect, even in retrospect.

Tabular Presentations

2.1 DRUGS AND CONGRESSES

Number of drugs with pharmacological designation of tranquilizer (T) or energizer (E) in clinical use for the treatment of schizophrenia (S), depression (D) or anxiety/insomnia (A/I) referred to at first seven CINP Congresses. The figure in the Congress column designates the total number of references made to the drug during the seven Congresses.

The pharmacological designation of the drugs is based on Earl Usdin and Daniel H. Efron's *Psychotropic Drugs and Related Compounds* published by the Public Health Service, U.S. Department of Health, Education and Welfare (Public Health Service Publication No. 1589) in 1967.

DRUG NAME	CLASS	USE	CONGRESSES (1-7)
Acepromazine	T		2
Acetophenazine	T	S	2
Adiphenine	T		1
Amitriptyline	E	D	55
Amphetamine PO_4	E		132
Amphetamine SO_4	E	D	1
Anisoperidone	T		1
Bemegride	E		6
Benactyzine	T		20
Benzperidol	T		1
Butaperazine	T	S	7
Captagon	E		1
Captodiame	T	A/I	2
Carphenazine	T	S	3
Chlordiazepoxide	T	A/I	65
Chlorpromazine	T	S	209
Chlorprothixene	T	S	12
Clopenthixol	T	S	3
Clothiapine	T		3
Deanol	E		8
Deserpidine	T	S	2
Desipramine	E	D	43
Diazepam	T	A/I	29
Dibenzepin	E	D	7
Dimethacrine	E		1
Doxepin	E	D	4
Etryptamine	E		1
Flupentixol	T		1
Fluphenazine Decanoate	T	S	41
Fluphenazine Enanthate	T	S	2
Glutethimide	T	A/I	1
Haloperidol	T	S	18
Hydroxyphenamate	T		18
Hydroxyzine	T	A/I	10
Imipramine	E	D	128
Iproniazid	E	D	52
Isocarboxazide	E	D	12
Isoniazid	E		5
Mebanazine			7

DRUG NAME	CLASS	USE	CONGRESSES (1-7)
Mefaxamide	E		5
Melitracen(e)	E		2
Mephenesin	T	A/I	4
Meprobamate	T	A/I	58
Mesoridazine	T	S	2
Methamphetamine	E	D	7
Methaqualone	T	A/I	1
Methophenazine	T		4
Methylpentynol	T		6
Methylphenidate	E		7
Nialamide	E	D	16
Nicotinamide	E		2
Nicotinic Acid	E		6
Nortriptyline	E	D	5
Opipramol	E		7
Oxanamide	T	A/I	2
Oxazepam	T	A/I	5
Oxypertine	T		16
Pargyline	E	D	6
Pemoline	E		2
Perazine	T		2
Perphenazine	T	S	24
Phenaglycodol	T	A/I	1
Phenelzine	E	D	16
Phenmetrazine	E		2
Phenyltoloxamine	T		2
Phenytoin	T		5
Pipradrol	E		4
Prochlorperazine	T	S	9
Proheptatriene	T		3
Promazine	T	S	3
Promethazine	T	A/I	10
Propericiazine	T		2
Prothipendyl	T		3
Protriptyline	E	D	5
Reserpine	T	S	129
Thalidomide	T		1
Thiethylperazine	T		1
Thioproperazine	T	S	12
Thioridazine	T	S	36
Thiothixene	T	S	5
Triflouperazine	T	S	21
Triflupromazine	T	S	7
Trimepramine	E	D	7
Trimeprazine	T		1
Triperidol	T		3
Tybamate	T	A/I	6

(Based on draft by J-F. Dreyfus)

2.2 DRUGS AND MANUFACTURERS

By the late 1960's there were sixty-five companies which manifactured and/or marketed more than two psychotropics. Of these sixty-five companies four manifactured/marketed ten or more psychotropics. (Note: In this group only one had more than fifteen.)

COMPANIES	*DRUGS*
A & H	Bemegride, Fencamfamine, Perphenazine
Abbot	Deserpidine, Ectylurea, Ethchlorvynol, Isoniazid, Methamphetamine, Pemoline, Trioxazine, Pargyline, Procaine
Astra	Promazine, Promethazine, Prothipendyl
Ayerst	Acepromazine, Benactyzine, Captodiame, Clopenthixol Meprobamate, Phendimetrazine, Prothipendyl
Bayer	Butaperazine, Chlormethazanone, Chlorpromazine, Methotrimeprazine, Prochlorperazine, Promazine, Promethazine, Propericiazine, Trimeprazine
Bohringer	Doxepin, Pemoline, Phenmetrazine, Reserpine
Byk-Gulden	Fluphenazine Dihydrochloride, Mephenesin, Melitracene
Ciba	Adiphenine, Captodiame, Glutethimide, Indamine, Methoxy-propanediol, Methylphenidate, Reserpine, Syrosingopine
Clin-Byla	Acepromazine, Benzperidol, Fluanisone, Propiomazine
Dorsey	Clothiapine, Dibenzepin, Pyrovalerone
Dumex	Benactyzine, Chlorpromazine, Imipramine N-Oxide
Farmitalia	Chlorpromazine, Prochlorperazine, Promethazine, Trimepramine
Geigy	Carbamazepine, Desipramine, Imipramine, Opipramol, Phen-metrazine
Harvey	Ethchlorvynol, Hydroxyzine, Isoniazid, Nialamide
Homburg	Captagon, Homophenazine, Prothipendyl
ICI	Benactyzine, Mebanazine, Meprobamate
Ives	Petrichloral, Propericiazine, Thioproperazine, Trimepramine
Janssen	Anisoperidone, Butropipazone, Dehydrobenzperidol, Floropipamide, Fluanisone, Haloperidol, Meperidide, Methylperidol, Spiroperidol, Triperidol
Kabi	Emylcamate, Meprobamate, Pipradrol
Key	D-Amphetamine Sulphate, Mephenesin, Reserpine
Lakeside	Desipramine, Fencamfamine, Mephenoxalone, Pheniprazine
Lannett	Isoniazid, Mephenesin, Phenytoin, Reserpine
Lederle	Mephenoxalone, Meprobamate, Methotrimeprazine, Methoxy-promazine, Metaxalone
Leo	Haloperidol, Methylpentynol, Trimeprazine
Lepetit	Diethadione, Meprobamate, Methocarbamal, Promazine, Reserpine
Lilly	Deserpidine, Isoniazid, Methamphetamine, Nicotinic Acid, Nortriptyline, Phenaglycodol, Reserpine

COMPANIES	*DRUGS*
Lind. & Reimer	Dehydrobenzperidol, Floropipamide, Haloperidol, Triperidol
Lundbeck	Amytriptyline, Captodiame, Chlorprothixene, Clopenthixol, Melitracene
M&B	Chlorpromazine, Methotrimeprazine, Methoxypromazine Maleate, Prochlorperazine, Propericiazine, Promethazine, Trimeprazine, Trimepramine, Thioproperazine
Maney	Benactyzine, Chlorpromazine, Reserpine
McNeil	Benzperidol, Dehydrobenzperidol, Haloperidol, Methamphetamine, Triperidol
Medial	Amphetamine Sulphate, Mephenoxalone, Methocarbamal
Medimpex	Dehydrobenzperidol, Diphenazine, Methophenazine, Trioxazine
Medo-Chem	D-Amphetamine, Methylpentynol, Pemoline
Merck	Amytriptyline, Benactyzine, Chlorprothixene, Emylcamate, Protriptyline, Perphenazine, Reserpine
Merrell	Azacyclonol, Diethylpropione, Isoniazid, Oxanamide, Pipradrol, Thalidomide,
Natl. Drug	Diethylpropione, Fluorophenothiazine, Promoxolane
Nordmark	D-Amphetamine, Dehydrobenzperidol, Diphenazine
Oryx	Dehydrobenzperidol, Floropipamide, Triperidol
Parke, Davis	Isoniazid, Pentazol, Piperazine, Phenytoin, Promethazine, Reserpine,
Pfizer	Benzquinamide, Buclizine, Doxepin, Hydroxyzine, Isoniazid, Nialamide, Rescinnamine, Thiothixene, Xanthiol
Pharmacia	Pemoline, Propiomazine, Rescinnamine
Pierrel	Meprobamate, Phenaglycodol, Pipradrol, Promazine
Pitman-Moore	D-Amphetamine, Piperacetazine, Reserpine
Rhone-Poulenc	Chlorpromazine, Ethylisobutrazine, Methiomeprazine, Metho-trimeprazine, Methoxypromazine, Prochlorperazine, Promazine, Promethazine, Propericiazine, Thioproperazine, Trimeprazine, Trimepramine
Riker	Acetylcarbromal, Butaperazine, Deanol, Ethamivan, Reserpine
Robins	Butaperazine, Doxapram, Mephenoxalone, Metaxalone, Methocarbamol
Roche	Amitriptyline, Diazepam, Chlordiazepoxide, Chlorprothixene, Iproniazid, Isocarboxazide, Isoniazid, Methyprylon, Pivalylbenz-hydrazine
Sandoz	Methyltryptamine, Piperidochlorpromazine, Thiethylperazine, Thioridazine
Schering	Acetophenazine, Fluphenazine Dihydrochloride, Isoniazid, Methylpentynol, Perphenazine
Searle	Amiphenazole, Butropipazone, Haloperidol, Pipamazine, Thiopropazate
Shinogi	Methotrimeprazine, Methoxpromazine Maleate, Prochlorperazine, Promethazine, Thioproperazine

COMPANIES	DRUGS
SKF	Amphetamine Sulphate, Chlorpromazine, D-Amphetamine, Fluorophenothiazine, Methamphetamine, Methiomeprazine, Methotrimeprazine, Prochlorperazine, Promethazine, Propericiazine, Prothipendyl, Tranylcypromine, Trifluoperazine, Triflupromazine, Trimeprazine, Thioproperazine, Reserpine
Squibb	Benanserin, Fluphenazine Decanoate, Fluphenazine Dihydrochloride, Fluphenazine Enanthate, Isoniazid, Reserpine, Thiazenone, Triflupromazine
Sterling	Chlormethazone, Isoniazid, Oxypertine
Strasen	Aminophenyl pyridone, Amphetamine Phosphate, Benzperidol,
Tropon	Clorprothixene, Flupentixol, Meprobamate, Nortriptyline, Phenyltoloxamine
Tutag	Mephenesin, Methoxypropanediol, Reserpine,
U.S. Vit.	Ethamivan, Isoniazid, Nylidrin
UCB	Buclizine, Dehydrobenzperidol, Dixyrazine, Hydroxyzine
Upjohn	Benzphetamine, Ectylurea, Etryptamine, Methyl-tryptamine, Reserpine, Triflupromazine
Wallace & Tiernan	Methaqualone, Meprobamate, Tybamate
Wander	Dibenzepin, Phenelzine, Pyrovalerone,
Warner	Amitriptyline, Captodiame, Chlorprothixene, Modaline, Prazepam, Phenelzine, Thymoxyalkylamine
Wyeth	Carphenazine, Chlorethiazol, Iprindole, Meprobamate, Oxazepam, Promazine, Promethazine, Propiomazine

2.3 FOUNDERS

The country representation and nature of work of each of the thirty-three Founders are as follows:

SURNAME	COUNTRY	WORK
Arnold	Austria	Clinician
Baruk	France	Clinician
Booij	The Netherlands	Clinician
Bovet	Italy	Basic Scientist
Bradley	United Kingdom	Basic Scientist
Brill	United States	Clinician (1)
Brodie	United States	Basic Scientist (2)
Cameron	Canada	Clinician
Delay	France	Clinician
Delgado	Peru	Clinician
Denber	United States	Clinician
Deniker	France	Clinician
Faurbye	Denmark	Clinician
Flugel	Germany	Clinician
Gozzano	Italy	Clinician
Hippius	Germany	Clinician
Hoff	Austria	Clinician
Hoffer	Canada	Clinician
Kline	United States	Clinician
Laborit	France	Clinician (3)
Lewis	United Kingdom	Clinician
Odegard	Norway	Clinician
Osmond	Canada	Clinician
Radouco-Thomas	Switzerland	Basic Scientist
Rees	United Kingdom	Clinician
Rothlin	Switzerland	Basic Scientist (4)
Shepherd	United Kingdom	Clinician
Stoll	Switzerland	Clinician
Tellez-Carrasco	Venezuela	Clinician
Thuillier	France	Clinician (5)
Trabucchi	Italy	Basic Scientist
Van der Horst	The Netherlands	Clinician
Van Rhyn	The Netherlands	Clinician

(1) Psychiatrist working as Deputy Commissioner of Mental Health (New York State)

(2) Organic chemist, working as Division Chief of the National Heart Institute of the National Institute of Health of the United State Public Health Service

(3) A surgeon in the French Navy from 1945 to 1950, working in clinical research at Val de Grace (military hospital)

(4) Pharmacologist, working as Scientific Director of Sandoz Laboratories

(5) Clinician, working in clinical and basic research

2.4 MEMBERSHIP

CINP Membership by 1970 with members' name, year of election to membership and country. N/A means the year of election to membership could not be verified.

NAME/YEAR	COUNTRY	NAME/YEAR	COUNTRY
Allert N/A	Germany	Clouet N/A	USA
Amdisen N/A	Denmark	Coirault N/A	France
Angst 1964	Switzerland	Cole 1958	USA
Ansell N/A	UK	Cook 1962	USA
Arnold 1957	Austria	Coppen 1968	UK
Axelrod 1958	USA	Cornu 1966	Switzerland
Bailly N/A	France	Corson 1970	USA
Balestrieri 1964	Italy	Costa 1966	USA
Ban 1962	Canada	Crammer N/A	Denmark
Baruk 1957	France	Crane N/A	USA
Battegay 1966	Switzerland	Cuenca N/A	Spain
Bein 1958	Switzerland	Davies 1962	Australia
Benesova 1970	Czechoslovakia	De Albaquerque-Fortes N/A	Brazil
Bente N/A	Germany	De Barahona-Fernandez N/A	Portugal
Berger 1966	USA	De Boor N/A	Germany
Bickel 1968	Switzerland	De Oliveira N/A	Brazil
Biel N/A	USA	Degkwitz N/A	Germany
Bignami N/A	Italy	Delay 1957	France
Bobon D. N/A	Belgium	Delgado 1957	Peru
Bobon J. N/A	Belgium	Denber 1957	USA
Bohacek 1966	Yugoslavia	Deniker 1957	France
Boissier N/A	France	Detre 1968	USA
Booij 1957	Netherlands	Dews 1962	USA
Bordeleau N/A	Canada	Di Mascio N/A	USA
Böszörményi 1962	Hungary	Dick 1968	Switzerland
Bovet 1957	Italy	Dille N/A	USA
Bradley 1957	UK	Domenjoz 1962	Germany
Brill 1957	USA	Domino 1966	USA
Brimblecombe 1964	UK	Downing N/A	USA
Brodie 1957	USA	Eccles N/A	Australia
Broussolle N/A	France	Edelstein 1968	Israel
Brugmans N/A	Belgium	Elkes 1960	USA
Brunaud 1962	France	Engelhardt 1962	USA
Buckett 1970	UK	Essman 1968	USA
Bunney 1970	USA	Estrada-Robles N/A	Mexico
Buser 1964	France	Everett 1962	USA
Cameron 1957	Canada	Faurbye 1957	Denmark
Carlsson 1958	Sweden	Fazio N/A	Italy
Carranza N/A	USA	Feer 1970	Switzerland
Carvalhal N/A	Brazil	Feldberg N/A	UK
Cazzullo 1958	Italy	Fieve 1970	USA
Cerletti N/A	Switzerland	Fink 1958	USA
Ciurezu N/A	Romania	Fisher 1966	USA

NAME/YEAR	COUNTRY	NAME/YEAR	COUNTRY
Flament 1962	Belgium	Ingvar N/A	Sweden
Fleischhauer N/A	Switzerland	Irwin N/A	USA
Flügel 1957	Germany	Isbell 1958	USA
Folch-Pi 1958	USA	Itil 1962	USA
Forrest 1968	USA	Itoh N/A	Japan
Fragoso-Mendes N/A	Portugal	Jacob 1964	France
Freedman, A.M. 1960	USA	Jacobsen N/A	Denmark
Freedman, B.Z. 1968	USA	Janke 1970	Germany
Freyhan N/A	USA	Janssen 1964	Belgium
Gantt 1958	USA	Janzarick 1962	Germany
Garattini 1958	Italy	Jarvik 1962	USA
Gatti N/A	Italy	Jenner N/A	UK
Gayral N/A	France	Jouvet 1968	France
Gerle 1958	Sweden	Joyce N/A	Switzerland
Gershon 1968	USA	Joyce-Basseres 1966	France
Giberti 1962	Italy	Julou 1962	France
Ginestet 1964	France	Jung N/A	Switzerland
Giurgea 1970	Belgium	Jus 1962	Poland
Glowinski 1968	France	Kalinowsky N/A	USA
Goldman N/A	USA	Kanig 1962	Germany
Goldstein 1970	USA	Karczmar 1970	USA
Goldwurm N/A	Italy	Kety 1958	USA
Gottfries 1962	Sweden	Keup N/A	Germany
Gozzano 1957	Italy	Key N/A	UK
Greenblatt N/A	USA	Kido N/A	Japan
Grof 1968	Canada	Kielholz N/A	Switzerland
Gross N/A	Austria	Killam 1962	USA
Grossman 1968	USA	King 1966	Hong Kong
Guy N/A	USA	Kingstone 1970	Canada
Guyotat 1958	France	Kirkegaard N/A	Denmark
Haase 1962	Germany	Klerman N/A	USA
Hall N/A	UK	Kletzkin 1970	USA
Hamilton N/A	UK	Kline 1957	USA
Harrer 1966	Austria	Knopp 1968	USA
Heimann 1962	Germany	Kobayashi 1962	Japan
Heinrich 1962	Germany	Kornetsky 1962	USA
Helmchen 1964	Germany	Kramer N/A	USA
Herz 1966	Germany	Kranz N/A	Germany
Hippius 1957	Germany	Kreiskott 1966	Germany
Hoch 1958	USA	Kryspin-Exner N/A	Austria
Hoff 1957	Austria	Kuhn 1958	Switzerland
Hoffer 1957	Canada	Kunkel N/A	Germany
Hoffman 1964	Austria	Kurland 1958	USA
Hoffmeister 1966	Germany	Labhardt N/A	Switzerland
Holden N/A	UK	Laborit 1957	France
Hole N/A	Germany	Lader 1964	UK
Holliday 1958	USA	Ladewig 1970	Switzerland
Horita N/A	USA	Lajtha 1962	USA
Idestrom N/A	Sweden	Lambert C. 1964	UK

NAME/YEAR	COUNTRY	NAME/YEAR	COUNTRY
Lambert P. 1958	France	Peron-Magnan N/A	France
Lassenius N/A	Sweden	Petersen N/A	Denmark
Launay 1962	France	Petkov 1968	Bulgaria
Lechat 1962	France	Pfeiffer N/A	USA
Lehmann 1958	Canada	Pichler 1958	France
Lemperiere 1962	France	Pichot 1958	France
Lesse N/A	USA	Pletscher 1958	Switzerland
Leuner 1962	Germany	Pöldinger 1964	Switzerland
Levine 1970	USA	Polvan N/A	Turkey
Levy N/A	France	Prange 1970	USA
Lewis 1957	UK	Quadbeck 1962	Germany
Lienert 1962	Germany	Radouco-Thomas 1957	Switzerland
Loew N/A	Switzerland	Rafaelsen N/A	Denmark
Longo 1966	Italy	Randrup 1966	Denmark
Lopez-Ibor N/A	Spain	Ravn 1962	Denmark
Lucas-Brasseres 1966	France	Ray 1970	USA
Lundquist 1962	Sweden	Rees 1957	UK
Lunn 1958	Denmark	Rennert N/A	Germany
Malitz 1958	USA	Revol N/A	France
Mangoni 1966	Italy	Richter N/A	UK
Martis N/A	Italy	Rickels 1958	USA
Matussek 1964	Germany	Roos 1966	Sweden
Maxwell C. 1970	UK	Rosic 1970	Yugoslavia
Maxwell D.R. N/A	USA	Rossi 1966	Italy
May N/A	USA	Roth L.J. N/A	USA
McDonald N/A	USA	Roth M. 1964	UK
Mercier N/A	France	Rothlin 1957	Switzerland
Meriategui 1962	Peru	Rothman 1958	USA
Merlis 1962	USA	Salva N/A	Spain
Meyer 1962	Germany	Sarro N/A	Spain
Mirsky 1966	USA	Sartorius 1966	Switzerland
Moller N/A	Denmark	Sarwer-Foner 1962	Canada
Montagu N/A	UK	Sayers N/A	Switzerland
Montserrat N/A	Spain	Schmitt N/A	Germany
Morselli 1970	France	Schou N/A	Denmark
Munkvad N/A	Denmark	Schulze N/A	Germany
Musacchio N/A	USA	Scotto N/A	France
Nahunek 1970	Czechoslovakia	Shagass 1964	USA
Nodine N/A	USA	Shaw 1970	UK
Oberholzer N/A	Switzerland	Shepherd 1957	UK
Odegard 1957	Norway	Sheth N/A	India
Oliverio 1968	Italy	Silverstone 1970	UK
Osmond 1957	Canada	Simon 1966	France
Overall 1968	USA	Simpson 1966	USA
Pare N/A	UK	Sirnes N/A	Norway
Paykel 1968	UK	Sjöström N/A	Sweden
Pekkarinen N/A	Finland	Sloane 1958	USA
Pepeu 1968	Italy	Smith 1966	USA
Perier N/A	France	Smythies 1962	UK

NAME/YEAR	COUNTRY	NAME/YEAR	COUNTRY
Solti N/A	Hungary	Utena N/A	Japan
Spiegelberg N/A	Germany	Valdecasas N/A	Spain
St. Laurent N/A	Canada	Valzelli N/A	Italy
Steinberg 1958	UK	Van Der Horst 1957	Netherlands
Stille N/A	Germany	Van Praag 1968	Netherlands
Stolerman N/A	UK	Van Rhyn 1957	Netherlands
Stoll 1957	Switzerland	Van Rossum 1966	Netherlands
Stromgren N/A	Denmark	Vencovsky 1966	Czechoslovakia
Sulser 1970	USA	Verdeaux 1962	France
Summerfield N/A	UK	Vianna N/A	Brazil
Sutter 1958	France	Villeneuve 1968	Canada
Szara 1966	USA	Vinar 1966	Czechoslovakia
Taeschler N/A	Switzerland	Voelkel N/A	Germany
Tedeschl N/A	USA	Vojtechovsky 1966	Czechoslovakia
Teller N/A	USA	Volmat N/A	France
Tellez Carrasco 1957	Venezuela	Von Kerekjarto N/A	Germany
Temkov N/A	Bulgaria	Von Schlichtegroll 1964	Germany
Terranova 1962	Italy	Votava 1962	Czechoslovakia
Tesarova 1970	Czechoslovakia	Waelsch N/A	USA
Tetreault N/A	Canada	Watt N/A	UK
Theobald N/A	Switzerland	Wheatley 1966	UK
Thesleff 1962	Sweden	Wijesinghe N/A	Ceylon
Thuillier 1957	France	Wikler N/A	USA
Todrick N/A	UK	Wilhelm N/A	USA
Trabucchi 1957	Italy	Wilson 1964	Ireland
Uhlenhuth N/A	USA	Winkelman N/A	USA
Ulett 1962	USA	Wirth 1958	Germany
Unna N/A	USA	Wittenborn N/A	USA
Usdin N/A	USA		

2.5 EXECUTIVES

Country representation of the forty-two members serving as Officers and the offices held by the Officers in the first seven Executives:

MEMBER	*COUNTRY*	*1957 1958*	*1958 1960*	*1960 1962*	*1962 1964*	*1964 1966*	*1966 1968*	*1968 1970*
Arnold	Austria				S			
Bente	Germany					FC		C
Boissier	France							C
Bovet	Italy	C						
Bradley	United Kingdom	FC	FC	FC		T	T	T
Cameron	Canada	C						
Cerletti	Switzerland							VP
Cole	United States					S	S	S
Costa	United States							C
Cuenca	Spain							C
Davies	Australia							C
deBoor	Germany	C		S				
Delay	France	VP			PE	P	PP	
Delgado	Peru	C						
Denber	United States	S	S					
Deniker	France	FC	FC	FC	FC	S	S	S
Eccles	Australia	C						
Feldberg	United Kingdom	C						
Freyhan	United States			S	S	FC	FC	FC
Garattini	Italy							C
Gozzano	Italy	C						
Hippius	Germany						FC	FC
Hoch	United States	VP	PE	P	PP			
Hoff	Austria	VP		PE	P	PP		
Ingvar	Norway	C						
Jacobsen	Denmark							PE
Janssen	Belgium							C
Jung	Switzerland	C						
Jus	Poland							C
Ketty	United States	C						
Lehmann	Canada						PE	P
Radouco-Thomas	Switzerland	S	S					
Rennert	Germany							VP
Rothlin	Switzerland	P	P	PP				
Schou	Denmark							C
Shepherd	United Kingdom	VP						
Steinberg	United Kingdom							VP
Stoll	Switzerland	T	T					
Thuillier	France			T	T			
Valdecasas	Spain					PE	P	PP
Votava	Czechoslovakia							C
Waelsch	United States	C						

Offices: C=Councillor, FC=First Councillor, P=President, PE=President Elect, PP=Past President, S=Secretary, T=Treasurer, VP=Vice Pesident

Country profile of the first seven Executives:

FIRST EXECUTIVE (21 Officers)

COUNTRY (rank order)	*OFFICERS (n)*
Switzerland	4
United States	4
United Kingdom	3
France	2
Italy	2
Australia	1
Austria	1
Canada	1
Germany	1
Norway	1
Peru	1

SECOND EXECUTIVE (7 Officers)

COUNTRY (rank order)	OFFICERS (n)
Switzerland	3
United States	2
France	1
United Kingdom	1

THIRD EXECUTIVE (8 Officers)

COUNTRY (rank order)	OFFICERS (n)
France	2
United States	2
Austria	1
Germany	1
Switzerland	1
United Kingdom	1

FOURTH EXECUTIVE (7 Officers)

COUNTRY (rank order)	OFFICERS (n)
France	3
Austria	2
United States	2

FIFTH EXECUTIVE (7 Officers)

COUNTRY (rank order)	OFFICERS (n)
United States	2
Austria	1
France	1
Germany	1
Spain	1
United Kingdom	1

SIXTH EXECUTIVE (7 Officers)

COUNTRY (rank order)	OFFICERS (n)
United States	2
Canada	1
France	1
Germany	1
Spain	1
United Kingdom	1

SEVENTH EXECUTIVE (20 Officers)

COUNTRY (rank order)	OFFICERS (n)
Germany	3
United States	3
Denmark	2
Spain	2
United Kingdom	2
Australia	1
Belgium	1
Canada	1
Czechoslovakia	1
Francee	1
Italy	1
Poland	1
Switzerland	1

2.6 PROGRAMS

FIRST CONGRESS (Rome, September 1958)

Methods and analysis of drug-induced behaviour in animals (First Symposium)

Methods and analysis of drug-induced abnormal mental states in men (Second Symposium)

Comparison of abnormal behavioural states induced by psychotropic drugs in animals and man (Third Symposium)

Comparison of drug-induced and endogenous psychoses in man (Fourth Symposium)

The impact of psychotropic drugs on the structure, function and future of psychiatric services: (a) In the hospitals (First plenary session)

The impact of psychotropic drugs on the structure, function and future of psychiatric services: (b) In extra-mural clinics (Second plenary session)

The present state of neurochemistry (Third plenary session)

Experimental studies in animals (Communications – Section 1)

Reports on investigations in normal human subjects and theoretical papers (Communications – Section 2)

Clinical and therapeutic reports (Communications - Section 3)

SECOND CONGRESS (Basel, July 1960)

Psychophysiology and psychopharmacology (Opening Session)

Problems arising from the generalized use of psychotropic drugs (Opening Session)

The problem of antagonists to psychotropic drugs (First Symposium)

The effects of psychotropic drugs on conditioned responses in animals and man (Second Symposium)

The influence of specific and non-specific factors on the clinical effects of psychotropic drugs (Third Symposium)

Measurement of changes in human behaviour under the effects of psychotropic drugs (Fourth Symposium)

Biochemical mechanisms related to the site of action of psychotropic drugs (Fifth Symposium)

THIRD CONGRESS (Munich, September 1962)

Methods of comparison of behaviour changes with drugs in animals and man (First Symposium)

Effectiveness of drugs in relationship to psychological and social forms of treatment (Second Symposium)

Ten years of psychopharmacology: Critical assessment of the present and future (Third Symposium)

Biochemical mechanisms of drug action (Round Table Conference)

Drug action on microstructures (Round Table Conference)

Clinical and experimental studies with new drugs (Communications)

(General Communications)

FOURTH CONGRESS (Birmingham, September 1964)

The mode of action of psychotropic drugs and its implications for the pathophysiology of psychotic disturbances (Part I)

Experimental and clinical biochemistry (Working Group 1)

Experimental and clinical neurophysiology (Working Group 2)

Psychology and experimental psychopathology (Working Group 3)

Pharmacological and clinical action of neuroleptic drugs (Working Group 4)

Pharmacological and clinical action of antidepressant drugs (Working Group 5)

Dynamics and significance of psychopharmacological intervention in psychiatry (Working Group 6)

Individual Communications (Part II)

FIFTH CONGRESS (Washington, March 1966)

Research methodologies in psychopharmacology; issues of research approval, research design, and statistical approaches to the analyses of data (1st Symposium)

Pharmacological and clinical differences in the actions of sedative-hypnotic, tranquilizer and neuroleptic drugs (2nd Symposium)

Drug effects on memory and learning (3rd Symposium)

Drug abuse and drug dependence (4th Symposium)

Mechanisms of action of psychotropic drugs at both the clinical and pharmacologic level (5th Symposium)

Anticholinergic drugs and brain function in animals and man (6th Symposium)

The use of psychotomimetic agents as treatments in psychiatry including relevant basic research on the effects of such drugs in man (7th Symposium)

Drug combinations, their effects at both the animal and clinical levels (8th Symposium)

Clinical, institutional and other milieu factors influencing drug responses (9th Symposium)

Side effects of drug toxicity including behavioral toxicity (10th Symposium)

Identification of specific therapeutic indications for psychoactive drugs (11th Symposium)

Animal test models relevant to the clinical actions of drugs (12th Symposium)

Classical conditioning and psychopharmacology (13th Symposium)

Drugs as tools in the study of mental illness (14th Symposium)

Individual Communications

SIXTH CONGRESS (Tarragona, April 1968)

Turnover rate of neuronal monoamines: Pharmacological implications (Main Lecture)

Recent advances in neurophysiology (Main Lecture)

Importance of drug metabolism and kinetics for pharmacological and clinical effects (Interdisciplinary Sessions A)

Insufficiencies and needs in psychopharmacology – Criteria of drug selection (Interdisciplinary Session B)
  Neuroleptics (I)
  Tranquilizers (II)
  Antidepressants (III)

Influence of psychotropic drugs on sleeping behavior in animals and humans (Interdisciplinary Session C)

Behaviour studies in animals (Free communications A)
Neuropharmacology (Free communications B)
Monoamines (Free communications C)
Drug metabolism (Free communications D)
Methods of clinical evaluation (Free communications E)
Neuro-psychopharmacology (Free communications F)
Neuroleptics (Free communications G)
Antidepressives (Free communications H)

SEVENTH CONGRESS (Prague, August 1970)

Clinical and pharmacological aspects of lithium therapy (1st Symposium)
Amine precursors in the treatment and study of affective disorders (2nd Symposium)
Methods of evaluation of anxiolytics (minor tranquilizers) (3rd Symposium)
Pharmacological and therapeutic aspects of amphetamine and hallucinogen abuse (4th
    Symposium)
Influence of drugs on social behaviour (5th Symposium)
Effects of drugs on interpersonal processes (Psychodynamics, drugs and psychotherapy, etc.)
    (6th Symposium)
Special questions: placebo, drug combinations, subjects in new drug trials (7th Symposium)
The role of putative central transmitters in behaviour and drug action (8th Symposium)

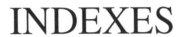

INDEXES

DRUG INDEX

NAME INDEX

PHOTO INDEX

SUBJECT INDEX